Reconstructive Surgery: Advanced Techniques

Reconstructive Surgery: Advanced Techniques

Editor: Marvin Trey

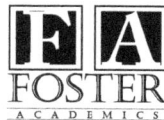

FOSTER
ACADEMICS

www.fosteracademics.com

www.fosteracademics.com

FA
FOSTER
ACADEMICS

Cataloging-in-Publication Data

Reconstructive surgery : advanced techniques / edited by Marvin Trey.
        p. cm.
Includes bibliographical references and index.
ISBN 978-1-63242-812-7
1. Surgery, Plastic. 2. Surgery, Plastic--Technique. 3. Transplantation of organs, tissues, etc.
4. Operations, Surgical. I. Trey, Marvin.
RD118 .R43 2019
617.95--dc23

Foster Academics,
118-35 Queens Blvd., Suite 400,
Forest Hills, NY 11375, USA

ISBN 978-1-63242-812-7 (Hardback)

Contents

Preface

The type of surgery which is meant to restore the form and function of the body is known as reconstructive surgery. It may include simple techniques, such as primary closure and dressings, as well as complex skin grafts, free flaps and tissue expansion. It does not include cosmetic surgery, which is concerned merely with the purpose of improving a person's physical appearance and the removal of one's signs of aging. Some of the branches of surgery under which reconstructive surgeries often take place include pediatric surgery, podiatric surgery and gynaecological surgery. Biomaterials are used in reconstructive surgery for correcting or replacing damaged body parts. A successful implantation can be achieved through an anatomical, biochemical, pathological and physiological understanding of the condition. This book covers in detail some existing theories and innovative concepts revolving around reconstructive surgery. It includes some of the vital pieces of work being conducted across the world, on various topics related to reconstructive surgery. The extensive content of this book provides the readers with a thorough understanding of the subject.

This book is a result of research of several months to collate the most relevant data in the field.

When I was approached with the idea of this book and the proposal to edit it, I was overwhelmed. It gave me an opportunity to reach out to all those who share a common interest with me in this field. I had 3 main parameters for editing this text:

1. Accuracy – The data and information provided in this book should be up-to-date and valuable to the readers.

2. Structure – The data must be presented in a structured format for easy understanding and better grasping of the readers.

3. Universal Approach – This book not only targets students but also experts and innovators in the field, thus my aim was to present topics which are of use to all.

Thus, it took me a couple of months to finish the editing of this book.

I would like to make a special mention of my publisher who considered me worthy of this opportunity and also supported me throughout the editing process. I would also like to thank the editing team at the back-end who extended their help whenever required.

Editor

Acute effects of remote ischemic preconditioning on cutaneous microcirculation - a controlled prospective cohort study

Robert Kraemer[1][*][†], Johan Lorenzen[2][†], Mohammad Kabbani[1], Christian Herold[1], Marc Busche[1], Peter M Vogt[1] and Karsten Knobloch[1]

Abstract

Background: Therapeutic strategies aiming to reduce ischemia/reperfusion injury by conditioning tissue tolerance against ischemia appear attractive not only from a scientific perspective, but also in clinics. Although previous studies indicate that remote ischemic intermittent preconditioning (RIPC) is a systemic phenomenon, only a few studies have focused on the elucidation of its mechanisms of action especially in the clinical setting. Therefore, the aim of this study is to evaluate the acute microcirculatory effects of remote ischemic preconditioning on a distinct cutaneous location at the lower extremity which is typically used as a harvesting site for free flap reconstructive surgery in a human in-vivo setting.

Methods: Microcirculatory data of 27 healthy subjects (25 males, age 24 ± 4 years, BMI 23.3) were evaluated continuously at the anterolateral aspect of the left thigh during RIPC using combined Laser-Doppler and photospectrometry (Oxygen-to-see, Lea Medizintechnik, Germany). After baseline microcirculatory measurement, remote ischemia was induced using a tourniquet on the contralateral upper arm for three cycles of 5 min.

Results: After RIPC, tissue oxygen saturation and capillary blood flow increased up to 29% and 35% during the third reperfusion phase versus baseline measurement, respectively (both p = 0.001). Postcapillary venous filling pressure decreased statistically significant by 16% during second reperfusion phase (p = 0.028).

Conclusion: Remote intermittent ischemic preconditioning affects cutaneous tissue oxygen saturation, arterial capillary blood flow and postcapillary venous filling pressure at a remote cutaneous location of the lower extremity. To what extent remote preconditioning might ameliorate reperfusion injury in soft tissue trauma or free flap transplantation further clinical trials have to evaluate.

Trial registration: ClinicalTrials.gov: NCT01235286

Keywords: Remote ischemic preconditioning, cutaneous microcirculation, free flap, soft tissue

Background

In several medical specialties, reduction of ischemia/reperfusion injury is a major topic. In trauma surgery, soft tissue defects after trauma due to accidents or due to operative trauma are quite common. In plastic and reconstructive surgery, on the other hand, soft tissue coverage is commonly performed using local or free flaps. Despite remarkable progress in surgical techniques and postoperative free flap monitoring devices over the last decades, free flap surgery is still associated with a significant morbidity. Current scientific literature reports a total loss rate of microsurgically transferred free flaps in one to five percent [1,2]. The main reasons are either persistent postoperative ischemia and hypoxia or transient ischemia associated with ischemia reperfusion injury [3]. Reducing or preventing soft tissue or free flap necrosis by conditioning tissue tolerance against ischemia is paramount in development of new treatment strategies. Current scientific literature demonstrates a possible induction of ischemic tolerance of

* Correspondence: kraemer.robert@mh-hannover.de
† Contributed equally
[1]Plastic, Hand and Reconstructive Surgery, Hannover Medical School, Carl-Neuberg-Strasse 1, 30625 Hannover, Germany
Full list of author information is available at the end of the article

several tissues by application of stressors including sublethal ischemia, hyperthermia, hypothermia, drugs and growth factors [4,5].

Applying brief periods of sublethal ischaemia to the target tissue with subsequent reperfusion is a simple method of ischemic tolerance induction, which is called ischemic preconditioning (IP). The aim of IP is to increase the resistance of the tissue against the subsequent deleterious ischemia reperfusion injury [4]. Nitric oxide (NO) as well as adenosine release has been shown to regulate endothelial function and increase blood flow in ischemic preconditioning settings [6]. However, direct IP produces trauma to major vessels and direct stress to the target organ.

Remote ischemic preconditioning (RIPC) is a further development of IP where ischemia followed by reperfusion of one organ is believed to protect remote organs either due to a systemic release of biochemical messengers in the circulation or activation of nerve pathways, also resulting in a secondary release of messengers that have a protective effect. This protects the target tissue without trauma to major vessels or direct stress to the target organ. In animal models, RIPC performed at the limb, gut, mesenteric, kidney or skeletal muscle reduced myocardial infarct size [7].

Furthermore, ischemic preconditioning has already been shown to be effective in flap surgery, demonstrated by an ameliorated survival of tissue in a porcine latissimus dorsi flap model [8].

A considerable number of experimental studies confirmed successful IP in flap surgery [9-11]. Since the introduction of IP to flap surgery, various procedures have been discussed such as the ideal time point of IP application, the duration of the IP cycle and the total number of cycles to apply.

Although the efficiency of IP has been demonstrated numerously in experimental in-vivo models, 'classical' IP has rarely been used in the clinical setting to target ischaemia- and reperfusion-associated complications [12].

A recent clinical trial among patients suffering from myocardial infarction demonstrated an increased myocardial salvage after prehospital remote ischaemic conditioning. To date, no scientific investigation has evaluated the acute microcirculatory effects of RIPC on cutaneous soft tissue in order to potentially attenuate the ischemia-reperfusion-injury during soft tissue traumatization or free flap transplantation in a perioperative clinical setting. Therefore, we hypothesized that intermittent remote ischemic preconditioning is able to immediately effect cutaneous microcirculation at a distinct cutaneous location at the lower extremity at a potential adipocutaneous free flap location

Methods

The research was carried out in accordance with the Declaration of Helsinki (2000) of the World Medical Association and was approved by the Institutional Ethics Committee in October 2010. The study was registered at ClinicalTrials.gov with the identifier number NCT01235286.

Written consent was obtained from each study subject prior to commencement of the investigation.

The study is reported according to the STROBE-guidelines (Strengthening the Reporting of Observational Studies in Epidemiology) [13].

Study design and setting

The study was designed as a prospective, controlled cohort study.

Data assessment was performed at the Department of Plastic, Hand and Reconstructive Surgery, Medical School Hannover, Germany between May and September 2010 using combined Laser-Doppler and photospectrometry (Oxygen-to-see, Lea Medizintechnik, Germany) which is regularly used for free flap microcirculatory monitoring at our department to determine postoperative free flap microcirculation. In order to determine changes of microcirculation resulting from remote ischemic preconditioning at a representative location for soft tissue traumatization and free flap transfer, we chose a distinct area for microcirculatory assessment at the anterolateral aspect of the thigh in the means of an ALT- (anterolateral thigh-) flap. A standardized location for microcirculatory assessment was determined on the left leg of each participant between the proximal and distal third of a drawn line between the anterior superior iliac spine and the lateral aspect of the Patella.

The healthy subjects had to rest before starting data assessment in a horizontal position for 15 minutes. The probe was taped on the left upper leg in a standardized manner after localizing the measuring point. A blood pressure cuff was applied on the contralateral upper arm. Baseline data was assessed over 5 minutes before starting remote ischemia. Three circles of a five minute ischemia were applied at the contralateral right upper arm at suprasystolic levels. Parameters of microcirculation were assessed continuously over time. Microcirculation during the reperfusion phase was ascertained over 10 minutes after first and second remote ischemia and 15 minutes after the third remote ischemia.

Participants

Study population and recruitment

Eligibility criteria were healthy male and female subjects aged 18 to 35 years. Measurements were performed at the Department of Plastic, Hand and Reconstructive Surgery, Medical School Hannover, Germany. Healthy subjects were recruited from the Medical School Hannover.

Exclusion criteria were soft tissue inflammation or osteomyelitis, peripheral arterial occlusive disease,

vasculitis, chronic kidney or liver disease, cardiac dysfunction, arterial hypotension and any type of vasoactive medication, i.e. ß-blockers, calcium channel blockers, nitroglycerin or equal.

The study population was a consecutive series of participants defined by the aforementioned selection criteria.

Variables
Determination of vital parameters of microcirculation
The determination of hemoglobin and the principle of blood flow measurement are combined in the O2C system. The optical method for measuring both, blood flow by Laser-Doppler technique and hemoglobin oxygenation and hemoglobin concentration in tissue by spectrometric techniques, has been described in detail elsewhere [14]. The local oxygen supply parameters, blood flow, oxygen saturation of hemoglobin, and the relative postcapillary venous filling pressures were recorded by an optical fiber probe. The fiber probe incorporates both the laser Doppler method and the broadband light spectrometry technique. The probe we used assessed data in 2 and 8 millimeters depth of the free flap regarding:

- capillary blood flow [arbitrary units AU]
- tissue oxygen saturation [%]
- relative postcapillary venous filling pressure [AU]

Bias
Structural measurement bias was avoided by standardisation of environmental factors during assessment of microcirculatory data, i.e. assessment by the same examiner, uniform subject's position during measurement, ambient light and temperature standardisation. Artefacts from microcirculatory measurements were tried to be avoided by fixation of the measurement probe on the same distinct location at the left upper leg of each subject.

The outcome variable selection bias was avoided by presenting all assessed microcirculatory variables in the paper that represent separate factors of microcirculation. Also, insignificant measures were presented. Literature retrieval biases were prevented by independent literature research through the National Library of Medicine. Funding bias was eliminated by disclosure of any financial support of any author of the paper.

Statistical analysis
Repeated measures ANOVA and a Bonferroni-Holm-procedure as standard in multiple t-tests of statistical analysis were applied for comparison of baseline pre-ischemic vs. post-ischemic microcirculatory changes. A p-value less than 0.05 was considered to indicate statistical significance. The SPSS statistical software package

16.0 for Windows (SPSS Inc., Chicago, Ill, USA) was used for statistical analysis.

Results
Participants' descriptive data
A total number of 27 healthy subjects (25 males, 2 females) were enrolled in the evaluation of microcirculatory effects of remote ischemic preconditioning at the Department of Plastic, Hand and Reconstructive Surgery, Medical School Hannover, Germany.

Mean subject's age was 24 ± 4 years. Mean body-mass-index was 23.3 ± 3.0. All subjects were healthy non-smokers without any history of arterial hypertension, diabetes mellitus or vascular disease. Two thirds of the participants performed sports activities on a regular basis.

Microcirculatory analysis
Capillary blood flow
Cutaneous capillary blood flow increased by 16% during the first reperfusion phase at the anterolateral thigh, which reached statistical significance during the first minute after the first remote ischemia (126 ± 71 Arbitrary Units [AU] vs. 146 ± 67 AU; p = 0.001; Figure 1).

After ascending undulation of the microcirculatory blood flow during second and third remote reperfusion, the peak blood flow was reached straight after the third remote ischemia with an increase versus baseline measurement by 35% (126 ± 71 AU vs. 170 ± 73 AU; p = 0.001).

Postcapillary venous filling pressure
Cutaneous postcapillary filling pressure at the anterolateral thigh decreased statistically significant 5 minutes after the second remote ischemia by 16% versus baseline (48 ± 19 AU vs. 41 ± 17 AU; p = 0.028; Figure 2).

Tissue oxygen saturation
Tissue oxygen saturation assessed at the anterolateral thigh increased three minutes after remote ischemia reaching statistical significance eleven minutes after the second remote ischemia with an increase by 19% versus baseline measurement (46 ± 10% vs. 55 ± 12%; p = 0.021; Figure 3). The highest tissue oxygen saturation was detected 10 minutes after the third remote ischemia showing an increased oxygen saturation by 29% versus baseline measurement (46 ± 10% vs. 59 ± 8%; p = 0.001).

Discussion
Key results
We hypothesized that remote ischemic preconditioning (RIPC) is able to immediately affect cutaneous microcirculation at a potential fasciocutaneous free flap location at the anterolateral thigh (ALT-) region in a human in-vivo setting. This prospective controlled clinical study could demonstrate a significant increase of cutaneous oxygen saturation at the anterolateral thigh (ALT) skin territory, a

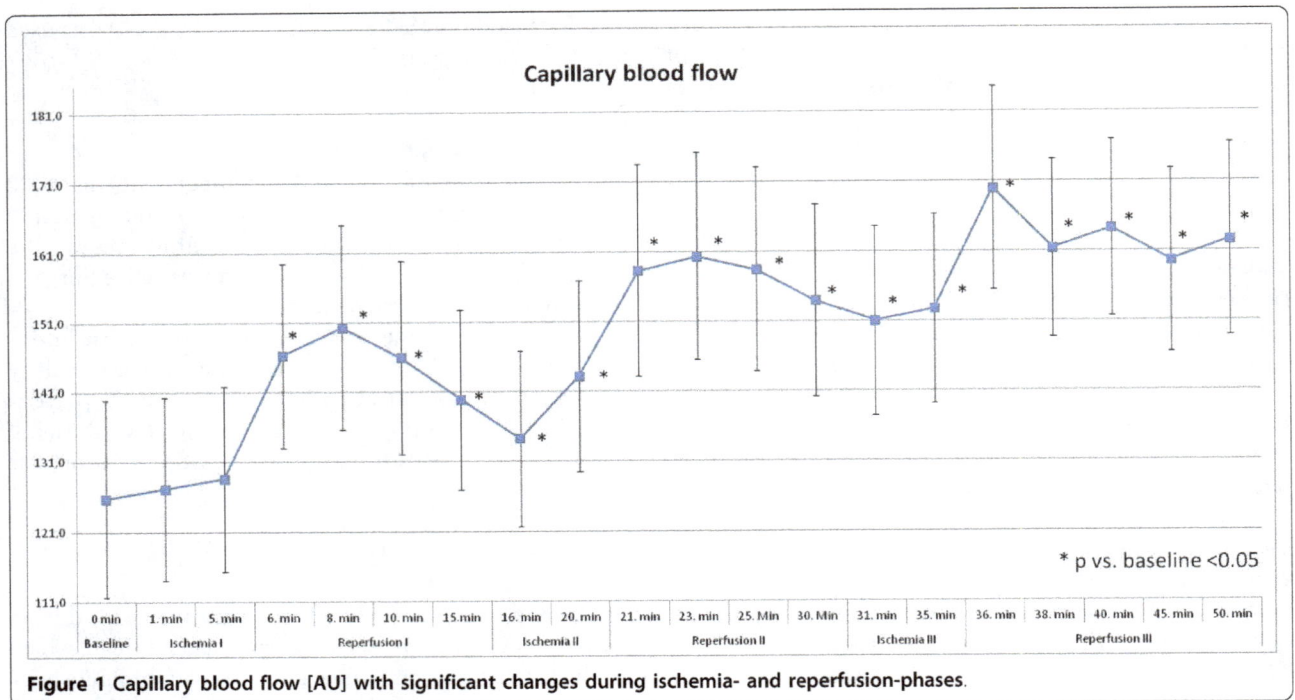

Figure 1 Capillary blood flow [AU] with significant changes during ischemia- and reperfusion-phases.

significant increase of the cutaneous capillary blood flow as well as a statistical significant decrease of the postcapillary filling pressure as a marker of venous stasis during reperfusion phases immediately after RIPC. Therefore, our primary hypothesis was supported. These results should be discussed in detail.

In trauma and reconstructive surgery, tissue survival is paramount. In spite of tremendous progress in surgical techniques notably in reconstructive microsurgery, soft tissue still is endangered by both the lack of reoxygenation and the reoxygenation-associated inflammation due to reperfusion injury, especially in soft tissue trauma as

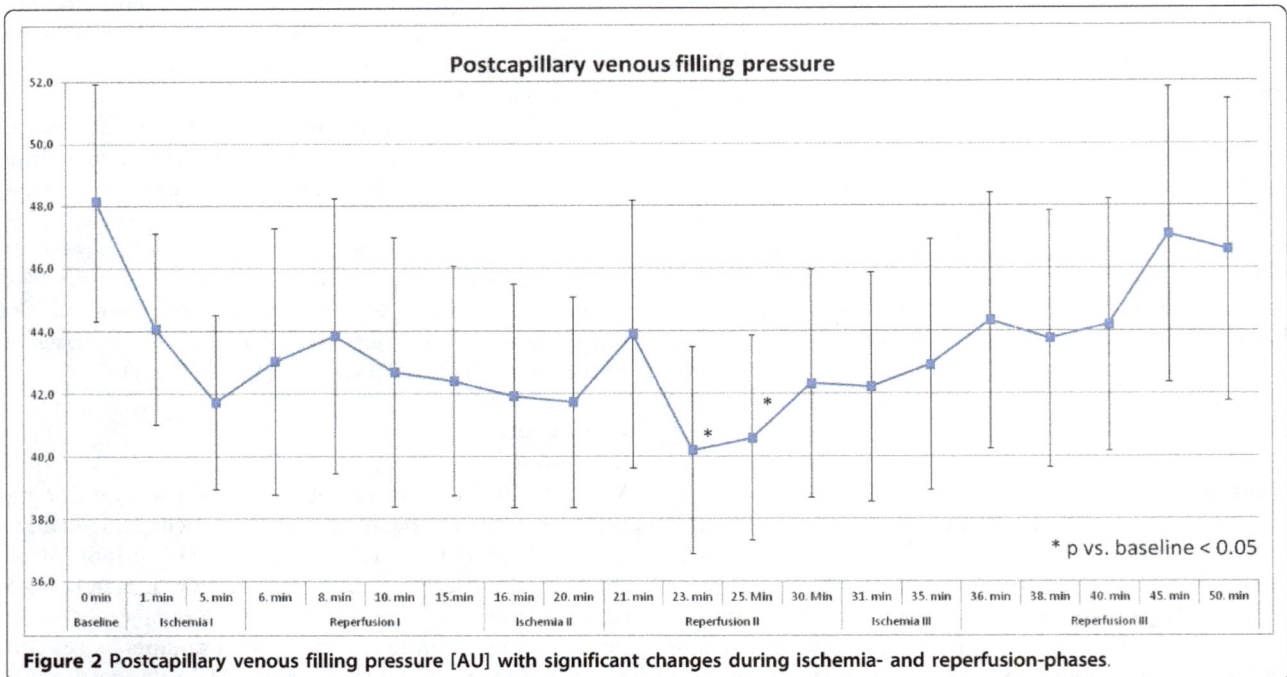

Figure 2 Postcapillary venous filling pressure [AU] with significant changes during ischemia- and reperfusion-phases.

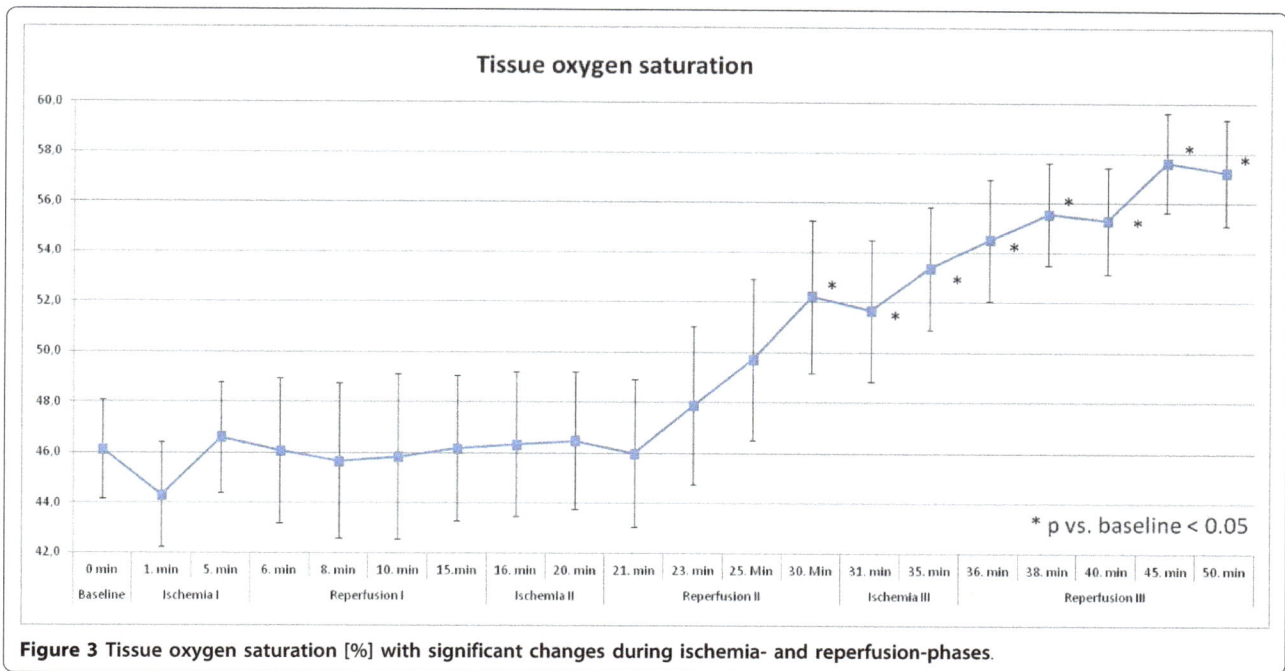

Figure 3 Tissue oxygen saturation [%] with significant changes during ischemia- and reperfusion-phases.

well as in free flap failure [15]. In order to reduce the deleterious effects of ischemia and reperfusion injury, several methods of ischemia tolerance induction were developed including sublethal ischemia, hyperthermia, hypothermia, drugs and growth factors [4,5].

In plastic and reconstructive surgery, effects of ischemic preconditioning were also evaluated in free flap transplantation leading to a significant reduction of muscle flap necrosis supposedly by increasing the critical ischemia time of the free flap's soft tissue.

With the aim of reducing the number of additional procedures and the invasiveness of the individual preconditioning measures, remote ischemic preconditioning (RIPC) was introduced. The ameliorating effect of RIPC was attributed to regulation of endothelial protection, whereas other studies about the mechanisms of preconditioning effects on muscle and musculocutaneous flaps disclosed a decrease of capillary no-reflow, attenuation of arteriolar vasospasm and an increase of blood flow response [11,16-18]. Furthermore, if ischemic preconditioning is applied directly before critical soft tissue ischemia, it protects both against the leukocytic inflammatory reperfusion injury and against microcirculatory dysfunction. On the other hand, ischemic preconditioning performed 24 hours or more before critical soft tissue ischemia acts anti-inflammatory, but is not capable of improving the microcirculation [19]. The short-term microcirculatory assessment in our study was performed straight after remote ischemia to detect acute cutaneous microcirculatory effects of remote ischemic preconditioning. The intention of this study was not to evaluate the protective effects of

RIPC on soft tissue in general over days after trauma or operation, but to detect whether RIPC has effects on cutaneous microcirculation and if so what kind of effects these might be. No other study before has demonstrated microcirculatory effects of RIPC on skin which should also be considered to be an important body organ that must be protected against ischemia in several settings.

Although it is generally accepted that IP increases flap survival by enhancing microvascular perfusion, the molecular and microcirculatory mechanisms are still not completely understood. The noninvasive application of a tourniquet at the hindlimb to induce IP was introduced by Kuentscher et al. and demonstrated to be as effective as the invasive clamping of the flap's pedicle itself, including both adipocutaneous and muscle flaps [20].

Recently, remote ischemic preconditioning demonstrated a modulation of hepatic microcirculation with consecutive reduction of the effects of ischemic reperfusion injury in an in-vivo animal model. RIPC in that setting significantly increased red blood cell velocity, sinusoidal flow and sinusoidal perfusion along with decreased neutrophil adhesion and cell death. For remote preconditioning the tourniquet was tightened around the limb until no flow was detected. The procedure involved 5 minutes of ischemia followed by 5 minutes of reperfusion. This was repeated four times [21]. Regarding myocardial perfusion, Hooele et al. could not find an effect of RIPC on coronary microvascular resistance or coronary flow in humans [22]. Nevertheless, Thielmann et al. found that myocardial injury after coronary artery bypass grafting was reduced by RIPC [23]. Zimmermann et al. demonstrated RIPC as protective from acute kidney injury in patients following cardiac surgery. In that study remote ischemic preconditioning was applied by an automated thigh tourniquet consisting of three 5-minute intervals of lower extremity ischemia separated by 5-minute intervals of reperfusion. Within 48 hours after surgery there was a significant both absolute and relative risk reduction due to preconditioning [24]. Another recent trial found no evidence that remote ischemic preconditioning provided protection of kidney function in children undergoing operation for complex congenital heart disease. Four cycles of five minutes RIPC were applied in that study [25].

The clinical and experimental data about RIPC in current literature remains confusing. An equal microcirculatory effect of RIPC on different kinds of tissue obviously is not mandatory demonstrated in several studies. A dose effect dependency can still not be included in RIPC because of the fact that there is still a non-equivalent effect apparent in different trials with identical dosages of RIPC. The main reason for this heterogeneous scientific data could be the indisputable heterogeneity of clinical studies concerning with RIPC, especially in terms of methodology and cohorts [26]. Thus, basic scientific research on RIPC is mandatory and must include investigations on healthy cohorts. For this reason, we included only young, healthy subjects in our study and focused our investigation on immediate and short-term effects of RIPC on a currently scientifically non-investigated body area.

Current scientific data demonstrate that three cycles of IP are significantly superior to one or two cycles, regardless of whether the cycles were 5 min or 10 min [27]. According to that current literature, remote ischemia in our study was applied at the contralateral upper arm including five minutes of ischemia with ten and finally fifteen minutes of reperfusion over three circles leading to an increase of cutaneous oxygen saturation at the anterolateral thigh skin territory, a significant increase of the capillary blood flow as well as a statistical significant decrease of the postcapillary filling pressure as a marker of venous stasis.

As our study elucidated the short term results of RIPC and documented the beneficial effect of the intermittent, repetitive component of RIPC on microcirculation, further studies should now focus on intermediate and long term effects of RIPC on cutaneous microcirculation. Another field of application of RIPC should also be part of further investigations calling muscular microcirculation as ischemia of muscle does not necessarily lead to muscle necrosis, but can lead to progressive microvascular dysfunction at an early stage with consecutive microcirculatory impairment as a vicious circle up to a compartment syndrome [28]. Therefore, an increase of cutaneous oxygen saturation and capillary blood flow as well as a decrease of venous stasis as immediate effects of RIPC, which we

demonstrated in our study, might also be beneficial in reoxygenation-associated inflammation due to reperfusion injury in muscular trauma or surgery.

Limitations

This study enrolled 27 healthy subjects for microcirculatory assessment of RIPC. In spite of the cohort size, statistical analysis found significant changes of microcirculation. Nevertheless, further studies have to evaluate the correlation of the microcirculatory parameters and RIPC in a clinical setting before and after extended soft tissue traumatization or elective free flap transplantation.

Conclusion

Remote ischemic preconditioning effects cutaneous tissue oxygen saturation, arterial capillary blood flow and postcapillary venous filling pressure at a distinct location of the lower extremity. Although, current scientific literature indicates that remote preconditioning is a systemic phenomenon, only a few studies have focused on the elucidation of its mechanisms of action. To what extent early and late remote preconditioning might influence the reperfusion injury of free flap transplantation, further clinical trials have to evaluate both in the means of microcirculatory assessment and clinical assessment of soft tissue necrosis due to traumatization or partial or total flap loss in free flap transplantation as end points of these studies.

Author details
[1]Plastic, Hand and Reconstructive Surgery, Hannover Medical School, Carl-Neuberg-Strasse 1, 30625 Hannover, Germany. [2]Department of Nephrology, Hannover Medical School, Carl-Neuberg-Strasse 1, 30625 Hannover, Germany.

Authors' contributions
RK, JL, KK, PMV conceived of the study, participated in its design and coordination and helped to draft the manuscript. MK carried out the data assessment. CH, MB participated in the design of the study, drafted the manuscript and performed the statistical analysis. All authors read and approved the final manuscript.

Competing interests
The authors declare that they have no competing interests.

References
1. Lorenzo AR, Lin CH, Lin CH, Lin YT, Nguyen A, Hsu CC, Wei FC: **Selection of the recipient vein in microvascular flap reconstruction of the lower extremity: Analysis of 362 free-tissue transfers.** *J Plast Reconstr Aesthet Surg* 2011, **64**(5):649-55, Epub 2010 Aug 21.
2. Nahabedian MY, Momen B, Manson PN: **Factors associated with anastomotic failure after microvascular reconstruction of the breast.** *Plast Reconstr Surg* 2004, **114**:74e82.
3. Moran SL, Serletti JM: **Outcome comparison between free and pedicled TRAM flap breast reconstruction in the obesepatient.** *Plast Reconstr Surg* 2001, **108**:1954e60, [discussion:61e2].
4. Cleveland JC Jr, Meldrum DR, Rowland RT, Banerjee A, Harken AH: **Preconditioning and hypothermic cardioplegia protect human heart equally against ischemia.** *Ann Thorac Surg* 1997, **63**:147e52.

5.   Friehs I, Moran AM, Stamm C, Choi YH, Cowan DB, McGowan FX, del Nido PJ: **Promoting angiogenesis protects severely hypertrophied hearts from ischemic injury.** *Ann Thorac Surg* 2004, **77**:2004e10, [discussion: 11].

6.   Koti RS, Seifalian AM, McBride AG, Yang W, Davidson BR: **The relationship of hepatic tissue oxygenation with nitric oxide metabolism in ischemic preconditioning of the liver.** *FASEB J* 2002, **16**:1654-1656.

7.   Kharbanda RK, Mortensen UM, White PA, Kristiansen SB, Schmidt MR, Hoschtitzky JA, Vogel M, Sorensen K, Redington AN, MacAllister R: **Transient limb ischemia induces remote ischemic preconditioning in vivo.** *Circulation* 2002, **106**:2881.

8.   Mounsey RA, Pang CY, Boyd JB, Forrest C: **Augmentation of skeletal muscle survival in the latissimus dorsi porcine model using acute ischemic preconditioning.** *J Otolaryngol* 1992, **21**:315e20.

9.   Adanali G, Ozer K, Siemionow M: **Early and late effects of ischemic preconditioning on microcirculation of skeletal muscle flaps.** *Plast Reconstr Surg* 2002, **109**:1344e51.

10. Zhang F, Oswald T, Holt J, Gerzenshtein J, Lei MP, Lineaweaver WC: **Regulation of inducible nitric oxide synthase in ischemic preconditioning of muscle flap in a rat model.** *Ann Plast Surg* 2004, **52**:609e13.

11. Kinnunen I, Laurikainen E, Schrey A, Laippala P, Aitasalo K: **Effect of acute ischemic preconditioning on blood-flow response in the epigastric pedicled rat flap.** *J Reconstr Microsurg* 2002, **18**:61e8.

12. Scheufler O, Andresen R, Kirsch A, Banzer D, Vaubel E: **Clinical results of TRAM flap delay by selective embolization of the deep inferior epigastric arteries.** *Plast Reconstr Surg* 2000, **105**:1320e9.

13. Vandenbroucke JP, von Elm E, Altman DG, Gøtzsche PC, Mulrow CD, Pocock SJ, Poole C, Schlesselman JJ, Egger M, STROBE initiative: **Strengthening the Reporting of Observational Studies in Epidemiology (STROBE): explanation and elaboration.** *Ann Intern Med* 2007, **147(8)**: W163-94.

14. Frank KH, Kessler M, Appelaum K, Dümmler W: **The erlangen micro-lightguide spectrophotometer EMPHO I.** *Phys Med Biol* 1989, **34**:1883-1900.

15. Menger MD, Pelikan S, Steiner D, Messmer K: **Microvascular ischemia-reperfusion injury in striated muscle: significance of "reflow paradox".** *Am J Physiol* 1992, **263**:H1901e6.

16. Pang CY, Yang RZ, Zhong A, Xu N, Boyd B, Forrest CR: **Acute ischaemic preconditioning protects against skeletal muscle infarction in the pig.** *Cardiovasc Res* 1995, **29**:782e8.

17. Wang WZ, Anderson G, Maldonado C, Barker J: **Attenuation of vasospasm and capillary no-reflow by ischemic preconditioning in skeletal muscle.** *Microsurgery* 1996, **17**:324e9.

18. Wang WZ, Anderson G, Firrell JC, Tsai TM: **Ischemic preconditioning versus intermittent reperfusion to improve blood flow to a vascular isolated skeletal muscle flap of rats.** *J Trauma* 1998, **45**:953e9.

19. Adanali G, Ozer K, Siemionow M: **Early and late effects of ischemic preconditioning on microcirculation of skeletal muscle flaps.** *Plast Reconstr Surg* 2002, **109**:1344e51.

20. Küntscher MV, Schirmbeck EU, Menke H, Klar E, Gebhard MM, Germann G: **Ischemic preconditioning by brief extremity ischemia before flap ischemia in a rat model.** *Plast Reconstr Surg* 2002, **109**:2398e404.

21. Tapuria N, Junnarkar SP, Dutt N, Abu-Amara M, Fuller B, Seifalian AM, Davidson BR: **Effect of remote ischemic preconditioning on hepatic microcirculation and function in a rat model of hepatic ischemia reperfusion injury.** *HPB (Oxford)* 2009, **11(2)**:108-17.

22. Hoole SP, Heck PM, White PA, Khan SN, O'Sullivan M, Clarke SC, Dutka DP: **Remote ischemic preconditioning stimulus does not reduce microvascular resistance or improve myocardial blood flow in patients undergoing elective percutaneous coronary intervention.** *Angiology* 2009, **60(4)**:403-11, Epub 2008 Dec 23.

23. Thielmann M, Kottenberg E, Boengler K, Raffelsieper C, Neuhaeuser M, Peters J, Jakob H, Heusch G: **Remote ischemic preconditioning reduces myocardial injury after coronary artery bypass grafting with crystalloid cardioplegic arrest.** *Basic Res Cardiol* 2005, **105**:657-664.

24. Zimmerman RF, Ezeanuna PU, Kane JC, Cleland CD, Kempananjappa TJ, Lucas FL, Kramer R: **Ischemic preconditioning at a remote site prevents acute kidney injury in patients following cardiac surgery.** *Kidney Int* 2011, **80(8)**:861-7, Epub 2011 Jun 15.

25. Pedersen KR, Ravn HB, Povlsen JV, Schmidt MR, Erlandsen EJ, Hjortdal VE: **Failure of remote ischemic preconditioning to reduce the risk of postoperative acute kidney injury in children undergoing operation for complex congenital heart disease: A randomized single-center study.** *J Thorac Cardiovasc Surg* 2011.

26. Peters J: **Remote ischaemic preconditioning of the heart: remote questions, remote importance, or remote preconditions?** *Basic Res Cardiol* 2011, **106(4)**:507-9, Epub 2011 May 5.

27. Zahir KS, Syed SA, Zink JR, Restifo RJ, Thomson JG: **Comparison of the effects of ischemic preconditioning and surgical delay on pedicled musculocutaneous flap survival in a rat model.** *Ann Plast Surg* 1998, **40**:422e8, [discussion: 8e9].

28. Zhang L, Bail H, Mittlmeier T, Haas NP, Schaser K: **Immediate microcirculatory derangements in skeletal muscle and periosteum after closed tibial fracture.** *J Trauma* 2003, **54(5)**:979-85.

Intraoperative use of enriched collagen and elastin matrices with freshly isolated adipose-derived stem/stromal cells: a potential clinical approach for soft tissue reconstruction

Ziyad Alharbi[1,2]*, Sultan Almakadi[1], Christian Opländer[1], Michael Vogt[3], Hans-Oliver Rennekampff[1] and Norbert Pallua[1]

Abstract

Background: Adipose tissue contains a large number of multipotent cells, which are essential for stem cell-based therapies. The combination of this therapy with suitable commercial clinically used matrices, such as collagen and elastin matrices (i.e. dermal matrices), is a promising approach for soft tissue reconstruction. We previously demonstrated that the liposuction method affects the adherence behaviour of freshly isolated adipose-derived stem/stromal cells (ASCs) on collagen and elastin matrices. However, it remains unclear whether freshly isolated and uncultured ASCs could be directly transferred to matrices during a single transplantation operation without additional cell culture steps.

Methods: After each fat harvesting procedure, ASCs were isolated and directly seeded onto collagen and elastin matrices. Different time intervals (i.e. 1, 3 and 24 h) were investigated to determine the time interval needed for cellular attachment to the collagen and elastin matrices. Resazurin-based vitality assays were performed after seeding the cells onto the collagen and elastin matrices. In addition, the adhesion and migration of ASCs on the collagen and elastin matrices were visualised using histology and two-photon microscopy.

Results: A time-dependent increase in the number of viable ASCs attached to the collagen and elastin matrices was observed. This finding was supported by mitochondrial activity and histology results. Importantly, the ASCs attached and adhered to the collagen and elastin matrices after only 1 h of *ex vivo* enrichment. This finding was also supported by two-photon microscopy, which revealed the presence and attachment of viable cells on the upper layer of the construct.

Conclusion: Freshly isolated uncultured ASCs can be safely seeded onto collagen and elastin matrices for *ex vivo* cellular enrichment of these constructs after liposuction. Although we observed a significant number of seeded cells on the matrices after a 3-h enrichment time, we also observed an adequate number of isolated cells after a 1-h enrichment time. However, this approach must be optimised for clinical use. Thus, *in vivo* studies and clinical trials are needed to investigate the feasibility of this approach.

Keywords: Adipose tissue-derived stem/stromal cells, Stromal vascular fraction, Liposuction, Fat grafting, Biomaterials, Collagen-based scaffolds, Regeneration and tissue engineering

* Correspondence: zalharbi@ukaachen.de
[1]Department of Plastic, Reconstructive and Hand Surgery - Burn Center, Medical Faculty, RWTH Aachen University, Pauwelsstr. 30, Aachen D-52074, Germany
[2]Division of Plastic Surgery, Specialist Surgery Center, King Abdullah Medical City, Mecca, Kingdom of Saudi Arabia
Full list of author information is available at the end of the article

Background

Adipose tissue stores a large number of multipotent cells, which are essential for stem cell-based therapies [1]. Stem and progenitor cells typically comprise approximately 3 to 7% of the cells in the uncultured stromal vascular fraction (SVF) from adipose tissue [1,2]. The term SVF is commonly used in the literature and refers to the cellular pellet without fat cells (i.e., mature adipocytes). This fraction can be obtained through an isolation process that uses collagenase secondary to liposuction (i.e., fat harvesting), resulting in a component that contains multiple cells: adipose-derived stem/stromal cells (ASCs). ASCs consist of endothelial cells, smooth muscle cells, fibroblasts and stem cells. [2]. Adipose-derived stem cells are adult self-renewing cells of mesenchymal origin that can differentiate not only into the adipogenic lineage but also into the osteogenic, chondrogenic, myogenic and neurogenic lineages *in vitro* [3,4].

We previously demonstrated that the method of liposuction influences the viability of the ASCs isolated from adipose tissue and the quantity of growth factors produced after cellular transplantation onto clinically used collagen and elastin matrices [5]. The results also indicated that collagen and elastin matrices could be used as *ex vivo* cellular carriers for tissue engineering. In this context, several studies investigated the safety of collagen and elastin matrices for keratinocyte and ASC cultivation [6]. Tissue engineering protocols that include a specific time period for the cultivation of ASCs require the use of a lab facility for as long as several days. Such protocols require Good Manufacturing Practicing (GMP) facilities and may be expensive. In contrast, the manual or automatic isolation of ASCs can be performed directly in the operating room (e.g., using a Cytori device). Thus, the direct transfer of ASCs onto available commercial matrices would be possible during a single operation. However, a short cultivation time (i.e., 1 to 3 hours) would be ideal for transplantation, particularly in a clinical setting with no access to further lab processing or GMP facilities.

The time required for *ex vivo* attachment of adipose-derived cells to collagen and elastin matrices before transplantation of the enriched construct to the patient during soft tissue reconstruction remains unknown. The results obtained in our previous study demonstrated that a significant number of cells attached to the collagen and elastin matrices after 24 hours of cultivation, regardless of the method of liposuction. However, this time is not realistic for a surgeon performing surgery under anaesthesia. Therefore, we compared the enrichment of collagen and elastin matrices with ASCs after short time periods (i.e., 1 h and 3 h) and long time periods (i.e., 24 h) to define a protocol that avoids delays in the operating room (Figure 1).

These time intervals were chosen to determine whether a 3-h time period is needed for cellular sedimentation onto the scaffolds or whether a 1-h sedimentation time is adequate for the cells to attach and migrate onto the collagen and elastin matrices prior to transplantation of the enriched construct in the operating room. We compared the results obtained using short cultivation times (1 and 3 h) with the results obtained using a 24-h cellular cultivation time, which was demonstrated to be a successful approach in our previous study [5]. We designed the experiment without the need for processing of the cells to simulate clinical conditions. Thus, for example, a patient could have a single operation that included the enrichment of the selected collagen-based matrix and split thickness skin transfer for multi-layer reconstruction of soft tissue defects.

Methods

Patients

Ten healthy patients (5 males and 5 females) between 27 and 59 years of age had elective liposuction (i.e., fat harvesting) in the Department of Plastic, Reconstructive and Hand Surgery – Burns Center at RWTH Aachen University Hospital. Each patient signed the consent form. The protocol and the use of human material were approved by the ethics committee of the Faculty of Medicine at RWTH University in Aachen, Germany (Name in German: Ethik-Kommission des Universitätsklinikums Aachen, Votum Number: EK163/07). The experiments were conducted in compliance with the Declaration of Helsinki Principles.

Liposuction and centrifugation of the obtained lipoaspirate

Fat was harvested via tumescent liposuction, as described previously [5,7]. The harvesting cannula used in this study was the st'RIM cannula (Thiebaud Biomedical Devices, Margencel, France), which was developed by Guy Magalon for micro-lipografting. This cannula was 2 mm in diameter with a blunt tip and four 600-μm gauge orifices. After the liposuction procedure, the samples were centrifuged for 3 min at 3,000 rpm using a Sigma 2–16 K centrifuge (Osterode am Harz, Germany). After centrifugation, the purified lipoaspirate was immediately used in experiments (Figure 1).

Isolation of ASCs from lipoaspirate

Isolation of the cellular pellet was performed as described previously [5]. Briefly, the purified lipoaspirate was transferred into a sterile tube and normal saline was added to remove cell debris and blood. A second centrifugation process was then completed for 10 min at $300 \times g$. The extracellular matrix was digested with 0.075% collagenase I (Biochrom, Berlin, Germany) for 45 min at 37°C. The digested tissue solution was subsequently filtered using a

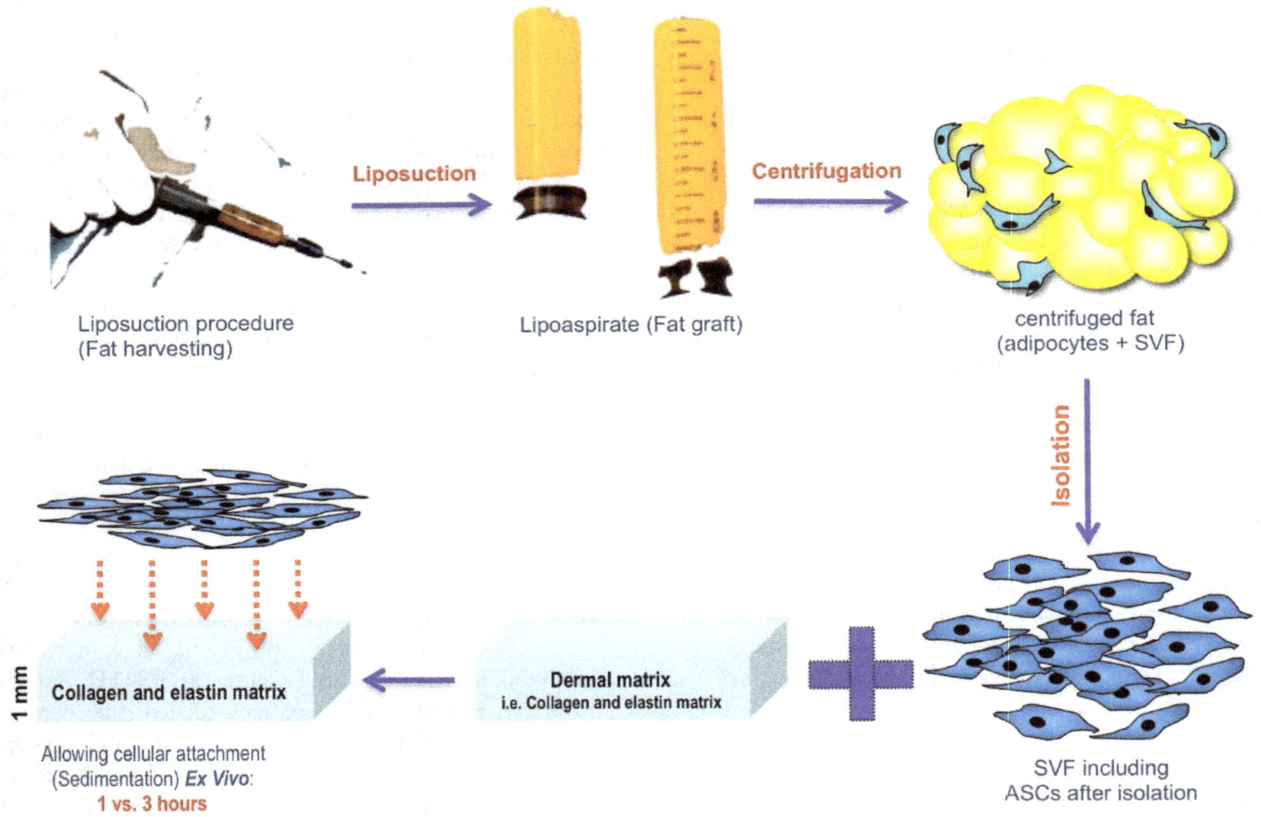

Figure 1 An illustration of the described approach. After isolation of cells from adipose tissue secondary to liposuction, the obtained adipose-derived stem/stromal cells were directly transferred to the collagen and elastin matrix without additional cell culture steps. The cells were incubated on top of the material for different clinically relevant time periods (i.e., 1 and 3 h) for cellular matrix enrichment. For comparison, the cells were incubated with the matrices for 24 h.

250 μm filter (Neolab, Heidelberg, Germany). The pellet was resuspended in 30 ml of a NaCl solution and centrifuged for another 10 min at 300 × g to obtain the SVF, which contained the ASCs. The pellet was then resuspended in DMEM/F12 supplemented with 100 U/ml of penicillin and 100 μg of streptomycin, without foetal calf serum or proliferation factors. The isolated cells were not cultured or passaged prior to direct transplantation onto the collagen and elastin matrix.

Incubation of ASCs on collagen and elastin matrices to assess cellular adherence

Circular 1 mm thick pieces of non–cross-linked native bovine collagen and elastin matrix containing type I, III, and V collagen derived from bovine skin were used (Matriderm® sheet; MedSkin Solutions Dr. Suwelack AG, Billerbeck, Germany). A circular punch biopsy device measuring 0.8 cm in diameter was used to cut the matrix into small pieces, which were placed into 48-well culture plates. The isolated cells were added to 48-well culture plates lined with collagen and elastin matrix at a density

of 50,000 cells per well and incubated at 37°C with 5% CO_2 for 1, 3 or 24 h. The collagen and elastin matrix that was incubated with the isolated cells was separated after a 1-, 3- or 24-h incubation period (Figure 1). The matrices were washed carefully with normal saline (0.9% NaCl) and transferred into a clean culture Plate. A 270 μl volume of DMEM/F12 supplemented with 100 U/ml penicillin and 100 μg/ml streptomycin was added, and 30 μl of the alamarBlue® resazurin reagent (AbD Serotec, Oxford, UK), was subsequently delivered to each well. This assay can be used to detect the metabolic activity of cells using a fluorescence spectrometer. The medium/alamarBlue® mix was repeated and carefully removed from the well after 2 hours at 37°C and 5% CO_2. The samples were then measured at room temperature using a Fluostar Optima fluorescence spectrometer (BMG Labtech, Offenburg, Germany), with an excitation wavelength of 540 nm and an emission wavelength 590 nm. We avoided measuring the matrix itself to avoid the influence of the matrix on fluorescence. The alamarBlue® reagent was added to the medium without cells as a negative control.

Analysis of cellular attachment and migration by histology

Cell-loaded pieces of collagen and elastin matrix were histologically investigated directly after cellular transplantation onto the matrix. The samples were fixed overnight in Lidi's 4% formalin (Merck, Darmstadt, Germany). The formalin was then removed by extensive washing, and the samples were dehydrated using an increasing gradient of isopropanol, embedded into paraplast, and cut into 15 μm sections. Staining was then performed using hematoxylin and eosin. Microscopic analyses of all samples were performed via light microscopy in our laboratory.

Analysis of cellular distribution on collagen and elastin matrices using two-photon microscopy

Two-photon microscopy using an FV1000MPE microscope (Olympus Corp., Tokyo, Japan) attached to a pulsed Ti-Sapphire laser (MaiTai DeepSee, SpectraPhysics, Santa Clara, CA, USA) was performed to visualise the 3D-structure of the collagen and elastin matrices, including the organisation of the isolated cells within the matrix. Hoechst 33342 was added for vital staining of the nuclei. The enriched collagen and elastin matrices were also stained with fluorescein diacetate (FDA) to image the isolated cells in combination with Hoechst 33342 for nuclei staining. The enriched collagen and elastin matrix was then visualised using the non-linear optical effect of second harmonic generation (SHG). Hoechst was excited at 730 nm and detected at 418–468 nm. Series of subsequent 1024 × 1024 pixel xy-frames were then obtained in 1 mm z-steps for structural 3D reconstruction using Imaris Software (Bitplane, Zurich, Switzerland).

Statistical analysis

Data analysis was performed using Prism® software, version 5.01c (GraphPad, La Jolla, CA, USA). A Gaussian distribution of the values was assessed using the D'Agostino & Pearson omnibus normality test. One-way repeated measures ANOVA was performed followed by an appropriate post-hoc multiple comparison test (i.e., Tukey method). Differences for which $p < 0.05$ were considered statistically significant.

Results

Assessment of ASC adherence to collagen and elastin matrices

The relative viability and adherence rates of the isolated adipose-derived cells on the collagen and elastin matrices were tested using the alamarBlue-assay® after different enrichment times on the matrices (i.e., 1 h, 3 h, and 24 h). A significantly larger number of viable cells were attached to the collagen and elastin matrices after a 3-h enrichment time (mean: 1,551 and SD: 790; median: 1615 and range: 284.5-2,972) than after a 1-h incubation time (mean: 791.4 and SD: 471.3; median: 882.5 and

range: 219.5-1,856) (Figure 2). The observed cellular viability and adhesion rates were 3- to 4-fold higher after a 24-h incubation (mean: 5,120 and SD: 2,070; median: 5,368 and range: 1,267-7,947). However, it should be noted that freshly isolated uncultured ASCs attached and adhered to the collagen and elastin matrices after only 1 h of incubation, indicating that this approach is clinically relevant.

Analysis of cellular attachment and migration using histology

Cell-loaded pieces of collagen and elastin matrix were investigated histologically 1, 3 and 24 hours after seeding the ASCs onto the matrices. After a 1-h incubation, the seeded ASCs were observed on the upper layer of the matrices (Figure 3). Cells that were incubated on the collagen and elastin matrices for 3 h exhibited small cytoplasmic fragments deeper in the matrices. ASCs incubated on the collagen and elastin matrices for 24 hours exhibited the same migration process into the middle layer.

Visualisation of the 3D structure of collagen and elastin matrices to assess morphology and attachment of seeded ASCs

The enriched collagen and elastin matrices were investigated after a 1-h enrichment time via two-photon microscopy using autofluorescence to reveal the collagen and elastin structures. Based on the results we obtained using two-photon microscopy with a 24-h time point in our previous study [5], we concentrated on early time

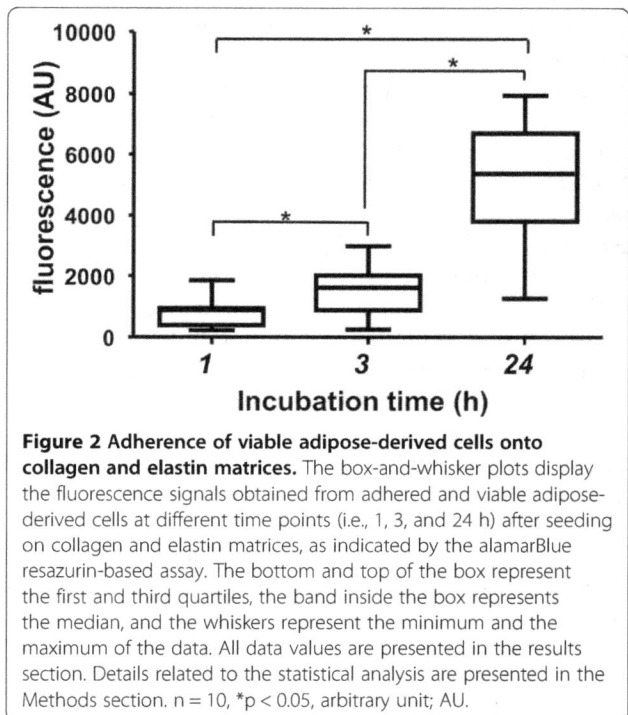

Figure 2 Adherence of viable adipose-derived cells onto collagen and elastin matrices. The box-and-whisker plots display the fluorescence signals obtained from adhered and viable adipose-derived cells at different time points (i.e., 1, 3, and 24 h) after seeding on collagen and elastin matrices, as indicated by the alamarBlue resazurin-based assay. The bottom and top of the box represent the first and third quartiles, the band inside the box represents the median, and the whiskers represent the minimum and the maximum of the data. All data values are presented in the results section. Details related to the statistical analysis are presented in the Methods section. n = 10, *p < 0.05, arbitrary unit; AU.

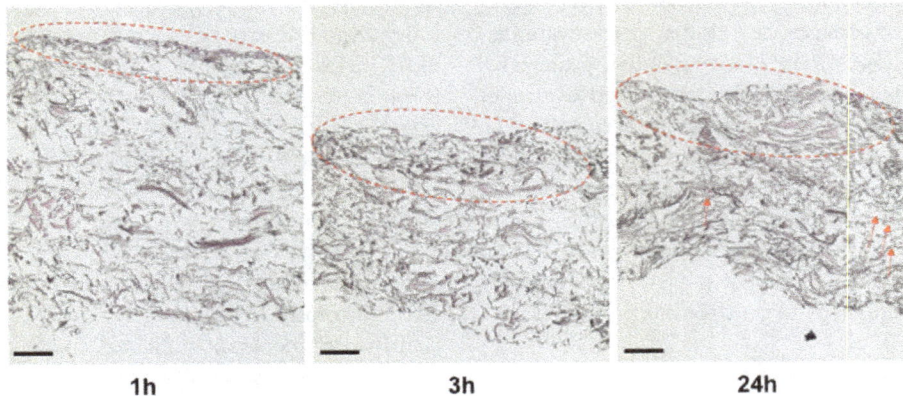

1h   **3h**   **24h**

Figure 3 Histology of enriched collagen and elastin matrices. This figure shows representative histology images of the collagen and elastin matrices, which were incubated with freshly isolated adipose-derived stem/stromal cells for the indicated time periods (scale bar is 200 μm).

points. Viable cells with visible cytoplasm and nuclei were observed on the 3D structure of the collagen and elastin matrix (Figure 4). The previously discussed metabolic activity tests and histological investigations demonstrated that a number of isolated cells attached to the collagen and elastin matrices after 1 h. The green colour indicates the cytoplasmic portion of cells, which was stained with FDA, and the blue colour shows the nuclei, which were stained with Hoechst 33342. The spatial distribution of the cells is also shown (Figure 4).

Discussion

The clinical applicability of adipose-derived stem cell therapy has been investigated extensively during the last decade, and interesting results have been obtained with respect to regeneration and wound healing, as well as reconstruction and rejuvenation [4]. One advantage of this approach is that adipose tissue represents an easily available and accessible source of mesenchymal stem cells that are supported by abundant stromal cells and growth factors [5]. However, it is essential to determine the applicability of this approach, particularly with respect to legal issues. In some countries, including Germany, any patient materials that leave the operating room for stem cell processing and future re-injection must be processed in GMP facilities. These facilities are expensive and difficult to find. In contrast, autologous transplantation of ASCs in a single session would overcome this problem. Several previous studies investigated the effect of enriching fat grafts with the SVF in a clinical setting [8]. However, it remains unclear whether the enrichment of a safe and biocompatible collagen and elastin matrix with autologous and freshly isolated ASCs is possible. In addition, the role of enrichment time in this approach has not been investigated. Studies addressing these issues could expand the use of soft tissue matrices in combination with ASCs.

Biocompatible matrices, such as collagen and elastin matrices, are currently used in combination with skin grafting as double-layer constructs to support the graft and the formation of a neodermis [9]. However, it must be determined not only whether such matrices are biocompatible but also whether they are cytocompatible. In our previously published study, we demonstrated that freshly isolated uncultured ASCs adhere to collagen and elastin matrices *ex vivo* in only 24 hours. This result

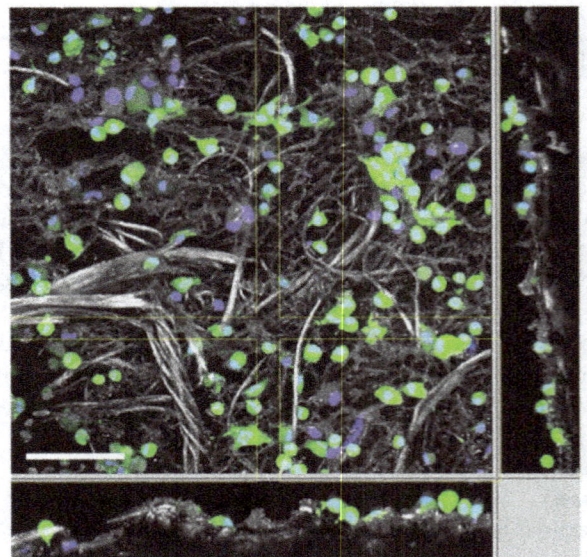

Figure 4 Two-photon microscopy of the enriched collagen and elastin matrices. This figure shows a representative two-photon microscopy image of a collagen and elastin matrix, which was incubated with freshly isolated adipose-derived stem/stromal cells for only 1 h. The green colour indicates the cytoplasm of viable cells, which was stained using fluorescein diacetate (FDA), the blue colour indicates the cell nuclei, which were stained using Hoechst 33342, and the grey colour indicates the collagen and elastin structure (scale bar is 100 μm).

indicates that these biocompatible materials are also cytocompatible and appropriate for use with mesenchymal stem cells immediately after their isolation.

However, a 24-h enrichment time is too long to be implemented in the operating room. Thus, a shorter enrichment time of the selected scaffolds with the stem cells is required. We investigated different time intervals to determine whether a 3-h or 1-h cellular sedimentation time on the scaffolds is sufficient to support cellular attachment and migration onto the collagen and elastin matrices prior to transplantation of the enriched construct in the operating room. We compared the results obtained using these short cultivation times (i.e., 1 and 3 h) with the results obtained using a 24 h cellular cultivation time.

In this study, we observed that cellular enrichment on the collagen and elastin matrices after 3 h is improved compared to that observed after 1 h. These results were supported by mitochondrial activity results, which indicate viability, and histological analysis [10-13]. In addition, we demonstrated that enrichment of a collagen and elastin matrix with cells obtained from adipose tissue is possible after a 1-h *ex vivo* enrichment time. This conclusion was also supported by two-photon microscopy results, which revealed the presence and attachment of viable cells on the upper layer of the construct. However, penetration depth is limited based on the employed material, tissue or scaffold (e.g., for collagen and elastin matrices up to 150 μm).

Protocols must be defined for clinical use. Such protocols should include the ideal time for cellular enrichment on the selected biocompatible and cytocompatible matrices, the number of isolated adipose cells per square meter, the proportions of specific cellular elements, including stem cells, in the total population, the commitment of those stem cells toward adipogenic conversion or conversion into other lines *in vivo* and the factors important for control of the environment, including factors that support nutrition and angiogenesis. These factors must be investigated *in animal models* before this type of therapy can be applied in a clinical setting. The fate of ASC-enriched collagen and elastin matrices after transplantation can only be determined *in vivo* in clinical trials. However, prior to clinical trials, it is also necessary to optimise this approach. Specifically, the type of isolated cells that adhere to the matrix must be characterised. The regenerative potential of these cells and the potential benefits for patients should also be addressed in future studies. As previously discussed, the use of the freshly isolated uncultured ASCs seeded directly onto biocompatible scaffolds during a single surgery avoids the need for GMP facilities. Thus, this approach would bridge the gap between the bench and the bedside.

Conclusion

Freshly isolated uncultured ASCs can be safely seeded onto collagen and elastin matrices after a liposuction procedure for *ex vivo* cellular enrichment of these constructs. Although we observed a significant number of transplanted cells on the matrices after a 3-h enrichment time, we could also observed an adequate number of isolated cells on the matrices after a shorter 1-h enrichment time. This finding was also supported by two-photon microscopy. However, it is necessary to optimise this approach for clinical use. Thus, *in vivo* studies and clinical trials are needed to investigate the feasibility of this approach.

Competing interests
The authors declare that they have no competing interests.

Authors' contributions
ZA drafted the manuscript, participated in study design and conducted the isolation procedure, in vitro procedures and helped in statistical analysis. CO performed the statistical analysis and assisted in histology. HR participated in the coordination of the study and helped to draft the manuscript. SA aided in the organisation of materials and assisted during surgery. MV performed the two-photon microscopy. NP participated in the study design, performed all liposuction procedures, funded this study and helped to draft the manuscript. All authors read and approved the final manuscript.

Acknowledgements
We thank MedSkin Solutions Dr. Suwelack AG in Billerbeck, Germany for supplying the Matriderm® sheets. This work was also supported by the two-photon microscopy facility, which is a core facility of the Interdisciplinary Center for Clinical Research (IZKF) Aachen within the Faculty of Medicine at RWTH Aachen University. We acknowledge the American Manuscript Editors for their extensive editing service of this manuscript. Finally, all authors acknowledge Prof. Hilgers and his team in the department of medical statistics at RWTH Aachen University for the revision of our statistical analysis.

Author details
[1]Department of Plastic, Reconstructive and Hand Surgery - Burn Center, Medical Faculty, RWTH Aachen University, Pauwelsstr. 30, Aachen D-52074, Germany. [2]Division of Plastic Surgery, Specialist Surgery Center, King Abdullah Medical City, Mecca, Kingdom of Saudi Arabia. [3]Two-Photon Microscopy Facility, Interdisciplinary Center for Clinical Research (IZKF), Medical Faculty, RWTH Aachen University, Aachen, Germany.

References
1. Fraser JK, Zhu M, Wulur I, Alfonso Z: **Adipose-derived stem cells.** *Methods Mol Biol* 2008, **449**:59–67.
2. Tholpady SS, Llull R, Ogle RC, Rubin JP, Futrell JW, Katz AJ: **Adipose tissue: stem cells and beyond.** *Clin Plast Surg* 2006, **33**(1):55–62.
3. Mizuno H: **Adipose-derived stem cells for tissue repair and regeneration: ten years of research and a literature review.** *J Nihon Med Sch* 2009, **76**(2):56–66.
4. Gimble JM: **Adipose tissue-derived therapeutics.** *Expert Opin Biol Ther* 2003, **3**:705–713.
5. Alharbi Z, Opländer C, Almakadi S, Fritz A, Vogt M, Pallua N: **Conventional vs. micro-fat harvesting: how fat harvesting technique affects tissue-engineering approaches using adipose tissue-derived stem/stromal cells.** *J Plast Reconstr Aesthet Surg* 2013, **66**(9):1271–1278.
6. Keck M, Haluza D, Lumenta DB, Burjak S, Eisenbock B, Kamolz LP, Frey M: **Construction of a multi-layer skin substitute: Simultaneous cultivation of keratinocytes and preadipocytes on a dermal template.** *Burns* 2011, **37**(4):626–630.

7. Coleman SR: **Structural fat grafts: the ideal filler?** *Clin Plast Surg* 2001, **28**:111–119.
8. Chang Q, Li J, Dong Z, Liu L, Lu F: **Quantitative volumetric analysis of progressive hemifacial atrophy corrected using stromal vascular fraction-supplemented autologous fat grafts.** *Dermatol Surg* 2013, **39**(10):1465–1473.
9. Jeon H, Kim J, Yeo H, Jeong H, Son D, Han K: **Treatment of diabetic foot ulcer using matriderm in comparison with a skin graft.** *Arch Plast Surg* 2013, **40**(4):403–408.
10. Walum E, Hansson E, Harvey AL: **In vitro testing of neurotoxicity.** *ATLA* 1990, **18**:153–179.
11. Li K, Wong D, Hiscott P, Stanga P, Groenewald C, McGalliard J: **Trypan blue staining of internal limiting membrane and epiretinal membrane during vitrectomy: Visual results and histopathological findings.** *Br J Ophthalmol* 2003, **87**:216–219.
12. Ahmed SA, Gogal RM Jr, Walsh JE: **A new Rapid and Simple Non-Radioactive assay to Monitor and Determine the proliferation of Lymphocytes: An Alternative to H3-thymidine incorporation assay.** *J Immunol Methods* 1994, **170**:211–224.
13. Alley MC, Scudiero DA, Monks A, Hursey ML, Czerwinski MJ, Fine DL, Abbott BJ, Mayo JG, Shoemaker RH, Boyd MR: **Feasibility of Drug Screening with Panels of Human Tumor Cell Lines Using a Microculture Tetrazolium Assay.** *Cancer Res* 1988, **48**:589–601.

Aortic bypass and orthotopic right renal autotransplantation for midaortic syndrome

Hao Zhang[†], Fang-da Li[†], Hua-liang Ren and Yue-hong Zheng[*]

Abstract

Background: Midaortic syndrome (MAS) is a rare vascular anomaly characterized by segmental narrowing of the distal descending thoracic or abdominal aorta. Renal or visceral arteries may also be affected to varying degrees. MAS is often associated with renovascular hypertension, and requires early intervention. When medical therapy and percutaneous interventions fail to control hypertension, surgical treatment is required. We report a case of MAS that failed to respond to bilateral renal artery stenting, but treated with aortic bypass and orthotopic right renal autotransplantation with good outcome.

Case presentation: A 31-year-old woman presented with headache and poorly controlled hypertension due to severe MAS. She had severe ostial stenoses of renal and visceral arteries. Her hypertension failed to respond to medical therapy (four drugs) and bilateral renal artery stenting. The implanted stent in the right renal artery rendered revascularization of the artery difficult. A one-stage revascularization was performed, which consisted of an aortoaortic bypass (between the suprarenal and infrarenal abdominal aorta) with a prosthetic graft, an orthotopic right renal autotransplantation and an aorto-left renal arterial bypass with autogenous saphenous vein grafts. Her recovery was uneventful. At 1-year follow-up, the patient remained well. Her hypertension improved. A postoperative computed tomography angiography showed that all the grafts were patent with no abnormalities at the anastomosis.

Conclusion: Multiple bypass surgery with reimplantation of autogenous vein graft onto the prosthetic graft is a feasible and effective procedure in renal artery revascularization for MAS. Orthotopic autotransplantation is the procedure of choice in complex renal artery reconstruction.

Keywords: Midarotic syndrome, Aortoaortic bypass, Renal artery stenting, Orthotopic renal autotransplantation, Hypertension

Background

MAS is a rare vascular anomaly characterized by segmental narrowing of the distal descending thoracic or abdominal aorta. The term midaortic syndrome (MAS) was originally used by Sen et al [1]. MAS may be congenital or caused by some acquired reasons, such as Takayasu's arteritis, neurofibromatosis and fibromuscular dysplasia [2]. Visceral and renal artery stenoses are usually attached to the syndrome. Proximal renal artery stenosis may occur in up to 80% of cases, and visceral arteries may be stenosed

in at least 30% of cases [2,3]. MAS is often associated with refractory hypertension. If left untreated, most patients would die by the age of 40 as a result of complications from hypertension [3]. Computed tomography angiography offers convenient, fast and sharp images, and it is a useful tool in diagnosing MAS. Treatments for MAS include medical management, endovascular therapy, bypass grafting, and patch aortoplasty [2,4]. Kim et al introduced a novel treatment for midaortic syndrome, in which a tissue expander was used to induce longitudinal growth of the normal distal abdominal aorta and iliac arteries in a 3-year-old girl [5]. The goals of treatment for MAS are to normalize the blood pressure, avoid any complications of the hypertension, and preserve the renal function as much as possible. Invasive measures are favored when medical

---
* Correspondence: yuehongzheng@yahoo.com
[†]Equal contributors
Department of Vascular Surgery, Peking Union Medical College Hospital, Peking Union Medical College and Chinese Academy of Medical Sciences, No, 1 Shuaifuyuan, Dongcheng district, Beijing 100730, P.R China

management is insufficient or there is impending end-organ damage [3].

The present report involves a case of severe MAS affecting the renal and visceral arteries. She had undergone stenting for bilateral renal artery stenoses at another hospital. The patient successfully underwent a one-stage revascularization with an orthotopic right renal autotransplantation in our hospital. Since very few technical reports on orthotopic renal autotransplantation in MAS revascularization are found in the literature, the present report would add significant value.

Case presentation

A 31-year-old Chinese woman presented with headache and poorly controlled hypertension. Her blood pressure was 170/100 mm Hg in the brachial artery and 150/90 mm Hg in the thigh. She had a history of hypertension for about 20 years and her medical therapy comprised four antihypertensive medications (hydrochlorothiazide, amlodipine, arotinolol, irbesartan). Two years previously, she was diagnosed with Takayasu's arteritis and had undergone stenting for bilateral renal artery stenoses at another hospital. However, her arterial hypertension failed to improve. In the present admission, laboratory investigations revealed that a blood urea nitrogen level of 26.2 mg/dl, serum creatinine level of 4.9 mg/dl and erythrocyte sedimentation rate of 7 mm/h. Technetium-99m-diethylenetriaminepentacetic acid (99mTc-DTPA) renogram revealed decreases in the renal blood flow and the glomerular filtration rate (GFR). The GFR of the left and right kidney were 20.4 ml/min and 12.1 ml/min, respectively (total GFR 32.5 ml/min). Computed tomography angiography showed marked narrowing of the abdominal aorta, stents in bilateral renal arteries, well-established arc of Riolan, and ostial stenoses of the superior mesenteric artery and the celiac artery. Her right kidney was significantly atrophied (Figure 1). The thoracic aorta and its branches were normal.

Finally, an open repair was required for relief of her hypertension and preservation of the renal function. An aortoaortic bypass (between the suprarenal and infrarenal abdominal aorta) with a Gore-Tex® ring reinforced tube (16 mm diameter, WL Gore & Associates Inc, USA), an orthotopic right renal autotransplantation and an aorto-left renal arterial bypass with autogenous saphenous vein grafts were performed. The operation was performed through an arch incision below the costal margin under general anesthesia. We obtained a satisfactory exposure through appropriate division and traction. The aorta coarctation extended approximately 7 cm. After heparinization, the descending aorta was clamped and the prosthetic graft was anastomosed to the aorta in an end-to-side fashion. The autogenous saphenous vein grafts were harvested. To revascularize the right renal

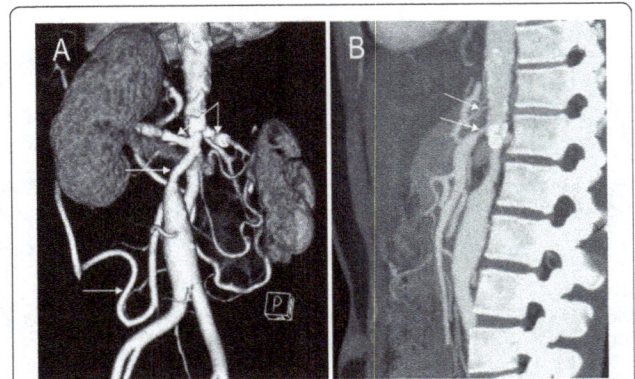

Figure 1 Preoperative imaging showing multiple arterial stenoses. A, Posteroanterior view of three-dimensional computed tomography angiography showing coarctation of the abdominal aorta (middle arrow), bilateral renal artery stents (two upper arrows) and arc of Riolan (lower arrow). **B**, Superior mesenteric artery stenosis (lower arrow) and celiac artery stenosis (upper arrow).

artery, we performed an *ex vivo* right renal artery repair and orthotopic autotransplantation. The right renal artery and vein were detached and the kidney was cold perfused with University of Wisconsin (UW) solution at 4°C. The ureter was left intact. The proximal stenosis containing the stent was resected. The right kidney was then re-implanted into its original fossa. Then the right renal artery was reconstructed with the autogenous vein graft and re-implanted onto the prosthetic graft. And the right renal vein was re-implanted onto the inferior vena cava (Figure 2). The ischemic time for the right kidney was 1 hour and 45 minutes. The right kidney was fixed to the surrounding tissues to prevent

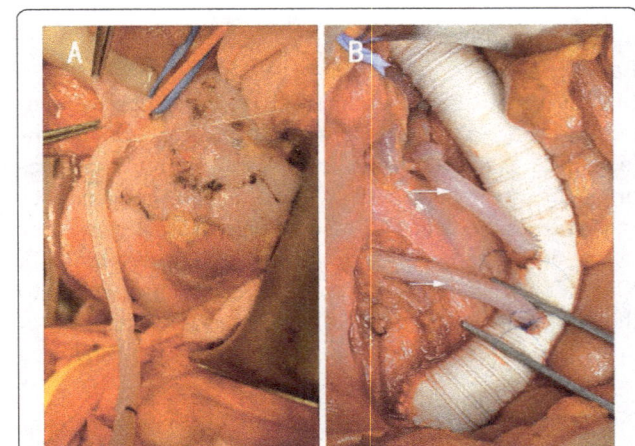

Figure 2 Cold perfusion of the right kidney and multiple bypass surgery. A, Cold perfusion of the right kidney with University of Wisconsin solution. **B**, Autogenous saphenous vein bypasses connect the left (upper arrow) and right (lower arrow) renal arteries to the prosthetic graft.

migration or kinking. Next, the proximal stenosis of the left renal artery containing the stent was resected and the artery was re-implanted onto the prosthetic graft in an end-to-side fashion with autogenous saphenous vein graft.

The postoperative course was uneventful. Postoperative anticoagulant therapy consisted of low molecular weight heparin (4000 U/twice a day) for 2 weeks. The therapy was then switched to clopidogrel (75 mg/day) for 3 months and aspirin (100 mg/day) for 6 months.

Evaluation at one year showed that the patient was well, still on nifedipine on a daily basis, and had a blood pressure of 140/90 mmHg. 99mTc-DTPA renogram revealed that the GFR of the left and right kidney were 53.7 ml/min and 10.1 ml/min, respectively (total GFR 63.8 ml/min). The computed tomography angiography showed that all the grafts were patent and there were no abnormalities at the anastomosis (Figure 3).

Discussion

We performed a one-stage revascularization for the patient. Percutaneous interventions are effective in relieving

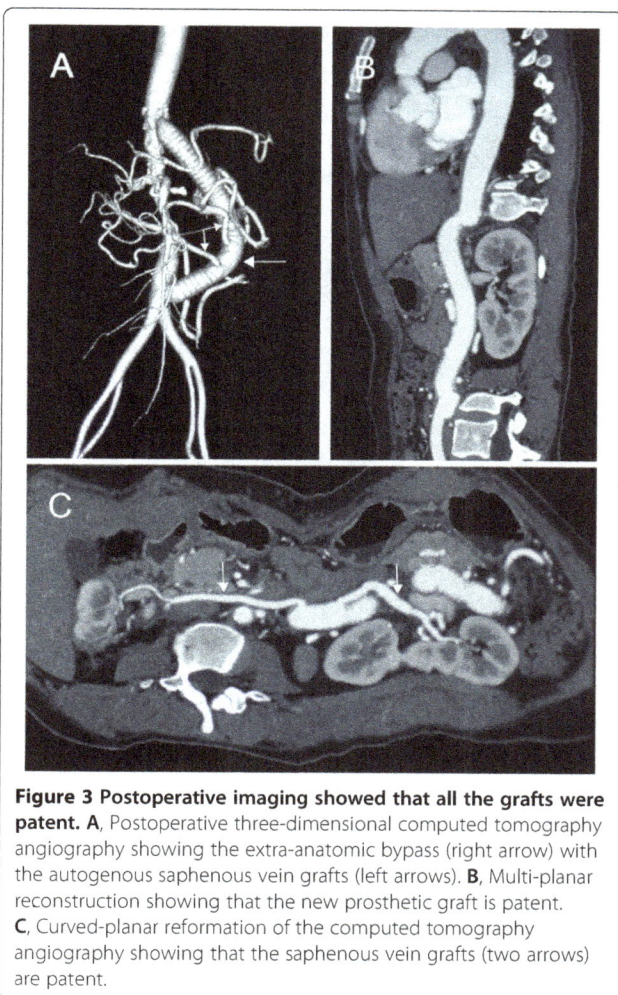

Figure 3 Postoperative imaging showed that all the grafts were patent. A, Postoperative three-dimensional computed tomography angiography showing the extra-anatomic bypass (right arrow) with the autogenous saphenous vein grafts (left arrows). **B**, Multi-planar reconstruction showing that the new prosthetic graft is patent. **C**, Curved-planar reformation of the computed tomography angiography showing that the saphenous vein grafts (two arrows) are patent.

obstruction of the renal arteries. However, renal artery stenting has not generally been effective in treating Takayasu's disease because of the severe vessel fibrosis [6]. In this patient, the symptoms of hypertension did not improve from renal artery stenting. In cases of complex disease affecting the renal or visceral arteries, bypass surgery is preferred [4]. Thus, severe stenoses of the visceral arteries and renal arteries in this patient justified an aggressive reconstructive approach. We previously reported a case of a 15-year-old boy with marked narrowing of the descending aorta, the orifice of the celiac artery and the superior mesenteric artery. The boy successfully underwent a bypass surgery [7].

To get a better exposure of the abdominal aorta and renal arteries, an arch incision was used below the costal margin. Nonetheless, reconstruction remained difficult because the right renal artery lied behind the inferior vena cava and the short right renal vein; moreover, the stenosis containing the stent needed resection, which rendered the reconstruction more difficult. Thus, right renal autotransplantation was indicated [8]. The preoperative renogram showed that the total GFR was 32.5 ml/min with the left kidney contributing 20.4 ml/min and the right kidney contributing 12.1 ml/min. To preserve the kidney function, right renal autotransplantation was preferred to a right radical nephrectomy. Multiple bypass surgery with reimplantation of the autogenous vein grafts onto the prosthetic graft was performed in bilateral renal artery revascularization. This anastomotic technique has been proved effective in our previous case report [7]. As the well-developed arc of Riolan provided enough flow to the superior mesenteric artery, the patient did not show any intestinal ischemic symptoms. Superior mesenteric artery revascularization did not appear to be necessary.

Postoperative hypertension in patients with MAS involves multiple systems [9]. In this patient, reduced arterial compliance and atrophied right kidney are expected to contribute to postoperative hypertension. The postoperative renogram revealed that left renal function was significantly improved and evaluation at one year showed that the patient's blood pressure was satisfactory. Long-term follow-up of patients with operated MAS has shown that surgery does not offer a lasting cure and the rate of recurrence of hypertension is high and surgical re-intervention is often needed [10]. Long-term complications of bypass surgery include anastomotic aneurysm, congestive heart failure, graft deterioration, abdominal aortic aneurysms, renal failure, and other cardiovascular events [11]. Thus, lifelong follow-up is mandatory.

Conclusion

We report a case of one-stage revascularization of severe MAS in a female patient who failed to respond to medical and endovascular therapy. In this case, multiple bypass surgery with reimplantation of autogenous vein grafts onto prosthetic graft is a feasible and effective procedure in renal artery revascularization. Besides, in cases of complex renal artery reconstruction, orthotopic autotransplantation may be the procedure of choice.

Consent

Written informed consent was obtained from the patient for publication of this case report and any accompanying images. A copy of the written consent is available for review by the Editor of this journal.

Abbreviations

MAS: Midaortic syndrome; GFR: Glomerular filtration rate; 99mTc-DTPA: Technetium-99m-diethylenetriaminepentacetic acid; UW: University of Wisconsin.

Competing interests

The authors declare that they have no competing interests.

Authors' contributions

HZ collected and analyzed the case and made substantial contributions to the writing of the manuscript. F-DL and H-LR contributed substantially to the process of analyzing the case and writing the manuscript. Y-HZ performed the operation and made the expert assistance in preparing the manuscript. All authors read and approved the final manuscript.

Acknowledgments

We would like to acknowledge Jean A Trejaut for revising the manuscript.

References

1. Sen PK, Kinare SG, Engineer SD, Parulkar GB: **The Middle Aortic Syndrome.** *Br Heart J* 1963, **25:**610–618.
2. Delis KT, Gloviczki P: **Middle aortic syndrome: from presentation to contemporary open surgical and endovascular treatment.** *Perspect Vasc Surg Endovasc Ther* 2005, **17:**187–203.
3. Porras D, Stein DR, Ferguson MA, Chaudry G, Alomari A, Vakili K, Fishman SJ, Lock JE, Kim HB: **Midaortic syndrome: 30 years of experience with medical, endovascular and surgical management.** *Pediatr Nephrol* 2013, **28**(10):2023–2033.
4. Stanley JC, Criado E, Eliason JL, Upchurch GR Jr, Berguer R, Rectenwald JE: **Abdominal aortic coarctation: surgical treatment of 53 patients with a thoracoabdominal bypass, patch aortoplasty, or interposition aortoaortic graft.** *J Vasc Surg* 2008, **48**(5):1073–1082.
5. Kim HB, Vakili K, Modi BP, Ferguson MA, Guillot AP, Potanos KM, Prabhu SP, Fishman SJ: **A novel treatment for the midaortic syndrome.** *N Engl J Med* 2012, **367**(24):2361–2362.
6. Connolly JE, Wilson SE, Lawrence PL, Fujitani RM: **Middle aortic syndrome: distal thoracic and abdominal coarctation, a disorder with multiple etiologies.** *J Am Coll Surg* 2002, **194**(6):774–781.
7. Liu Q, Song X, Liu C, Zheng YH: **Revascularization of midaortic dysplastic syndrome.** *J Vasc Surg* 2012, **55**(4):1166.
8. Novick AC, Jackson CL, Straffon RA: **The role of renal autotransplantation in complex urological reconstruction.** *J Urol* 1990, **143**(3):452–457.
9. Kenny D, Polson JW, Martin RP, Paton JF, Wolf AR: **Hypertension and coarctation of the aorta: an inevitable consequence of developmental pathophysiology.** *Hypertens Res* 2011, **34**(5):543–547.
10. Brown ML, Burkhart HM, Connolly HM, Dearani JA, Cetta F, Li Z, Oliver WC, Warnes CA, Schaff HV: **Coarctation of the aorta: lifelong surveillance is mandatory following surgical repair.** *J Am Coll Cardiol* 2013, **62**(11):1020–1025.
11. Taketani T, Miyata T, Morota T, Takamoto S: **Surgical treatment of atypical aortic coarctation complicating Takayasu's arteritis–experience with 33 cases over 44 years.** *J Vasc Surg* 2005, **41**(4):597–601.

4

Abdominal wall reconstruction with components separation and mesh reinforcement in complex hernia repair

Claire L Nockolds[1], Jason P Hodde[2] and Paul S Rooney[1*]

Abstract

Background: Abdominal closure in the presence of enterocutaneous fistula, stoma or infection can be challenging. A single-surgeon's experience of performing components separation abdominal reconstruction and reinforcement with mesh in the difficult abdomen is presented.

Methods: Medical records from patients undergoing components separation and reinforcement with hernia mesh at Royal Liverpool Hospital from 2009 to 2012 were reviewed. Patients were classified by the Ventral Hernia Working Group (VHWG) grading system. Co-morbidities, previous surgeries, specific type of reconstruction technique, discharge date, complications and hernia recurrence were recorded.

Results: Twenty-three patients' (15 males, 8 females) notes were reviewed. Median age was 57 years (range 20-76 years). Median follow-up at the time of review was 17 months (range 2-48 months). There were 13 grade III hernias and 10 grade IV hernias identified. Synthetic mesh was placed to reinforce the abdomen in 6 patients, cross-linked porcine dermis was used in 3, and a Biodesign® Hernia Graft was placed in 14. Complications included wound infection (13%), superficial wound dehiscence (22%), seroma formation (22%) and stoma complications (9%). To date, hernias have recurred in 3 patients (13%).

Conclusions: Components separation and reinforcement with biological mesh is a successful technique in the grade III and IV abdomen with acceptable rate of recurrence and complications.

Keywords: Hernia, Contamination, Infection, Components separation, Biologic graft, Mesh, Reinforcement

Background

Abdominal reconstruction using components separation in the presence of enterocutaneous fistula, stoma or infection is challenging. Large incisional hernias vary in their complexity and in the past it has been difficult to compare outcomes of the different reconstructive techniques.

In 2010, the Ventral Hernia Working Group (VHWG) devised a grading system to stratify a patient's risk of developing post-operative complications. Grade III hernias are potentially contaminated due to the presence of stoma, violation of the gastrointestinal tract or previous wound infection, while Grade IV hernias include hernias with a concomitant infected abdomen [1]. Houck et al [2] showed a 41% chance of re-infection and Iqbal et al [3] showed an increase in hernia recurrence after repair of Grade IV hernias. The grading system doesn't take into account the size or the complexity of the hernia, but it is generally established that complications increase along with the size and complexity of the defect.

The aims for surgery in these complex patients are to initially perform enteroclysis and, if possible, restore intestinal continuity before proceeding to the abdominal wall reconstruction. Different surgical techniques to reconstruct the abdominal midline are required depending on the complexity of the hernia. The repair is then reinforced with mesh [1].

Controversy still exists with regard to abdominal reconstruction, the types of mesh and the positioning of the mesh. We present our experience of abdominal reconstruction with components separation and abdominal wall

---

* Correspondence: Paul.Rooney@rlbuht.nhs.uk
[1]Royal Liverpool Hospital, Prescot Street, Liverpool, Merseyside, L7 8XP, UK
Full list of author information is available at the end of the article

reinforcement in the Grade III and Grade IV abdomen and hope to clarify some of these issues.

Methods
Study design
Approval for this retrospective audit was granted by the techniques and devices committee at Royal Liverpool Hospital where waiver of informed consent was granted. Patient consent was obtained to publish the surgery images contained in this manuscript. All review procedures were conducted according to the principles outlined in the Declaration of Helsinki. Medical records of 23 patients undergoing abdominal wall reconstruction at Royal Liverpool Hospital between 2009 and 2012 were retrospectively analysed. Patient co-morbidities, hernia classification, and previous surgeries were identified. Operative notes were studied and the surgical reconstruction technique was recorded. Length of stay, complications and recurrence were also noted.

Pre-surgical work-up
Preoperatively, all patients were assessed clinically. Their hernia was graded using the Ventral Hernia Working Group system, taking into account co-morbidities, presence of stoma, fistula or infection [1]. For patients presenting with fistulas, contrast studies were performed to confirm the fistula anatomy and a CT scan was obtained to assess the size of the hernia, extent of loss of domain, and to identify occult hernia defects so that the surgical technique could be planned (Figure 1).

Surgical technique
Laparotomy, adhesiolysis and restoration of intestinal continuity, if achievable, was performed. The abdominal midline was then reconstructed; the Rectus sheath was mobilised and the Ramirez technique of components separation [4] was used to close the midline depending on the individual patient and defect. Finally, the repair was reinforced with mesh with wide overlap [5], with the intent to situate it in a sublay position. In most cases, only one mesh was placed in the position noted (Table 1). When mesh was placed as both a sublay and onlay, a large piece of mesh was placed diagonally as a sublay, the corners were cut, and the cut pieces were used as an onlay over the lateral release of the component separation. Collatamp°G sponges were placed in some patients prior to closure as a means to reduce the risk of surgical site infection.

Post-operative care
Patients remained in the hospital following their surgery until they were ambulatory and their bladder and bowel functions were normal. Drains were left in for an average of 14 days and removed after discharge. Patients were

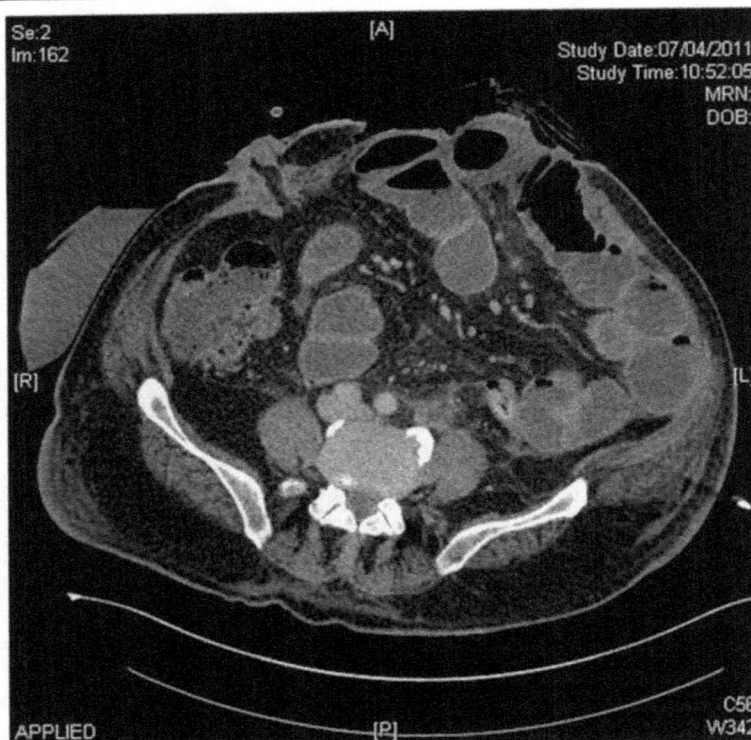

Figure 1 CT scan demonstrating a patient with a stoma and a large incisional hernia with loss of domain.

Table 1 Position of the mesh

Type of reconstruction	Grade III n = 13	Grade IV n = 10	Total n = 23
Onlay mesh	6	7	13
Sublay mesh	3	0	3
Sublay and onlay mesh	3	1	4
Inlay mesh	1	2	3

followed up regularly for the first 3 months and then were followed up on an as-needed basis.

Results

Twenty-three patients with complex medical histories (Table 2) underwent abdominal reconstruction with mesh reinforcement at Royal Liverpool Hospital between 2009 and 2012. A total of 13 patients presented with Grade III hernias and 10 patients presented with Grade IV hernias. Of these 23 patients, 15 had stomas at the time of presentation. Defect width ranged from 8 cm to 17 cm. Seven of the 10 patients (70%) with Grade IV hernias presented with an enterocutaneous fistula as compared to only one patient with a Grade III hernia. The enterocutaneous fistulas varied in their aetiology and ranged from complications secondary to Crohn's Disease to 4 patients having post-operative complications arising from appendectomy, post cystoproctectomy ileoconduit, superior mesenteric artery embolization, or parastomal hernia repair. The median day of discharge was 9 days for Grade III and 16.5 days for Grade IV hernias. Median follow up was 17 months. Baseline demographic information and follow-up information is presented in Table 3.

Of all patients studied, 14 (61%) needed components separation using the Ramirez technique (Figure 2) to help achieve midline closure. Rectus sheath mobilisation was performed in all patients to help re-approximate the

Table 2 Patient medical histories

Previous operations/medical problems	Grade III Hernia (n = 13)	Grade IV Hernia (n = 10)
Pelvic excenteration for anal SCC	2	0
Ileoanal pouch for ulcerative colitis	4	0
Subtotal colectomy for ulcerative colitis	2	3
Hartmans procedure for diverticular disease	1	0
Multiple operations for crohns disease	2	3
Incisional hernia repair	1	0
Laparotomy leading to enterocutaneous fistula (not crohns)	0	4

One patient with a Grade III hernia had multiple previous operations and is not included in the table.

Table 3 Results of patients undergoing abdominal wall reconstruction for Grade III and IV incisional hernias

Results	VHWG Grading		
	III	IV	Total
Number of cases	13	10	23
Median age (min-max)	59 (42-76)	51 (20-76)	57 (20-76)
Male: female	8:5	7:3	15:8
Stoma	8	7	15
Enterocutaneous fistula	1	7	8
Anastomosis	4	5	9
Median discharge day (min-max)	9 (3-70)	16.5 (7-60)	12 (3-70)
Median follow up, months (min-max)	14 (3-46)	18.5 (2-48)	17 (2-48)

midline. In 12/13 (92%) of patients with Grade III hernias and 8/10 (80%) of patients with Grade IV hernias the midline closure was achieved. Of the 15 patients who presented with stomas, 4 were reversed at the time of surgery. Of the 11 that were not reversed, 2 underwent pelvic excenteration for anal cancer; the others were complex patients in whom it was either not technically possible to anastomose or due to co-morbidities it was felt the leak rate would have been too high.

An abdominal wall reinforcement material was used to help reinforce the midline closure in all patients. Depending on the size of the defect, a 20×20 cm, 20×30 cm or 30×30 cm mesh was used. Synthetic mesh was placed in 6 patients, while a biologic graft was placed in 17. Details of the different materials used are presented in Table 4, and the different placement positions are described in Table 1. Of note, in the 3 cases where complete closure of the anterior sheath was not possible, the mesh position is described as an inlay. In 7 patients, 4 with Grade III hernias and 3 with Grade 4 hernias, Collatamp®G sponges were placed prior to closure as a means to reduce the risk of surgical site infection.

Postoperative surgical site complications are shown in Table 5 and included ischaemic stoma in 2 patients and prolonged seroma formation in 5 patients. The cause of the ischaemic stoma complications was thought to be related to a too-tight repair; both of these patients were treated with local refashioning of the stoma after a 3 month period of nutrition and control of wound sepsis.

Figure 3 demonstrates CT scan images of a complete rupture of a hernia repair and seroma formation above and below a sublay mesh. To address the significant number of seromas that form in these patients, we now seek to minimise seroma formation by routinely placing 2 -3 redivac drains above and below the anterior rectus sheath at the time of surgery and leave them for approximately 2 weeks or until the daily fluid output is less than 25 ml.

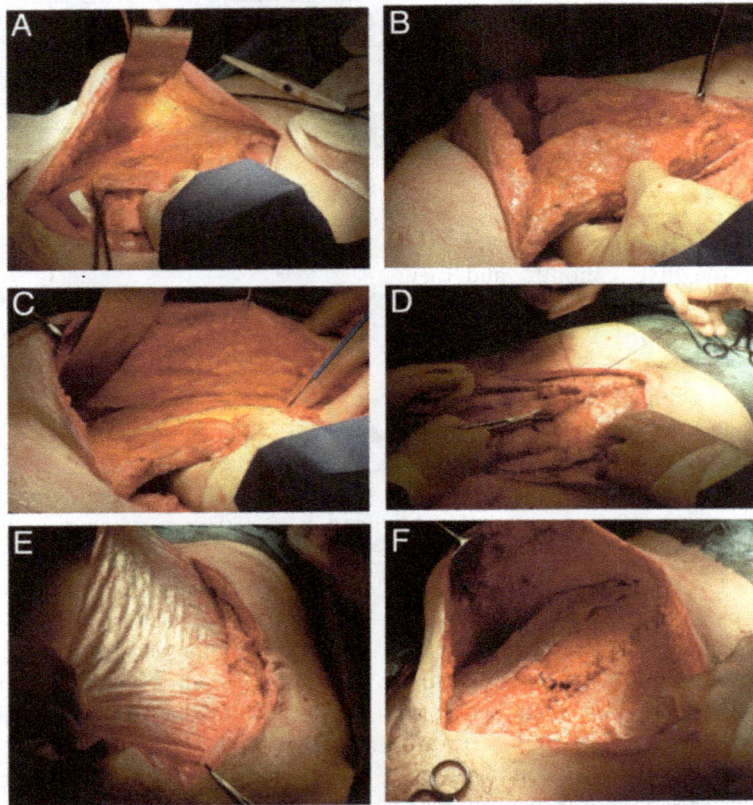

Figure 2 Ramirez technique of components separation using a sublay and onlay Biodesign mesh on a patient with a Grade 3 incisional hernia. A) Rectus sheath mobilised. **B)** Rectus sheath now free laterally. **C)** Sheath incised vertically, lateral to semilunaris. **D)** Posterior layer is closed. **E)** A sublay Biodesign graft is sutured in place. **F)** Remnants of graft are sutured over the lateral releasing incisions.

Discussion

Abdominal reconstruction in the contaminated or potentially-contaminated abdomen is challenging because of the high risk of re-infection and hernia recurrence. Surgical techniques, synthetic meshes, and biologic graft materials that allow for complete restoration of the midline fascia have been developed to improve outcomes in these patients. For example, in a study comparing suture repair of incisional hernia to mesh repair, it was found that "mesh repair results in a lower recurrence rate and less abdominal pain and does not result in more complications than suture repair" after long term follow-up [6]. In this series,

we demonstrate that components separation and midline reinforcement with a variety of graft materials in Grade III and Grade IV hernias is safe and feasible with low morbidity and a low risk of medium-term recurrence.

The VHWG classification was used in this study as we feel it identifies high risk patients and those in which we could consider to use a biological mesh. The European Hernia Society (EHS) have published their own classification which includes the location and size of the hernia defect; however the potential contamination and infection risk is not mentioned [4]. A combination of the VHWG and EHS classification would enable an incisional hernia

Table 4 Types of abdominal wall reconstruction

Type of reconstruction	Grade III n = 13	Grade IV n = 10	Total n = 23
Rectus sheath mobilised	13	10	23
Lateral release	7	7	14
Ultrapro prolene mesh	3	0	3
Proceed mesh	1	2	3
Biodesign hernia graft	8	6	14
Crosslinked porcine dermis	1	2	3

Table 5 Postoperative surgical site complications

	Biodesign n = 14	Synthetic mesh n = 6	Crosslinked porcine dermis n = 3
Seroma	4	1	0
Recurrence	1	1	1
Infection	2	1	0
Wound dehiscence	1	1	3
Ischaemic stoma	1	0	1

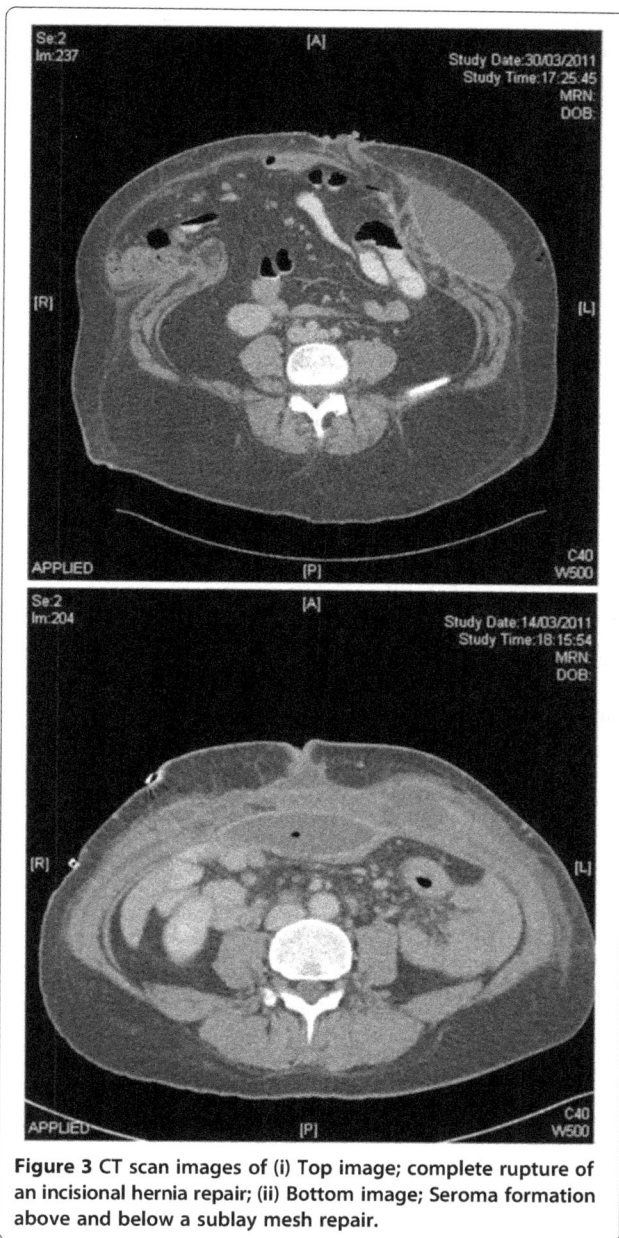

Figure 3 CT scan images of (i) Top image; complete rupture of an incisional hernia repair; (ii) Bottom image; Seroma formation above and below a sublay mesh repair.

to be fully described; however in our subgroup of patients, all with large, complex hernias, the emphasis was on the potential of contamination. In 7 patients, we determined that the risk of post-operative surgical site infection was so high that we opted to place Collatamp®G, a fully resorbable collagen "sponge" impregnated with high doses of fast-release gentamicin for local delivery of broad spectrum antibiotic, prior to abdominal wall closure.

Reconstituting the midline is an important step in the repair to reduce recurrence; we achieved this in 87% of all patients. A variety of reconstruction techniques have been

described in the literature [7,8]. The Ramirez technique is common and successfully allows separation of the abdominal wall components for rectus advancement and achieves closure of the midline in 80% of cases [8]. In larger or complex hernias it is sometimes necessary to adopt double-breasting of the fascia techniques [5] and other methods to gain more width. The importance of achieving midline closure has been demonstrated recently by Itani et al [9] who prospectively followed 80 patients undergoing Grade III or IV hernia repair using components separation and biologic mesh reinforcement and found the recurrence rate was increased if the midline wasn't closed. Similarly, another study of large incisional hernia repairs using polypropylene mesh showed a recurrence rate of 44% using an inlay bridging technique as compared to only 12% when an underlay reinforcement was used [10]. Reinforcing the reconstruction with mesh has also been shown to reduce recurrence rates [11]; the mesh can be placed as an onlay, sublay or inlay.

In this series, 7 out of 23 patients had the recommended sublay mesh; therefore the majority had midline closure and an onlay mesh. Sublay mesh was described by Rives in 1973 as a retromuscular or preperitoneal mesh [12] and is the preferred position because of reduced wound complications and low recurrence rates [7]. In patients who have undergone multiple surgery it is often not feasible to create space for a sublay mesh. If the midline can be closed, an onlay mesh [13] has been shown to be effective, with an 18.5% recurrence rate at 10 years [14]. We feel the most important step to reduce recurrence is to achieve midline closure regardless of the location of mesh reinforcement.

An inlay mesh or 'bridging mesh' is to be avoided if at all possible because serious complications, such as adhesion formation, fistulation and hernia recurrence, have been reported [7,15].

Various mesh types are available and can be classified as either biologic or synthetic. Within these two classifications, meshes can further be classified as either nonabsorbable or absorbable, and biologic meshes may also be classified as human-derived or animal-derived. While synthetic surgical meshes have been used successfully for many decades, complications associated with adhesion, erosion, persistent infection, persistent inflammation, fistula formation, seroma formation, and hematoma are common. Additionally, they are relatively contraindicated for use in Grade III and Grade IV hernias due to the risk of chronic infection. For example, Kapiris et al [15] reported 282 cases of seroma and hematoma formation in 3530 hernias (8%) repaired with polypropylene mesh using the transabdominal (TAPP) approach, and Bingener et al [16] noted adhesion formation in 35% of patients following laparoscopic ventral incisional hernias repair with polypropylene mesh.

Initially, we used synthetic mesh in 6 patients but more recently, we have chosen to use biologic graft materials in Grade III and Grade IV hernias due to recommendations made by the VHWG. Biologic mesh materials have been introduced to the market in an attempt to minimize the complications associated with synthetic materials. Examples of biologic surgical meshes include Peri-Guard® (Synovis), Permacol® (Covidien), AlloDerm® and Strattice® (Life Cell), and Biodesign® (Cook). Peri-Guard, Permacol, Strattice and Biodesign products are manufactured from collagen obtained from animal tissues, while AlloDerm is derived from human dermal tissue. The Peri-Guard and Permacol products have been cross-linked using chemical methods to minimize immunogenicity and to make them more resilient in the face of contamination. The Biodesign, Strattice and AlloDerm surgical mesh products are not cross-linked and are often associated with remodelling of new tissues.

While not specifically indicated for use in Grade III and Grade IV hernias, biologic meshes may minimize the adverse events seen with synthetic materials because they more closely recapitulate the natural tissue environment into which they are placed. These natural tissue meshes can be fabricated to integrate quickly with the patient's tissues, allow rapid angiogenesis to allow the patient to combat infection and stimulate the deposition of additional host connective tissue, optimizing tissue restoration in ways that synthetic mesh materials are unable. Additionally, in the contaminated abdomen, many of the biologic meshes do not have to be removed in the face of infection.

The most common post-operative complication that we experienced in our series with biologic graft materials was transient seroma formation following implant. While most of these seromas are associated with the level of complexity of the dissection and repair, they often resolve, but can cause patient discomfort and impair the healing process. In order to minimize the extent of seroma formation, we now routinely employ the use of 2-3 drains that are left in place above and below the graft reinforcement until daily fluid output is less than 25 ml. A study of 37 patients undergoing repair of enterocutaneous fistula and abdominal reconstruction reported an anastomotic leak in 4 out of 37 and a hernia recurrence rate of 32% [17], in our series there was no anastomotic leaks and a hernia recurrence rate of 12.5% in the enterocutaneous fistula patients (1 out of 8).

The low incidence of recurrence and complications in this series prevents us from clearly assessing the effect of mesh type or location on outcomes. A larger series examining these variables is warranted.

Conclusion

In this initial experience, utilising components separation and midline reinforcement with a biologic graft material in large, complex Grade III and Grade IV hernias is a safe and feasible alternative to traditional, non-reinforced hernia repair with a minimal recurrence rate and satisfactory results in medium-term follow-up.

Abbreviation
VHWG: Ventral hernia working group.

Competing interests
CN has no competing interests. JH is an employee of Cook Biotech. PR has participated as a preceptor and trainer for Cook and has received reimbursement from Cook for his activities. Cook Biotech provided funds to support the publication of this study, but otherwise played no role in the study design or implementation.

Authors' contributions
CN collected the data, prepared the manuscript, and contributed to the analysis and interpretation of the results. JH prepared the manuscript and contributed to the analysis and interpretation of the results. PR performed the surgical procedures, collected the data, and contributed to the analysis and interpretation of the results. All authors read and approved the final manuscript.

Acknowledgements
We thank Cook Biotech for providing funds to support the open-access publication of this study.

Author details
[1]Royal Liverpool Hospital, Prescot Street, Liverpool, Merseyside, L7 8XP, UK. [2]Cook Biotech Incorporated, 1425 Innovation Place, West Lafayette, IN 47906, USA.

References
1. Ventral Hernia Working Group, Breuing K, Butler CE, Ferzoco S, Franz M, Hultman CS, Kilbridge JF, Rosen M, Silverman RP, Vargo D: **ncisional ventral hernias: review of the literature and recommendations regarding the grading and technique of repair.** *Surgery* 2010, **148**:544–558.
2. Houck JP, Rypins EB, Sarfeh IJ, Juler GL, Shimoda KJ: **Repair of incisional hernia.** *Surg Gynecol Obstet* 1989, **169**:397–399.
3. Iqbal CW, Pham TH, Joseph A, Mai J, Thompson GB, Sarr MG: **Long-term outcome of 254 complex incisional hernia repairs using the modified Rives-Stoppa technique.** *World J Surg* 2007, **31**:2398–2404.
4. Muysoms FE, Miserez M, Berrevoet F, Campanelli G, Champault GG, Chelala E, Dietz UA, Eker HH, El Nakadi I, Hauters P, Hidalgo Pascual M, Hoeferlin A, Klinge U, Montgomery A, Simmermacher RK, Simons MP, Smietański M, Sommeling C, Tollens T, Vierendeels T, Kingsnorth A: **Classification of primary and incisional abdominal wall hernias.** *Hernia* 2009, **13**:407–414.
5. Arnaud J, Tuech J, Pessaux P, Hadchity Y: **Surgical treatment of postoperative incisional hernias by intraperitoneal insertion of Dacron mesh and an aponeurotic graft.** *Arch Surg* 1999, **134**:1260–1262.
6. Burger JW, Luijendijk RW, Hop WC, Halm JA, Verdaasdonk EG, Jeekel J: **Long-term follow-up of a randomized controlled trial of suture versus mesh repair of incisional hernia.** *Ann Surg* 2004, **240**:578–583. discussion 583-585.
7. Hughes LE: **Incisional hernia.** *Asian J Surg* 1990, **13**:69.
8. Ramirez OM, Ruas E, Dellon AL: **"Components separation" method for closure of abdominal-wall defects: an anatomic and clinical study.** *Plast Reconstr Surg* 1990, **86**:519–526.
9. Itani KMF, Rosen M, Vargo D, Awad SS, DeNoto G III, Butler CE: **Prospective study of single-stage repair of contaminated hernias using a biological porcine tissue matrix: The RICH Study.** *Surgery* 2012, **152**:498–505.
10. de Vries Reilingh TS, van Geldere D, Langenhorst B, de Jong D, van der Wilt GJ, van Goor H, Bleichrodt RP: **Repair of large midline incisional hernias with polypropylene mesh: comparison of three operative techniques.** *Hernia* 2004, **8**:56–59.
11. Luijendijk RW, Hop WC, van den Tol MP, de Lange DC, Braaksma MM, IJzermans JN, Boelhouwer RU, de Vries BC, Salu MK, Wereldsma JC,

Bruijninckx CM, Jeekel J: **A comparison of suture repair with mesh repair for incisional hernia.** *N Engl J Med* 2000, **343**:392–398.

12. Rives J, Lardennois B, Pire JC, Hibon J: **Large incisional hernias. The importance of flail abdomen and of subsequent respiratory disorders.** *Chirurgie* 1973, **99**:547–563.

13. Chevrel JP: **The treatment of large midline incisional hernias by "overcoat" plasty and prosthesis (author's transl).** *Nouv Presse Med* 1979, **8**:695–696.

14. Sailes FC, Walls J, Guelig D, Mirzabeigi M, Long WD, Crawford A, Moore JH Jr, Copit SE, Tuma GA, Fox J: **Synthetic and biological mesh in component separation: A 10-year single institution review.** *Ann Plast Surg* 2010, **64**:696–698.

15. Kapiris SA, Brough WA, Royston CM, O'Boyle C, Sedman PC: **Laparoscopic transabdominal preperitoneal (TAPP) hernia repair. A 7-year two-center experience in 3017 patients.** *Surg Endosc* 2001, **15**:972–975.

16. Bingener J, Kazantsev GB, Chopra S, Schwesinger WH: **Adhesion formation after laparoscopic ventral incisional hernia repair with polypropylene mesh: a study using abdominal ultrasound.** *JSLS* 2004, **8**:127–131.

17. Krpata DM, Stein SL, Eston M, Ermlich B, Blatnik JA, Novitsky YW, Rosen MJ: **Outcomes of simultaneous large complex abdominal wall reconstruction and enterocutaneous fistula takedown.** *Am J Surg* 2013, **205**:354–358.

5

Comparison of single and two-tunnel techniques during open treatment of acromioclavicular joint disruption

Zhiyong Hou[1*], Jove Graham[2], Yingze Zhang[1], Kent Strohecker[2], Daniel Feldmann[2], Thomas R Bowen[2], Wei Chen[1] and Wade Smith[3]

Abstract

Background: Coracoclavicular (CC) ligament reconstruction with semitendinosus tendon (ST) grafts has become more popular and has achieved relatively good results; however optimal reconstruction technique, single-tunnel or two-tunnel, still remains controversial. This paper is to compare the clinical and radiographic data of allogenous ST grafting with single- or two-tunnel reconstruction techniques of the AC joint.

Methods: The outcomes of 21 consecutive patients who underwent anatomical reduction and ST grafting for AC joint separation were reviewed retrospectively. Patients were divided into two groups: single-tunnel group (11) and two-tunnel group (10). All patients were evaluated clinically and radiographically using a modified UCLA rating scale.

Results: The majority of separations (18 of 21) were Rockwood type V, with one each in type III, IV and VI categories. The overall mean follow-up time was 16 months, and at the time of the latest follow-up, the overall mean UCLA rating score was 14.1 (range 8–20).
The percentage of good-to-excellent outcomes was significantly higher for patients with the two-tunnel technique than for those with the one-tunnel technique (70% vs. 18%, respectively, p = 0.03). Within the single-tunnel group, there was no statistically significant difference in percentage of good-to-excellent outcomes between patients with vs. without tightrope augmentation (17% vs 20%, p > 0.99). Similarly, within the two-tunnel group, there was no significant difference in the percentage of good-to-excellent outcomes between the graft only and augment groups (67% vs. 75%, p > 0.99).

Conclusion: Anatomical reduction of the AC joint and reconstruction CC ligaments are crucial for optimal joint stability and function. Two-tunnel CC reconstruction with an allogenous ST graft provides superior significantly better radiographic and clinical results compared to the single-tunnel reconstruction technique.

Keywords: Acromioclavicular joint, Single-tunnel, Two-tunnel, Reconstruction, Augmentation

Background

Acromioclavicular (AC) joint injuries are among the most commonly occurring problems in the young and active patient population. Higher-grade AC joint injuries (Rockwood types III through VI) represent failure of the coracoclavicular (CC) ligament complex, which is formed by the conoid and trapezoid ligaments. This complex has been termed the primary suspensory structure of the upper limb [1,2]. In the literature, the incidence of traumatic AC joint separation varies from 3 to 4 per 100,000 people with 25-52% of these occurring during sporting activities, and they are also one of the most common shoulder injuries seen in orthopaedic traumatology [2-5]. For certain Rockwood type III AC joint separations and all type IV, V, and VI injuries, surgical treatment has been recommended to prevent disabling pain, weakness, and deformity [6-8]. Although more than 60 surgical techniques have been reported, the frequency of failure to maintain reduction after surgical treatment remains high [9,10].

* Correspondence: drzyhou@gmail.com
[1]Department of Orthopaedic Surgery, Third Hospital of Hebei Medical University, Shijiazhuang, Hebei 050051, China
Full list of author information is available at the end of the article

Recently, CC ligament reconstruction with tendon grafts has become more popular and has achieved relatively good results [11,12]. Biomechanical studies focusing on an anatomic reconstruction of the CC ligament complex using tendon grafts have reported promising potential for this technique [13-15]. Semitendinosus tendon (ST) grafting and anatomic reconstruction can be imitated, providing stability to the clavicle that is very close to that provided by the intact ligaments [13]. However, optimal reconstruction technique, single-tunnel or two-tunnel, still remains controversial. Anatomical two-tunnel reconstruction with tendon grafts or synthetic materials seems appealing because it has been shown by biomechanical studies to restore the original two ligaments (the conoid and trapezoid) and to produce an ultimate failure load that is equivalent to that of native CC ligaments [13-15]. However, it is technically difficult and theoretically increases the risk of fracture [16].

The purpose of this retrospective study was to analyze the clinical and radiographic data of allogenous ST tendon grafting with single- or two-tunnel reconstruction techniques of the CC ligaments. We hypothesize that anatomic reconstruction of the AC joint disruption using two-tunnel reconstruction technique results in a satisfying clinical function and provides stable fixation.

Methods

Between June 2003 and January 2009, twenty-three patients underwent open operation for AC joint reconstruction with ST allograft at our institution. In the earlier study period before 2007, we mostly used single-tunnel technique, and after 2007 mostly the two-tunnel technique. For analysis we divided patients into two groups: single-tunnel group and two-tunnel group. Patient data were collected retrospectively, including gender, age at the time of surgery, injury mechanism, classification according to Rockwood, and surgical technique. Patients with at least 12 months of clinical follow-up were included in this study. Patients were excluded if they had a previous shoulder injury, arthritis, or an associated neurological deficit on the side of injury.

The procedure was performed with the patient in the beach chair position under general anesthesia in combination with an interscalene block. An anterior delto-pectoral approach was utilized with saber incision, The AC joint, the lateral end of the clavicle, and the coracoid process were exposed. Subperiosteal detachment of the deltotrapezial fascia from the clavicle was performed. The distal end of the clavicle was resected 8 to 10 mm using an oscillating saw. For the single-tunnel technique, a 6-mm drill hole was made about 1.5-2 cm medial to the remaining end of the clavicle superior to inferior in a 300 posterior to anterior angle. A ST allograft was prepared by placing a whipstitch (Arthrex #2 Fiberwire

suture, Naples, FL, USA) on either end. After reducing the distal clavicle down to the acromion anatomically, the ST graft was introduced around the base of the coracoid and then both ends of the graft up through the clavicle hole. The graft was then mechanically tensioned and a 5.5 mm Bio-tenodesis screw was placed down through the center of the ST graft fixing it to the clavicle. The free ends of the graft were then passed underneath the clavicle and tied to themselves for additional fixation (Figure 1). If using a tightrope augment (Arthrex Fiberwire No. 5, Naples, FL, USA), a guide was used to place a pin from a point medial to the lateral tunnel, to the base of the coracoid. A 4.5 mm reamer was then used to create a tunnel through the clavicle and coracoid. The tight rope device was placed through the clavicular and then coracoid tunnel and endobutton secured against inferior cortex of coracoid. The tight-rope was then tied after fixation of the graft. Later in the series, a single clavicular tunnel was utilized for both the graft and tight-rope. The graft was placed around the coracoid and through the clavicular tunnel and tightrope device (Figure 2).

For the two-tunnel technique, the same delto-pectoral approach was used. Two holes were drilled in the clavicle to reconstruct each of the two CC ligaments, trapezoid and conoid ligaments. The lateral tunnel is created as in the single-tunnel technique. The medial tunnel is located 4.5 cm medial to the AC joint. A 5.5 mm tunnel is reamed like the medial tunnel. A single ST graft was prepared and looped under the coracoid. The lateral free end was brought up through the lateral tunnel, and the medial free end through the medial tunnel. The AC joint is reduced, and the grafts fixed into the tunnels with 5 mm biotenodesis screws and the graft tied to itself (Figure 3). If using tightrope augment, a guide pin is placed between the two graft tunnels, from midline, through the clavicle and base of coracoid. A 4.5 mm tunnel is reamed over the guide wire and the Tight-rope device placed through the clavicle and coracoid and secured to the inferior cortex of the

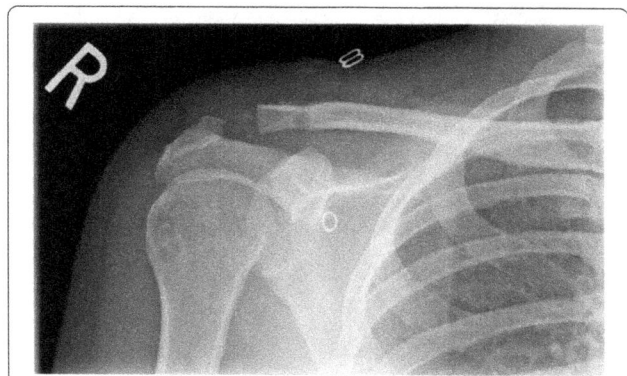

Figure 1 ST allograft reconstruction of the AC joint with single-tunnel technique.

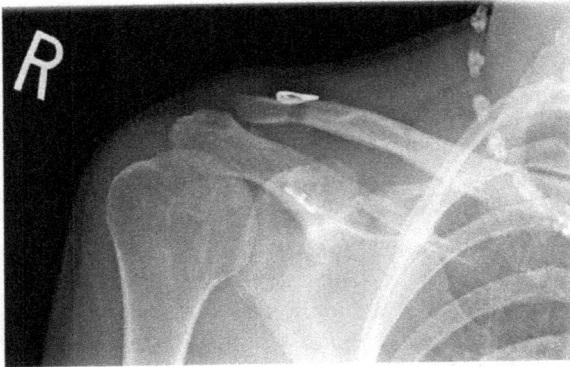

Figure 2 ST Allograft with tightrope augment reconstruction of the CC joint with single-tunnel technique.

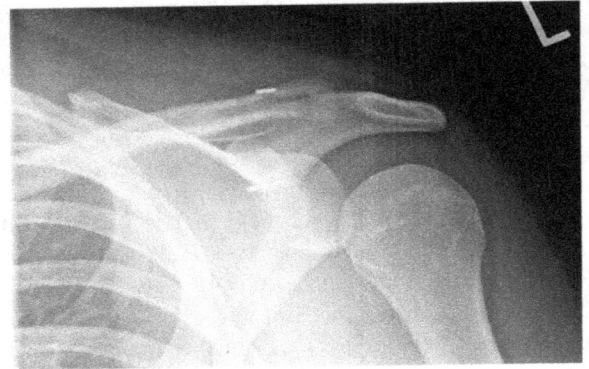

Figure 4 ST Allograft with tightrope augment reconstruction of the CC joint with two-tunnel technique.

coracoid. The device is tightened and tied after graft fixation (Figure 4). After reconstruction, attention was directed to repair of the deltotrapezial interval. This was performed in a pants-over-vest fashion using #1 or #2 non-absorbable sutures in an interrupted fashion. A layered closure was then performed. A drain was not utilized.

All patients were placed in a sling immobilizer post-op for 4 to 6 weeks. Gentle pendulums and Codman's were begun post-op day 1. At 4 weeks therapy was begun with passive motion and cuff isometrics. Resistive program started at 8 weeks. Patients were generally allowed to return to manual work and athletics at 4 to 6 months depending on level of rehabilitation. Contact sports not prior to six months. All patients were evaluated clinically and radiographically using a modified UCLA rating scale [5,17], which reflects three parts: maintenance of reduction, objective evaluation of the patient's function, and complications secondary to operation. In the radiological evaluation, the roentgenographic rating was determined by the degree of displacement of the AC joint, which

was evaluated by measuring the relation between the acromion and the clavicle on the anteroposterior view for vertical displacement (reduced = 4 points, subluxed = 2 points, dislocated = 0 points). In the physical evaluation, range of motion (ROM), pain, weakness, and complications were recorded. Finally, patients were asked their overall satisfaction with the postoperative result, with 0 points for dissatisfaction or unsure and 2 points for satisfaction.

Table 1 shows the relative weight given to each category of the rating scale and describes the criteria by which a patient was assigned an overall final result of excellent, good, fair, or poor.

Percentages of good-to-excellent outcomes and maintenance of reduction (reduced or subluxed) were compared between the two reconstruction procedures (single vs. two-tunnel), and between augmentation techniques (with vs. without tightrope). Because of the relatively small sample sizes, Fisher's exact test was used in place of chi-square testing at a significance level of $p < 0.05$. All analysis was performed using SAS statistical software (SAS 9.2, Cary, NC). Waiver of patient consent was granted by Institutional Review Board of Geisinger Medical Center for retrospective chart review.

Results

From the initial 23 patients who were surgically treated, two patients were lost to follow up and were excluded. Table 2 summarizes the demographics and injury characteristics of the 21 patients remaining in the study. The majority of fractures (18 of 21) were Rockwood type V, with one fracture each in type III, IV and VI categories. Most of those patients had received primary unsuccessful conservative care and switched to operative management, and one patient underwent a failed Weaver-Dunn procedure.

The overall mean follow-up time was 16 months, and at the time of the latest follow-up, the overall mean UCLA rating score was 14.1 (range 8–20). Eleven (52%) patients

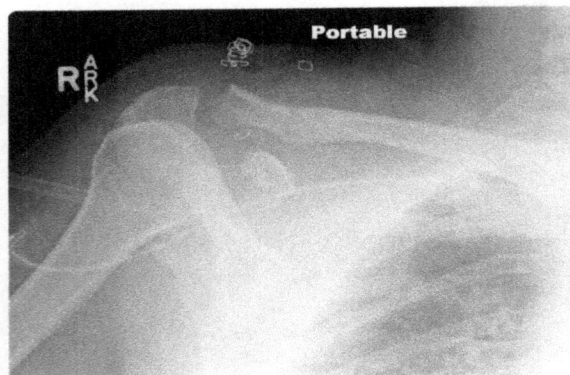

Figure 3 ST allograft reconstruction of the CC joint with two-tunnel technique.

Table 1 The modification of the UCLA rating scale[8.17]

Category	Points
Maintenance of reduction	
Reduced	4
Subluxion	2
Dislocation	0
Range of motion	
Full	2
Improved from preoperative	1
No change from preoperative	0
Strength	
Normal	2
Improved from preoperative	1
Unimproved from preoperative	0
Pain	
None	4
With strenuous activity	3
With moderate activity	2
With mild activity	1
All the time	0
Weakness	
None	2
With strenuous activity	1
All the time	0
Change in occupation	
Same or more strenuous	2
Less strenuous	0
Complication	
None	2
Minor/resolved	1
Major/affected outcome	0
Patient satisfaction	
Yes	2
No or unsure	0

Results: excellent, 18–20; good, 15–17; fair, 12–14; poor, ≤ 11.

Table 2 Demographic and injury characteristics, by single-tunnel and two-tunnel group

Parameter	Single-tunnel (11)	Two-tunnel (10)
Gender		
Male	6	9
Female	5	1
Mean age (range), years	37 (20–55)	42 (20–63)
Side of Fracture		
Right	5	8
Left	6	2
Mechanism of Injury		
Sporting	6	6
Traffic accident	4	2
Fall	1	2
Rockwood Classification		
C3	1	0
C4	0	1
C5	10	8
C6	0	1
Mean length of follow up (range), months	16 (12–38)	15 (12–40)

Table 3 summarizes the UCLA rating scale scores at last follow-up for the two groups (single- and two-tunnel), subdivided by augmentation type. The percentage of good-to-excellent outcomes was significantly higher for patients with the two-tunnel technique than for those with the one-tunnel technique (70% vs. 18%, respectively, $p = 0.03$). Within the single-tunnel group, there was no statistically significant difference in percentage of good-to-excellent outcomes between patients with vs. without tightrope augmentation (17% vs 20%, $p > 0.99$). Similarly, within the two-tunnel group, there was no significant difference in the percentage of good-to-excellent outcomes between ST-tightrope and ST-ST patients (75% vs. 67%, $p > 0.99$).

We noted that complications were observed in three of the 21 patients: two patients in the two-tunnel group had infection, and one patient in the single-tunnel group had a coracoid fracture. Calcification of the CC ligament occurred in one case, but it did not appear to cause symptoms, and was therefore not considered a complication. No patient had neurovascular or post-traumatic arthritis of the injured AC joint.

Discussion

Our data demonstrated that allogenous ST grafting with two-tunnel reconstruction technique of the AC joint yielded excellent or good clinical outcomes more frequently compared to single-tunnel reconstruction technique. These results also suggest that the materials used

rated the outcome as good to excellent, 3 (14%) rated it as fair, and 7 (33%) rated it as poor. Three of 21 patients underwent additional revision surgery for the failed CC ligament repair or reconstruction.

Of the 21 patients, eleven patients underwent allogenous ST grafting with single-tunnel reconstruction technique, and 6 of these received tightrope augmentation. Ten patients underwent allogenous ST grafting with two-tunnel reconstruction technique: four of these received one ST graft plus one tightrope graft ("ST-tightrope"), while the other six received two ST grafts ("ST-ST").

Table 3 Number of patients receiving single-tunnel vs. two-tunnel techniques, subdivided by augmentation type, with clinical outcome results based on modification of the UCLA rating scale

UCLA rating scale	Single-tunnel (n = 11)		Two-tunnel (n = 10)[*]	
	With augment	Without augment[^]	ST-tightrope	ST-ST[#]
Excellent	1	1	1	2
Good	0	0	2	2
Fair	2	1	1	1
Poor	3	3	0	1
Total	6	5	4	6
N(%) with excellent or good	1 (17%)	1 (20%)	3 (75%)	4 (67%)

*Two-tunnel group had significantly higher percentage of good-to-excellent outcomes than single-tunnel group, p = 0.03.
^No significant difference between with vs. without augmentation for single-tunnel group, p > 0.99.
#No significant difference between ST-tightrope vs. ST-ST for two-tunnel group, p > 0.99.

for augmentation in the two-tunnel reconstruction technique do not impact the clinical result. In this technique, one ST allograft combined with one tightrope graft construction can provide similar outcomes to using ST allograft in both tunnels. We also saw no significant differences between patients with and without tightrope augment in the single-tunnel technique group.

Based on well established anatomical ligament reconstruction in the knee injury, reconstructing the CC ligament using tendon graft for AC joint injury has become more popular because the construct is more physiologic, does not require implant removal and preserves the CA ligament [18,19]. ST tendon grafts are most common used for this procedure, which can be either autografts or allografts, and have achieved relatively good results [11-13,20,21]. The harvesting of an autogenous tendon may not result in long-term functional impairment but may still cause some morbidity associated with the donor site, and also create a second operative site during AC joint surgery [22]. Nicholas et al. [12] achieved excellent outcomes after fresh-frozen ST allograft reconstruction of the CC ligament; patients reported significant pain relief, return of normal strength and function, negligible loss of motion, and no loss of reduction on postoperative radiographs. Based on this information, the substitution of allograft material has become a routine procedure in our institution. The current surgical technique for the CC ligament reconstruction can be graft tendon passed though the clavicle with single tunnel or two tunnels technique [16,23], looped around the base of the coracoids [24], passed through a transosseous tunnel in the coracoids [25], or fixed to the base of coracoid using an anchor technique [6]. The CC ligament is stabilized by 2 sets of ligamentous structures: the conoid and trapezoid. Single-tunnel or two-tunnel reconstruction still remains controversial. Mazzocca et al. considered that each CC ligament has a separate function, and so each must be considered in reconstructive procedures [26]. Anatomical two-tunnel reconstruction with tendon grafts has yielded good

results because it restores the original 2 ligaments and produces an ultimate strength that is equivalent to that of native CC ligaments [14,15,23]. However, two-tunnel techniques are technically difficult, with increased risk of fracture, and sometimes are not possible in patients with a small clavicle [13,16]. This technique should be performed by an experienced arthroscopist [23]. Yoo et al. [16] reported that single-tunnel reconstruction has some advantages over two-tunnel techniques. They reconstructed CC ligaments in 21 patients using a single-tunnel ST autograft and achieved superior clinical result. 17 (81%) of the 21 patients maintained complete reduction, and only 1 patient (reportedly a manual laborer) had complete reduction loss. In our cohort, there was a statistically significant difference in percentages of good-to-excellent UCLA scores between the single-tunnel and two-tunnel groups. The two-tunnel group had better scores, with the caveat that we observed two cases of infection in the two-tunnel group which may be related to the greater length and complexity of this procedure as compared to the single-tunnel technique.

Anatomical two-tunnel reconstruction with ST tendon grafts or synthetic materials provided similar results. The tightrope system, consisting of one round clavicle titanium button and one long coracoid titanium button connected by non-absorbable sutures (No. 5 Ethibond suture), has been initially utilized for repair of acute syndesmosis disruptions. The application has been extended and previously described for AC joint dislocations [27,28]. It can be used as a single graft device or an augment for the other tendon graft construction. Two-tunnel reconstruction technique has been shown by biomechanical studies to restore the strength of the original two ligaments (the conoid and trapezoid) and result in significantly higher stability in the superoinferior as well as the anteroposterior plane when compared with the native CC ligaments [11,14,15,29]. Grafting materials for the two-tunnel technique use are variable, and may include two tendon grafts, two tightrope grafts, or one tendon with one tightrope grafts. Salzmann et al. [23] reported on 23 consecutive patients with the acute AC joint disruption who underwent two-tunnel anatomical reconstruction of CC ligaments using two flip-button tightropes. This procedure yielded satisfactory clinical function and provided a stable fixation at intermediate-term follow-up. In our two-tunnel group, most patients had good-to-excellent UCLA scores at last followup, and this result did not vary between the cases treated with one ST graft and one tightrope graft versus those treated with two ST grafts.

Augmentation has been shown to be beneficial during CC ligament reconstructions by biomechanical studies [30,31]. An effective augmentation must have biomechanical properties enabling it to shield the repair or reconstruction from excessive tensile force, ideally allowing early rehabilitation. It seems desirable for an augmentation to possess strength and stiffness similar to those of the intact CC ligament complex, thus protecting against physiologic loads while allowing for physiologic motion between the clavicle and coracoid. Tienen et al. [32] had good results with using an open modified Weaver-Dunn technique and AC joint augmentation with absorbable, braided suture in 21 paptients. The tightrope augmentation was initially described for acute AC joint dislocation and represented an excellent biological augmentation technique by Hernegger [27]. Scheibel et al. [33] also reported using a gracilis tendon reconstruction augmented with a tightrope achieved good and excellent results and maintained good reduction for acute AC joint dislocations with one year follow up. Recently, Yoo et al. [16] also reported a superior result by using the tightrope augment technique to protect the ST graft though the same tunnel during the healing period. They considered the tightrope augment was really important factor for their successful surgical procedure and good outcomes. However, in our one-tunnel group, although the sample size was small, we saw no significant difference between patients treated with and without tightrope augmentation. Both of them had a higher re-dislocation rate and achieved the inferior results comparing to the two-tunnel group. From our results, we cannot definitively state that tightrope augmentation is not important and effective for the CC complex reconstruction, but our results do provide strong evidence that the reconstruction technique (specifically the choice between one or two tunnels) largely impacts the radiographic and clinical outcomes.

The principal limitations of this study are the relative small sample size who met our inclusion criteria and the fact that we did not have preoperative functional scores. Thus, our conclusions are focused on the substantial difference in success rates we saw between the single-tunnel and two-tunnel groups (18% vs. 70%), and we have limited ability to assess and compare other aspects of the procedures. In addition, because this was an observational

study, our data did not permit an accurate assessment of the time to functional recovery. The two-tunnel technique became a standard technique at our institution at a later date than the single-tunnel technique, and so it is possible that surgeon experience may have played a role in the different outcomes among groups. However, we do not believe this confounding factor would be substantial enough to explain the large difference in the two groups that we observed.

Conclusion

Anatomical reduction the AC joint and biomechanical reconstruction CC ligaments are crucial for the optimal joint stability and function. Two-tunnel CC reconstruction with an allogenous ST graft provides superior radiographic and clinical results compared to single-tunnel reconstruction technique.

Abbreviations
CC ligament: Coracoclavicular ligament; ST tendon: Semitendinosus tendon; AC joint: Acromioclavicular joint; UCLA shoulder rating scale: University of California at Los Angeles shoulder rating scale; ROM: Range of motion.

Competing interests
The authors declare that they have no competing interests.

Authors' contributions
ZH and WS designed research; JG, KS and WC analyzed data and performed statistical analysis. All authors read and approved the final manuscript.

Author details
[1]Department of Orthopaedic Surgery, Third Hospital of Hebei Medical University, Shijiazhuang, Hebei 050051, China. [2]Department of Orthopaedic Surgery, Geisinger Medical Center, Danville, PA 17822, USA. [3]Mountain Orthopaedic Trauma Surgeons at Swedish, 701 East Hampden Avenue Suite 515, Englewood, CO 80113, USA.

References
1. Bosworth BM: **Acromioclavicular separation: New method of repair.** *Surg Gynecol Obstet* 1941, **73**:866–871.
2. Rockwood CA, Williams GR, Young DC: **Injuries to the Acromioclavicular Joint.** In *Fractures in Adults, Volume 2. Fourthth edition.* Edited by Rockwood CA, Green DP, Bucholz RW. Philadelphia: Lippincott-Raven Pub Publishers; 1996:1341–1413.
3. Horn JS: **The traumatic anatomy and treatment of acute acromioclavicular dislocation.** *J Bone Joint Surg Br* 1954, **36**:194–1201.
4. Lemos MJ: **The evaluation and treatment of the injured acromioclavicular joint in athletes.** *Am J Sports Med* 1998, **26**:137–144.
5. Lizaur A, Marco L, Cebrian R: **Acute dislocation of the acromioclavicular joint. Traumatic anatomy and the importance of deltoid and trapezius.** *J Bone Joint Surg Br* 1994, **76**:602–606.
6. Bannister GC, Wallace WA, Stableforth PG, Hutson MA: **The management of acute acromioclavicular dislocation. A randomised prospective controlled trial.** *J Bone Joint Surg Br* 1989, **71**:848–1850.
7. Fremerey RW, Lobenhoffer P, Ramacker K, Gerich T, Skutek M, Bosch U: **Acute acromioclavicular joint dislocation–operative or conservative therapy?** *Unfallchirurg* 2001, **104**:294–299.
8. Kumar S, Sethi A, Jain AK: **Surgical treatment of complete acromioclavicular dislocation using the coracoacromial ligament and coracoclavicular fixation: report of a technique in 14 patients.** *J Orthop Trauma* 1995, **9**:507–510.

9. Warren-Smith CD, Ward MW: Operation for acromioclavicular dislocation A review of 29 cases treated by one method. *J Bone Joint Surg Br* 1987, **69**:715–718.

10. Weaver JK, Dunn HK: Treatment of acromioclavicular injuries, especially complete acromioclavicular separation. *J Bone Joint Surg Am* 1972, **54**:1187–1194.

11. Jones HP, Lemos MJ, Schepsis AA: Salvage of failed acromioclavic acromioclavicular joint reconstruction using autogenous semitendinosus tendon from the knee: surgical technique and case report. *Am J Sports Med* 2001, **29**:234–237.

12. Nicholas SJ, Lee SJ, Mullaney MJ, Tyler TF, McHugh MP: Clinical outcomes of coracoclavicular ligament reconstructions using tendon grafts. *Am J Sports Med* 2007, **35**:1912–1917.

13. Costic RS, Labriola JE, Rodosky MW, Debski RE: Biomechanical rationale for development of anatomical reconstructions of coracoclavicular ligaments after complete acromioclavicular joint dislocations. *Am J Sports Med* 2004, **32**:1929–1936.

14. Lee SJ, Nicholas SJ, Akizuki KH, McHugh MP, Kremenic IJ, Ben-Avi S: Reconstruction of the coracoclavicular ligaments with tendon grafts: a comparative biomechanical study. *Am J Sports Med* 2003, **31**:648–655.

15. Mazzocca AD, Santangelo SA, Johnson ST, Rios CG, Dumonski ML, Arciero RA: A biomechanical evaluation of an anatomical coracoclavicular ligament reconstruction. *Am J Sports Med* 2006, **34**:236–246.

16. Yoo JC, Ahn JH, Yoon JR, Yang JH: Clinical results of single-tunnel coracoclavicular ligament reconstruction using autogenous semitendinosus tendon. *Am J Sports Med* 2010, **38**:950–957.

17. Guy DK, Wirth MA, Griffin JL, Rockwood CA Jr: Reconstruction of chronic and complete dislocations of the acromioclavicular joint. *Clin Orthop Relat Res* 1998, **347**:138–149.

18. Fu FH, Shen W, Starman JS, Okeke N, Irrgang JJ: Primary anatomic double-bundle anterior cruciate ligament reconstruction: a preliminary 2-year prospective study. *Am J Sports Med* 2008, **36**:1263–1274.

19. Stannard JP, Riley RS, Sheils TM, McGwin G Jr, Volgas DA: Anatomic reconstruction of the posterior cruciate ligament after multiligament knee injuries: a combination of the tibial-inlay and two-femoral-tunnel techniques. *Am J Sports Med* 2003, **31**:196–202.

20. LaPrade RF, Hilger B: Coracoclavicular ligament reconstruction using a semitendinosus graft for failed acromioclavicular separation surgery. *Arthroscopy* 2005, **21**:1277.

21. Tauber M, Gordon K, Koller H, Fox M, Resch H: Semitendinosus tendon graft versus a modified Weaver-Dunn procedure for acromioclavicular joint reconstruction in chronic cases: a prospective comparative study. *Am J Sports Med* 2009, **37**:181–190.

22. Yoo JC, Choi NH, Kim SY, Lim TK: Distal clavicle tunnel widening after coracoclavicular ligament reconstruction with semitendinous tendon: a case report. *J Shoulder Elbow Surg* 2006, **15**:256–259.

23. Salzmann GM, Walz L, Buchmann S, Glabgly P, Venjakob A, Imhoff AB: Arthroscopically assisted 2-bundle anatomical reduction of acute acromioclavicular joint separations. *Am J Sports Med* 2010, **38**(6):1179–1187.

24. Hessmann M, Gotzen L, Gehling H: Acromioclavicular reconstruction augmented with polydioxanonsulphate bands. Surgical technique and results. *Am J Sports Med* 1995, **23**:552–556.

25. Wolf EM, Pennington WT: Arthroscopic reconstruction for acromioclavicular joint dislocation. *Arthroscopy* 2001, **17**:558–563.

26. Mazzocca AD, Spang JT, Rodriguez RR, Rios CG, Shea KP, Romeo AA, Arciero RA: Biomechanical and radiographic analysis of partial coracoclavicular ligament injuries. *Am J Sports Med* 2008, **36**:1397–1402.

27. Hernegger GS, Kadletz R, Tight RV: The revolutionary anatomical Wxation in acromioclavicular joint dislocation VA case report. *Tech Shoulder Elbow Surg* 2006, **7**:86–88.

28. Quereshi F, Hinsche A, Potter D: Arthroscopic "TightRope" stabilization of Neer type 2 clavicle fractures. *Injury Extra* 2007, **38**:133–134.

29. Walz L, Salzmann GM, Fabbro T, Eichhorn S, Imhoff AB: The anatomic reconstruction of AC joint dislocations using two TightRope devices: a biomechanical study. *Am J Sports Med* 2008, **36**:2398–2406.

30. Bargren JH, Erlanger S, Dick HM: Biomechanics and comparison of two operative methods of treatment of complete acromioclavicular separation. *Clin Orthop Relat Res* 1978, **130**:267–272.

31. Fukuda K, Craig EV, An KN, Cofield RH, Chao EY: Biomechanical study of the ligamentous system of the acromioclavicular joint. *J Bone Joint Surg Am* 1986, **68**:434–440.

32. Tienen TG, Oyen JF, Eggen PJ: A modified technique of reconstruction for complete acromioclavicular dislocation: a prospective study. *Am J Sports Med* 2003, **31**:655–659.

33. Scheibel M, Ifesanya A, Pauly S, Haas NP: Arthroscopically assisted coracoclavicular ligament reconstruction for chronic acromioclavicular joint instability. *Arch Orthop Trauma Surg* 2008, **128**:1327–1333.

Lower extremity soft tissue reconstruction and amputation rates in patients with open tibial fractures in Sweden during 1998–2010

Ulrika Tampe[1], Rüdiger J Weiss[1], Birgit Stark[2], Pehr Sommar[2], Zewar Al Dabbagh[1] and Karl-Åke Jansson[1*]

Abstract

Background: The rates of soft tissue reconstruction and amputation after open tibial fractures have not been studied on a national perspective. We aimed to determine the frequency of soft tissue coverage after open tibial fracture as well as primary and secondary amputation rates.

Methods: Data on all patients (> = 15 years) admitted to hospital with open tibial fractures were extracted from the Swedish National Patient Register (1998–2010). All surgical procedures, re-admissions, and mechanisms of injury were analysed accordingly. The risk of amputation was calculated using logistic regression (adjusted for age, sex, mechanism of injury, reconstructive surgery and fixation method). The mean follow-up time was 6 (SD 3.8) years.

Results: Of 3,777 patients, 342 patients underwent soft tissue reconstructive surgery. In total, there were 125 amputations. Among patients with no reconstructive surgery, 2% (n = 68 patients) underwent amputation. In an adjusted analysis, patients older than 70 years (OR = 2.7, 95%, CI = 1.1-6) and those who underwent reconstructive surgery (OR = 3.1, 95% CI = 1.6-5.8) showed higher risk for amputation. Fixations other than intramedullary nailing (plate, external fixation, closed reduction and combination) as the only method were associated with a significant higher risk for amputation (OR 5.1-14.4). Reconstruction within 72 hours (3 days) showed better results than reconstruction between 4–90 days (p = 0.04).

Conclusions: The rate of amputations after open tibial fractures is low (3.6%). There is a higher risk for amputations with age above 70 (in contrast: male sex and tissue reconstruction are rather indicators for more severe soft tissue injuries). Only a small proportion of open tibial fractures need soft tissue reconstructive surgery. Reconstruction with free or pedicled flap should be performed within 72 hours whenever possible.

Keywords: Skeletal trauma, Tibial shaft fracture, Open fracture, Amputation, Lower extremity reconstruction, Limb salvage, Soft tissue injury

Background

Epidemiological studies have shown an incidence rate of 11.5 per 100,000 person-years for open long bone fractures [1]. A large proportion of these fractures are open tibial fractures [1-4]. Open tibial fractures are associated with a high rate of complications such as compartment syndrome, mal-union, non-union, osteomyelitis, and amputation [5,6]. Gustilo type III open fractures are the most severe, involving extensive soft-tissue trauma, and complex fracture patterns [7]. Some of these injuries can be managed with salvage procedures involving either a pedicled flap or microvascular free flap for coverage of soft tissue defects. An alternative to reconstruction of such severe injuries is amputation.

The choice of limb salvage vs. amputation has been a topic for discussion in many studies [6-10]. Both procedures are associated with complications. Sequelae after limb salvage include osteomyelitis, non-union, or flap loss [5,9].

Bosse et al. reported that patients with leg-threatening injuries had a similar clinical outcome after limb salvage compared with amputation at 2-years follow-up [8]. Others

* Correspondence: karl-ake.jansson@karolinska.se
[1]Department of Molecular Medicine and Surgery, Section of Orthopaedics and Sports Medicine, Karolinska Institutet at Karolinska University Hospital, SE-17176 Stockholm, Sweden
Full list of author information is available at the end of the article

have shown that limb salvage resulted in lower costs and higher utility compared with amputation [11]. Saddawi-Konefka et al. documented a trend towards limb salvage rather than amputation due to an improvement in surgical techniques for soft tissue reconstruction [6].

The recommended standard treatment for Gustilo type III open fractures is stabilization of the fracture and early soft tissue coverage (preferably within 72 hours). This concept was introduced by Godina [12] and has been further developed and evaluated [13-15].

So far, there have been no reports on a national level analysing the rates of limb salvage and amputation in patients with open fractures of the lower limbs. Therefore, we aimed to study the frequency of these surgical procedures in patients with open tibial fractures using Swedish national registries.

Methods
Source of data
Data were obtained from the Swedish National Patient Register [16], which covers more than 98% of all hospital admissions in Sweden [17]. A 10-digit national registration number for each individual in Sweden allows epidemiological studies on a nationwide basis. The Register includes e.g. data on diagnosis, surgical procedure codes, and demographic data for each hospital admission in Sweden. Diagnoses are coded according to the International Classification of Diseases (ICD). We extracted data from the Register on all hospital admissions and re-admissions of patients (> = 15 years of age) with the following diagnoses: open fractures of the proximal tibia (S82.11), the tibial shaft (S82.21), and the distal tibia (S82.31). No exclusions were made. The study period was 1998–2010. Fracture incidence rates per 100,000 person-years were calculated by using data from the Total Population Register.

Mechanisms of injury were collected from ICD E-codes and divided into 5 categories: fall on the same level, unspecified fall, fall from height, motor vehicle accident (MVA), and miscellaneous. Fall from height and MVA were considered as high energy mechanisms for the risk factor analysis. Fixation methods were grouped into 6 categories: intramedullary nail, plate, closed reduction/cast, external fixation, combination of external fixation and other definitive fixation, and miscellaneous. Reconstructive plastic surgical procedures were grouped into 3 categories: free flaps (ZZQ), pedicled flaps (ZZS), and skin graft only (ZZA00). Timing of free and pedicled flaps was registrered and analysed in categories: reconstruction within 72 hours (3 days), reconstruction within 4 to 90 days and reconstruction after 90 days. Amputations were analysed as follows: transfemoral amputation (NFQ19), knee disarticulation (NGQ09), and transtibial amputation (NGQ19). Ankle disarticulation and partial

foot amputation were regarded as one group (NHQ). Amputation was defined as early if performed within 3 months and late after 3 months. The etiology of amputation was registered as severe acute injury, infection/osteomyelitis, pseudarthrosis, high age and other/unknown. The study was approved by The Regional Ethical Review Board (2011/1280-32).

Statistics
The Welsh 2 Sample t-test was used to calculate differences for mechanisms of injury, sex, and mean age of the amputated as compared to the non-amputated patients. Amputation rate related to timing of reconstruction was analyzed with Fisher's exact test for count data. The differences between amputation rates after reconstructive procedures were calculated using Fisher's exact test for count data and Bon Ferroni correction. Logistic regression analysis was used to assess the risk of amputation within 3 months after the fracture. Odds ratios (ORs) and the associated 95% confidence intervals (CI) are presented. The crude results were adjusted for age, sex, mechanism of injury, and surgical procedure. Logistic regression with a binomial logit link function was applied. The results were considered statistically significant for p-values < =0.05. The statistical software used was R. R is available as free software, www.r-project.org.

Results
Patients
During the study period, 3,777 patients (67% males) were admitted to a Swedish hospital due to open tibial fractures (Table 1). The majority (3,704 patients, 98%) had a unilateral fracture and 73 patients had bilateral fractures (2%). Most fractures were located in the tibial shaft (60%). The mean age of the patients at admission was 47 (SD 20) years (males 42 [SD 20] and females 55 [SD 22]) (Figure 1). The mean follow-up time was 6 (SD 3.8) years.

The most common cause of injury was a MVA (43%), followed by a fall on the same level (21%). Fractures after MVA and falls from height were mainly seen in males (both 73%). Fractures after fall on the same level had a more even distribution (females, 55%) (Table 1). The mean age was higher for females in all age-groups (p < 0.01) (data not included).

During the study period, the incidence rate of open fractures was ranging between 2.8-3.4 per 100,000 person-years, and did not show any statistically significant change over time. The incidence rate was higher for males compared with females (p < 0.001) (Figure 2).

Surgical procedures
The most common fixation method was an intramedullary nail (32%) as the only method. Combinations of external fixation and other methods were used in 22% of

Table 1 Patients with open tibial fractures in Sweden during 1998-2010

	All patients		Males		Females	
	n	%	n	%	n	%
	3,777	100	2,537	67	1,240	33
Localization						
Proximal	540	14	329	61	211	39
Shaft	2,277	60	1,593	70	684	30
Distal	960	26	615	64	345	36
Mechanism of injury						
Fall on same level	791	21	359	45	432	65
Fall from height	414	11	304	73	109	27
Fall unspecified	229	6	138	60	91	40
Motor vehicle accident	1,631	43	1,191	73	440	27
Miscellaneous	712	19	544	76	168	24
Fixation method						
Intramedullary nail	1,212	32	850	70	362	30
Plate	325	9	188	58	137	42
Closed reduction, cast	145	4	78	54	67	46
External fixation	294	8	212	72	82	28
Combination external fixation and other methods	815	22	592	73	223	27
Miscellaneous	986	26	615	62	371	38

the patients. Plate as the only method was used in only 9% of the cases (Table 1).

A total of 342 patients (9%) underwent soft-tissue reconstructions. There were 102 free flaps and 83 pedicled flaps as some patients had more than one procedure. There were 166 patients treated with skin grafts only (Table 2). Reconstructive surgery with free or local flap

was performed within 3 days after the injury in 27 patients of whom no one was amputated within the study period. Between 4 and 90 days, there were 97 reconstructions of which 12 (12%) went to amputation. There was a significant difference in amputation rate between the two groups (p = 0.04). Approximately 50% of reconstructions with free or local flap were performed within 10 days, and

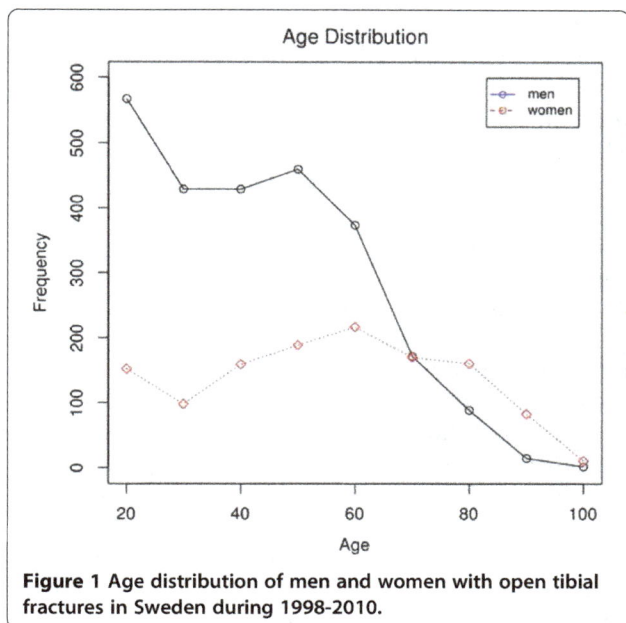

Figure 1 Age distribution of men and women with open tibial fractures in Sweden during 1998-2010.

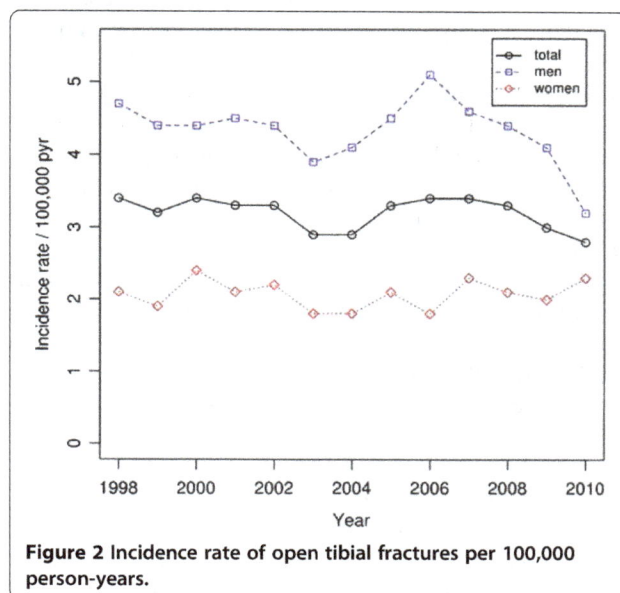

Figure 2 Incidence rate of open tibial fractures per 100,000 person-years.

Table 2 Surgical procedures after open tibial fractures among 3.777 patients, n = cases

	All patients	
	n	%
Flaps		
Total	342	100
Free flaps	102	30
Pedicled flaps	83	22
Skin graft only	166	48
Amputations		
Total	125	100
Transfemoral	30	24
Knee disarticulation	17	14
Transtibial	74	59
Ankle and foot	4	3

between day 4 and 7 there were 24 reconstructions, of which 3 went to amputation.

During the study period, 93 out of 3,777 patients underwent an amputation. In total, there were 125 amputations. The majority (59%) were transtibial amputations. At first admission, an amputation was performed in 43 patients. Early amputations were done in 63 patients and late amputations in 30 patients. Data showed that amputation was performed on day one in 28 patients. The etiology for an amputation within first admission was in 34 cases the acute injury; associated injuries like vascular damage (n = 11), severe open injuries, open foot injuries, nerve injuries, crush injuries, multiple fractures and dislocations. Other causes were acute infection (n = 2), patients with a high age (n = 13) and other/unknown reason (n = 2). In cases where amputation was performed later then first admission, the etiology was infection/osteomyelitis (n = 20), initial history of polytrauma with severe associated injuries (n = 8), pseudarthrosis (n = 6), and other/unknown reason (n = 8).

Amputated patients were older than non-amputated patients (p < 0.001). The mean age for amputated men was 51 (SD 20) years and for women 70 (SD 19) years. For non-amputated patients the mean age was 42 (SD 18) years for men and 55 (SD 21) years for women.

Patients who did not have soft tissue reconstruction had a lower amputation rate (2%) compared with patients who had reconstructive surgery (7%) (p < 0.001). No significant difference was seen between the three methods of tissue coverage regarding subsequent amputation (p = 0.44) (Table 3).

Risk factors for amputation

Logistic regression analysis with the outcome risk for amputation within 3 months after fracture showed higher risk for patients with male sex, age above 70 years

and in those who underwent reconstructive surgery. The mechanism of injury did not show any significant association. Regarding fixation methods, methods other than intramedullary nailing as the only method were associated with a significant higher risk for amputation (Table 4).

Discussion

We found that nearly 10% of all patients with open tibial fractures were reconstructed with a soft tissue flap in Sweden during 1998–2010. The overall risk of amputation in patients with open tibial fractures was low, ranging between 2-10%. Significant risk factors for amputation within 3 months after fracture were age above 70 years and soft tissue reconstruction, as an indicator of a severe injury.

The incidence rate of open tibial fractures per 100,000 person-years was stable during the study period, ranging between 2.8-3.4. This is in line with data from Court-Brown et al. who described an incidence rate of 3.4 per 100,000 person-years for open tibial shaft fractures in Edinburgh [18].

Open tibial fractures are often caused by high energy trauma. Motor vehicle accident was the most common mechanism of injury in our cohort and 2/3 of the fractures occured in males. This is in line with previous observations, as well as a sex difference where females mostly sustained low energy fractures due to simple falls and males were predominant in the group with higher energy trauma [1,18]. The age distribution for males was unimodal with the highest incidence at a younger age (around 20 years). For females this curve had a rather flat form but there was a bimodal tendency, with one peak around 20, and second peak around 60 years of age. We believe, as was shown in other publications, that the peak in younger age-groups represented high energy fractures and in higher ages low energy (osteoporotic) fractures [1,18]. The most common fixation method in this study was an intramedullary nail as only method. This is regarded as gold standard in shaft fractures. A combination of external fixation and other methods was the used in 22% of the cases. External fixation as an initial method that is later converted to nail or plate is commonly used in polytrauma or severe open injuries. The Gustilo-Anderson classification is often used for grading of open fractures [7]. Unfortunately this classification is not available in our national registers. The classification is graded in I-III, depending on the size of the skin laceration, the degree of contamination, the soft-tissue injury, and the fracture configuration. The Gustilo type IIIB injury has extensive soft-tissue damage with periosteal stripping and bone exposure with inadequate soft tissue for bone coverage, and thus often needs some kind of soft tissue reconstruction. In our cohort of nearly 4,000 patients with open tibial fracture, almost 9%

Table 3 Total number of amputations related to previous reconstructive surgery, n = patients

	No amputation	Total amputations		Early amputation <3 months		Late amputation >3 months	
	n	n	%	n	%	n	%
Flaps							
No flap	3,367	68	2	50	2	18	0.5
Free flap	93	9	9	3	3	6	6
Pedicled flap	76	7	10	3	4	4	5
Skin graft only	155	11	7	8	5	3	2
All reconstructions	315	25	7	13	4	12	4

Some patients have undergone several procedures.

obtained some type of flap or skin graft. Court-Brown et al. reported a prevalence of Type III fractures of 45% and almost 45% of these cases were graded as Type IIIB, which means totally 20% Type IIIB [18]. These numbers seem rather high compared to our population where only 9% of fractures were interpreted as Gustilo IIIB. This may reflect differences in the study cohorts, where our study included patients from all Swedish hospitals (around 50 emergency hospitals), and the material shown above from Edinburgh might be more selected.

We calculated the risk of amputation within 3 months and found age >70 years and the occurrence of flap surgery as independent risk factors. Higher age reasonably increases the risk for other diseases that lead to a poorer outcome for limb salvage. In this set-up, we have no data on co-morbidities. The Swedish Patient Register is valid for primary diagnoses to a great extent, especially for trauma and surgical procedures. When it comes to

comorbidities data are more unsecure [17]. We have considered this register not to be valid enough to perform statistical analyses on comorbidities.

We thought that mechanism of injury (an indicator of energy level) would be a risk factor for amputation. However, this was not the case in our cohort. This may indicate that low energy fractures diluted the effect by being present in the group of transport accidents. The subdivision of injury mechanisms in only 5 groups might not be sophisticated enough to show an association between energy level and amputation. Among fixation methods, all methods other than nailing as only method were associated with higher risk for amputation. A reason for this may be that nailing as early definitive treatment is mainly used in low energy fractures, Gustilo type I-II.

Reconstructive plastic surgery as a risk factor may indicate a more severe fracture Gustilo type III, ending in a higher amputation rate. In all cases with free flap

Table 4 Risk factors for amputation within 3 months in patients with open tibial fracture

		Crude			Adjusted		
		OR	95% CI	p	OR	95% CI	p
Sex	Men	1.0	ref		1.0	ref	
	Women	0.9	0.5-1.6	0.78	0.5	0.3-1.0	0.050
Age-group	15-60	1.0	ref		1.0	ref	
	61-70	1.4	0.6-2.9	0.45	1.6	0.6-3.5	0.27
	71-80	2.0	0.8-4.4	0.09	2.3	0.9-5.2	0.05
	≥81	5.8	2.9-10.7	<0.001	7.2	3.3-15.2	<0.001
Flap	No	1.0	ref		1.0	ref	
	Yes	2.8	1.4-5.0	0.001	3.0	1.5-5.6	0.001
Mechanism of injury Energy	Low	1.0	ref		1.0	ref	
	High	1.2	0.7-1.9	0.58	1.3	0.8-2.3	0.32
Fixation method	Nail	1.0	ref		1.0	ref	
	Plate	5.1	1.1-25.8	0.034	4.4	1.0-22.6	0.055
	Closed reduction	14.4	3.5-70.6	<0.001	12.1	2.9-60.3	<0.001
	External fixation	10.0	2.8-46.5	<0.001	6.6	1.8-31.3	<0.001
	Combination	6.2	2.0-27.4	0.0047	4.5	1.4-20.0	0.022
	Miscellaneous	12.9	4.6-53.8	<0.001	10.0	3.5-42.0	<0.001

CI = confidence interval, ref = reference value, adjusted for age, sex, reconstructive surgery, mechanism of injury and fixation method.

reconstructions, a substantial amount of lower limb soft tissue is damaged, exposing the fracture site. Extensive soft tissue deficiency should be considered as a negative prognostic sign for healing.

We could also differentiate the amputations as early (within 3 months) or late. Early amputations were seen in 63 patients and late amputations in 30 patients. Late amputations are considered to have a poorer outcome with more complications [9].

We found the amputation rate after free flap surgery similar to local flap surgery (9% and 10% respectively). For patients without flaps, the amputation rate was 2%. In a review by Saddawi-Konefka et al. the authors reported failure rates for pedicled flaps of 8% and 5% for free flaps [6]. In a study from the LEAP group, the authors found that pedicled flaps were associated with 4.3 times more wound complications requiring operative intervention than free flaps, in one sub-group of severe injuries [19]. Pedicle flaps might be constructed by tissue in the zone of injury affecting complication and amputation rate. This predisposing risk factor highlightened the important pre-operative decision making according to the reconstructive plastic ladder. Timing of flap surgery has earlier been shown to be of great importance for successful reconstruction [12]. Godina showed in his study that reconstruction within 72 hours (3 days) showed better results than reconstruction within 4–90 days or later. In this study results are similar. None of the patients that had reconstructive surgery within 3 days was amputated. The goal for most orthopedic and plastic surgeons is to perform reconstruction within 3 days and the time should not exceed one week [20]. We conclude that this goal is important to achieve whenever possible.

The amputation rate after attempted limb salvage varies between 4-40% in the literature [6,9,14,19,21]. There is an ongoing discussion about the decision between limb salvage and amputation in patients with severe lower limb trauma. We know that the complication rate is higher with attempted limb salvage, but self-reported results are similar after 2 years [9]. To evaluate complications is important, not only for prevention, but also for the possibility to give patients accurate information about lower limb reconstruction.

The major shortcomings of this study are the following: this is a register study with all it's advantages and disadvantages. No further investigation of medical records was performed. We have no data on the Gustilo classification, as this variable is not included in the Register. Comorbidities and injury mechanisms may not be valid enough to perform statistical analysis, as mentioned above. A further limitation is the relatively small amount of severe injuries that require reconstructive surgery. Therefore, more complex associations are difficult to detect statistically. However, the amputation rate and frequency of soft tissue coverage after open tibial fracture has not been studied previously on a national basis. Thanks to data obtained from Swedish registers, we have been able to study the epidemiology and outcome of open tibial fractures over a period of 13 years. This patient material covers nearly all hospital admissions in Sweden and we therefore consider the results representative for a population of 9 million inhabitants [17].

The number of patients in Sweden with a severe injury of the lower limb is low. In this material, only 13 limb reconstructions for open tibial fracture were performed every year. Knowledge about outcome of different treatment strategies is crucial to manage these patients properly and provide them with appropriate information on prognostic aspects. To be able to ensure best treatment, these patients with severe open tibial fractures should be treated at dedicated trauma units by multidisciplinary teams with both orthopedic and plastic surgeons. This information may therefore be important to health providers to plan the appropriate and cost-effective management of patients with these severe injuries.

In Sweden, a new fracture register has been developed recently in order to improve the quality of health care (www.registercentrum.se). This is promising because it is now possible to follow-up these uncommon and critical patients with severe injury of the lower limb.

Conclusion

The rate of amputations after open tibial fractures is low (3.6%). There is a higher risk for amputations with age above 70 (in contrast: male sex and tissue reconstruction are rather indicators for more severe soft tissue injuries). Only a small proportion of open tibial fractures need soft tissue reconstructive surgery. Reconstruction with free or pedicled flap should be performed within 72 hours whenever possible.

Competing interests
The authors declare that they have no competing interests.

Authors' contributions
UT and KÅJ: planning, data analysis, statistics, writing, and editing of the manuscript. RJW, BS, PS, and ZAD: planning and editing of the manuscript. All authors read and approved the final manuscript.

Acknowledgements
We thank "The Karolinska Trauma Fellowship 2011" and Dr. Stefan Israelsson Tampe for his support with the statistical analysis.

Author details
[1]Department of Molecular Medicine and Surgery, Section of Orthopaedics and Sports Medicine, Karolinska Institutet at Karolinska University Hospital, SE-17176 Stockholm, Sweden. [2]Department of Molecular Medicine and Surgery, Section of Plastic Surgery, Karolinska Institutet, Karolinska University Hospital, Stockholm, Sweden.

Lower extremity soft tissue reconstruction and amputation rates in patients with open tibial fractures...

39

References

1. Court-Brown CM, Rimmer S, Prakash U, McQueen MM: **The epidemiology of open long bone fractures.** *Injury* 1998, **29**(7):529–534.

2. Emami A, Mjoberg B, Ragnarsson B, Larsson S: **Changing epidemiology of tibial shaft fractures. 513 cases compared between 1971–1975 and 1986–1990.** *Acta Orthop Scand* 1996, **67**(6):557–561.

3. Howard M, Court-Brown CM: **Epidemiology and management of open fractures of the lower limb.** *Br J Hosp Med* 1997, **57**(11):582–587.

4. Weiss RJ, Montgomery SM, Ehlin A, Al Dabbagh Z, Stark A, Jansson KA: **Decreasing incidence of tibial shaft fractures between 1998 and 2004: information based on 10,627 Swedish inpatients.** *Acta Orthop* 2008, **79**(4):526–533.

5. Papakostidis C, Kanakaris NK, Pretel J, Faour O, Morell DJ, Giannoudis PV: **Prevalence of complications of open tibial shaft fractures stratified as per the Gustilo-Anderson classification.** *Injury* 2011, **42**(12):1408–1415.

6. Saddawi-Konefka D, Kim HM, Chung KC: **A systematic review of outcomes and complications of reconstruction and amputation for type IIIB and IIIC fractures of the tibia.** *Plast Reconstr Surg* 2008, **122**(6):1796–1805.

7. Gustilo RB, Mendoza RM, Williams DN: **Problems in the management of type III (severe) open fractures: a new classification of type III open fractures.** *J Trauma* 1984, **24**(8):742–746.

8. Bosse MJ, MacKenzie EJ, Kellam JF, Burgess AR, Webb LX, Swiontkowski MF, Sanders RW, Jones AL, McAndrew MP, Patterson BM, McCarthy ML, Travison TG, Castillo RC: **An analysis of outcomes of reconstruction or amputation after leg-threatening injuries.** *N Engl J Med* 2002, **347**(24):1924–1931.

9. Harris AM, Althausen PL, Kellam J, Bosse MJ, Castillo R: **Lower Extremity Assessment Project Study G. Complications following limb-threatening lower extremity trauma.** *J Orthop Trauma* 2009, **23**(1):1–6.

10. MacKenzie EJ, Bosse MJ, Castillo RC, Smith DG, Webb LX, Kellam JF, Burgess AR, Swiontkowski MF, Sanders RW, Jones AL, McAndrew MP, Patterson BM, Travison TG, McCarthy ML: **Functional outcomes following trauma-related lower-extremity amputation.** *J Bone Joint Surg Am* 2004, **86-A**(8):1636–1645.

11. Chung KC, Saddawi-Konefka D, Haase SC, Kaul G: **A cost-utility analysis of amputation versus salvage for Gustilo type IIIB and IIIC open tibial fractures.** *Plast Reconstr Surg* 2009, **124**(6):1965–1973.

12. Godina M: **Early microsurgical reconstruction of complex trauma of the extremities.** *Plast Reconstr Surg* 1986, **78**(3):285–292.

13. Cross WW 3rd, Swiontkowski MF: **Treatment principles in the management of open fractures.** *Indian J Orthop* 2008, **42**(4):377–386.

14. Gopal S, Majumder S, Batchelor AG, Knight SL, De Boer P, Smith RM: **Fix and flap: the radical orthopaedic and plastic treatment of severe open fractures of the tibia.** *J Bone Joint Surg (Br)* 2000, **82**(7):959–966.

15. Tielinen L, Lindahl JE, Tukiainen EJ: **Acute unreamed intramedullary nailing and soft tissue reconstruction with muscle flaps for the treatment of severe open tibial shaft fractures.** *Injury* 2007, **38**(8):906–912.

16. Socialstyrelsen. The National Board of Health and Welfare: **The Swedish Hospital Discharge Register.** http://www.sos.se.

17. Ludvigsson JF, Andersson E, Ekbom A, Feychting M, Kim JL, Reuterwall C, Heurgren M, Olausson PO: **External review and validation of the Swedish national inpatient register.** *BMC Public Health* 2011, **11**:450.

18. Court-Brown CM, Bugler KE, Clement ND, Duckworth AD, McQueen MM: **The epidemiology of open fractures in adults. A 15-year review.** *Injury* 2012, **43**(6):891–897.

19. Pollak AN, McCarthy ML, Burgess AR: **Short-term wound complications after application of flaps for coverage of traumatic soft-tissue defects about the tibia. The Lower Extremity Assessment Project (LEAP) Study Group.** *J Bone Joint Surg Am* 2000, **82-A**(12):1681–1691.

20. Nanchahal J, Nayagam D, Nayagam D, Khan U, Moran C, Barrett S, Sanderson F, Pallister I: *Standards for the management of open fractures of the lower limb.* 1st edition. published London: The British Orthopedic Association (BOA) and British Association of Plastic & Aesthetic Surgeons (BAPRAS); 2009:36–38.

21. Hoogendoorn JM, van der Werken C: **Grade III open tibial fractures: functional outcome and quality of life in amputees versus patients with successful reconstruction.** *Injury* 2001, **32**(4):329–334.

Primary flap reconstruction of tissue defects after sarcoma surgery enables curative treatment with acceptable functional results: a 7-year review

Jenny Fabiola López[1*], Kristiina Elisa Hietanen[1], Ilkka Santeri Kaartinen[1], Minna Tellervo Kääriäinen[1], Toni-Karri Pakarinen[2], Minna Laitinen[2] and Hannu Kuokkanen[1]

Abstract

Background: Sarcomas, a heterogeneous group of tumors, are challenging to treat and require multidisciplinary cooperation and planning. We analyzed the efficacy of flap reconstruction in patients with bone and soft tissue sarcoma.

Methods: Patient charts and operative records were retrospectively reviewed from January 2006 through October 2013 to identify sarcoma patient characteristics, postoperative complications, revisions, recurrences, and survival. Pedicled and/ or free flap reconstruction was performed in 109 patients. Flap selection was based on defect size, and exposure of anatomically critical structures or major orthopedic implants.

Results: Of 109 patients, 71 (65.1 %) were men, and mean age was 56.4 years. Tumors most frequently located in a lower extremity (38.7 %). Primary sarcomas comprised 79.2 % and recurrences occurred in 18.9 %. Wide resection was performed for 65.7 %, and there were 10 planned amputations combined with flap reconstruction. A total of 111 tumors received 128 flaps: 76 pedicled flaps, 42 free flaps, and 5 combined (10 total) pedicled + free-flaps. The success rate was 94 % for the pedicled flap group, 97 % for the free-flap group, and 100 % for the pedicle + free-flap group. Of 35 patients, 5 developed deep prosthetic infections. Only one amputation due to disease progression was performed. Satisfactory functional outcome was achieved in 69 %. Survival rate during a mean (standard deviation) 3(2) year follow-up was 83.5 %.

Conclusions: Primary flap reconstruction after sarcoma surgery satisfies oncologic goals. Large tumors in difficult areas can be removed and complete tumor resection achieved. Our findings indicate a high survival rate after sarcoma surgery utilizing flap reconstruction and a low recurrence rate.

Keywords: Sarcoma, Characteristics, Defect size, Flap reconstruction, Survival

Background

Soft tissue and bone sarcomas have characteristic patterns of biologic behavior on which staging and treatment protocols are based [1]. The international incidence rate ranges from 1.8-5 per 100,000 persons/year, with 11,410 new cases in 2013 [2]. The Finnish Cancer Registry reported an incidence of 0.7 and 1.4/100.000 persons/year for bone and soft tissue cancers [3].

Advances in the multimodal treatment approach of sarcoma patients have drastically improved survival and quality of life [4, 5]. Combined wide excision and adjuvant therapy remains the standard for local control without increased recurrence or mortality [6]. Nonetheless, recent studies demonstrated that narrower margins yield similar outcomes and complete tumor resection is the main aim for oncology surgeons [7–9].

Significant tissue defects may result from sarcoma excisions, with exposure of tendons, bones, joints, vessels, and prosthetic material, making substantial coverage crucial. Sarcoma patients require reconstructive procedures that

* Correspondence: jenny_lopez1978@hotmail.com
[1]Department of Plastic Surgery, Unit of Musculoskeletal Diseases, Tampere University Hospital, Pirkanmaa Hospital District, Teiskontie 35, PO BOX 2000, Tampere 33521, Finland
Full list of author information is available at the end of the article

provide quality vascularized tissue with a brief healing period, thus enabling adjuvant therapy.

Pedicled flaps are used most commonly to cover sarcoma defects and free flaps have gained popularity and provide fast healing, adequate functional results, and vascularized tissue coverage [10–12].

The benefits of primary tissue reconstruction for sarcoma patients, the most common postoperative complications, and the revision percentages remain unclear. The aim of this retrospective study was to analyze the results and benefits of primary tissue reconstruction in our multidisciplinary Sarcoma Unit.

Methods

The Tampere University Hospital Sarcoma Unit registry identified a total of 359 sarcoma patients from January 2006 through October 2013. This research was approved by the Tampere University Hospital Research Committee and a patient photography release consent form was obtained.

Flap reconstruction was performed in 109 of these patients. Patient charts were reviewed to determine demographic characteristics, comorbidities, pertinent laboratory results, and body mass index (BMI). Tumor information (location, pathology, and grade) was also collected. Surgical data included: resection type, hardware used, and defect size. Flap choice included tumor/defect size (defined through pathology specimen as length x width), tissue type, function, and donor site availability, among others. There were three reconstructive options: pedicled flaps, free flaps, and pedicled + free (as two separate) flaps. Pedicled flaps in our study were defined as true perforator flaps, such as propeller flaps, and local broad-based fasciocutaneous or muscle flaps. Using a two-team approach, the operating time included tumor resection, fixation, and reconstruction. Outcome analyses of postoperative complications and revisions were calculated. Early complications were defined as those occurring within the first 30 postoperative days. Postoperative pathologic margins were studied, as well as patient functionality. Finally, disease recurrence, progression, and patient survival were analyzed.

Data are presented as the mean (standard deviation) unless otherwise noted. Statistical analysis was performed using SPSS® version 22. For continuous variables, p values were calculated using the Kruskal-Wallis nonparametric test, and for the categorical variables, Fisher's exact test was used. Box plots were applied for defect size analysis, and the Kaplan-Meier test was used to analyze patient survival with Cox regression for individual variable analysis.

Results

A total of 109 sarcoma patients that underwent reconstruction were identified. Demographic information concerning comorbidities, age, BMI, and laboratory tests is provided in Table 1. The majority of patients (71, 65 %) were men. Mean patient age was 56.4 years and mean BMI was 26.22 kg/m^2. Age was significantly higher in the pedicled group and lower in the pedicled + flap group. The remaining demographic characteristics were not significantly different among the study groups.

Tumor localization and presentation (primary, recurrent, and metastatic) are shown in Table 2. There were more free-flap reconstructions for lower limbs and more pedicled flap reconstructions for thoracodorsal defects. Pedicled + free flaps were used more often for lower trunk reconstruction ($p = 0.02$). Lower trunk tumors were predominantly located in the pelvic and sacral regions. Free and pedicled flaps were used equally for head and neck, and lower trunk reconstruction. In the upper extremities, pedicled flaps were common, due to the versatility of pedicled radial forearm flaps.

The pathologic distribution of the tumors in this study is shown in Table 3. High grade tumors comprised 60.3 %, low grade 22.5 %, and intermediate 8.1 % (9 % not reported). Neoadjuvant therapy was performed in 16 patients (14 chemotherapy and 2 radiotherapy). Adjuvant therapy was distributed as follows: 22 patients received only chemotherapy, 23 received only radiotherapy, and 21 received both chemotherapy and radiotherapy. According

Table 1 Patient Characteristics

	Number (%)
Sex	
-Women	38 (34.8 %)
-Men	71 (65.1 %)
Comorbidities	
-Smoking	14 (12.8 %)
-Heart condition	27 (24.7 %)
-Diabetes	14 (12.8 %)
-Hypertension	38 (34.8 %)
Age (yr)	56.4 (20.5)
BMI (kg/m2)	26.2 (4.8)
Laboratory	
-Hb (g/L)	131 (18.7)
-WBC (mm^3)	7689 (2989)
-Platelets (µL)	293,981 (96997)
-Na (mEq/L)	138.9 (2.9)
-K (mEq/L)	3.95 (0.3)
-Creatinine (mg/dl)	0.42 (0.1)
-GFR (mL/min/1.73 m^2)	233.4 (105)
-INR (SU)	1.12 (0.1)

BMI (body mass index), Hb (hemoglobin), WBC (white blood count), Na (sodium), K (potassium), GFR (glomerular filtration rate), INR (international normalized ratio). Values expressed in number (n) and percentages (%) for categorical variables; and mean and standard deviation (SD) for continuous variables

Table 2 Tumor localization and presentation

Tumor Characteristics	Number (%)
Localization	
-Head and neck	8 (7,20 %)
-Thoracodorsal	23 (20,72 %)
-Abdominopelvic/ lumbosacral	27 (24,32 %)
-Upper extremity	10 (9,00 %)
-Lower extremity	43 (38,73 %)
Primary[a]	88 (79.2 %)
Recurrence	21 (18.9 %)
Metastasis	2 (1.8 %)

[a]2 patients had new primary tumors from distant sites

to Enneking's classification, surgical resections were performed as follows: wide (66 %), marginal (22 %), radical (8 %), and intralesional (3.6 %) [5]. In our series, planned pathologic wide margins were achieved in 94 % and planned marginal resections were accomplished in 96 %. This was possible despite the fact that 69 % of the tumors were T2 (>5 cm). Our multidisciplinary sarcoma team follows the Scandinavian Sarcoma Group Guidelines (SSG), which originally defined 'the wide cuff of healthy tissue' as 5 cm [8]. There has been a gradual shift towards accepting narrower margins that led the SSG to redefine wide margins as a 'cuff of 10 mm non-fascial tissue surrounding the tumor'. This opinion has gradually changed to accept even finer margins [8, 9]. In our series, R0 resections were obtained in 85 % of cases. Under the SSG policy, adjuvant radiotherapy is indicated if the margins are narrow and for all high-grade soft tissue sarcomas (STS) greater than 8 cm in size [9]. Additional surgery is not recommended unless there is a local recurrence after adjuvant radiotherapy. Adjuvant chemotherapy is given based on tumor

Table 3 Sarcoma pathology

Sarcoma Pathology	Number (%)
Rabdomyosarcoma	2 (1.8 %)
Ewing	3 (2.7 %)
MPNST	3 (2.7 %)
Synovial sarcoma	6 (5.4 %)
Hemagio-angiosarcoma	7 (6.3 %)
Dermatofibrosarcoma/fibrosarcoma	9 (8.1 %)
Osteosarcoma	12 (10.8 %)
Leiomyosarcoma	12 (10.8 %)
Liposarcoma	17 (15.3 %)
Chondrosarcoma	19 (17.1 %)
Undifferentiated Pleomorphic	21 (18.9 %)
TOTAL	111 (100 %)

[a]Values are expressed as number and percentage. MNSPT (malignant peripheral nerve sheath tumor)

grade, histology, age, and tumor size, and not based on the margins [13].

Reconstruction with metal implants was used for 29 % of the patients (endoprostheses, plates, and screws or spinal instruments) and surgical meshes for 18 % of the patients. Endoprosthetics were used in 14 patients. Autologous non-vascularized bone was used at the beginning of the study in three patients, but was replaced with vascularized bone due its clear benefits. The risk for infection was significant in patients who underwent endoprosthetic placement and bone grafting. In our study, muscular flaps were the preferred choice for prosthetic material coverage as they serve as an ideal vascular tissue barrier. In our experience, coverage with highly vascular tissue such as muscle is a safe method of protecting against infection and fistula formation. Additionally, muscular tissue provides volume to fill the dead space [14–17].

From a total of 111 defects, the distribution of the soft-tissue defect size varied from 4 cm [2] to 600 cm^2 (Fig. 1). Larger defects required combined reconstructions ($p = 0.004$).

Of 128 flaps, 42 were free, 76 pedicled, and 5 combined pedicled + free (10 total). The flaps comprised 39 % musculocutaneous, 36.5 % muscular, 18.6 % fasciocutaneous, and 5.6 % osteofasciocutaneous. The latissimus dorsi (LD) flap was most commonly performed in the free-flap group (62 %), 4 of which were neurovascular and 2 as a chimeric flap with scapular bone. An endoscopic LD harvest was performed in one case. An innervated (functional) free gracilis flap was also used for a brachial defect after a failed pedicled flap (Table 4).

The global mean operating time was 5.6(2.4) hr; 4.7(2.4) hr for the pedicled flap group (range 1–10.5), 6.6(1.8) hr for the free-flap group (2.5-11), and 7.7(0.8) hr for the pedicled + free flap group. Surgical time was greater in patients requiring two flaps ($p = 0.001$). Operative time was significantly lower for pedicled reconstructions ($p = <0.0001$ compared with free-flap reconstruction). In 11 patients, delayed reconstruction was performed due to patient condition and/or prolonged tumor resection.

The most frequent early complications encountered were: minor necrosis (30 %), delayed wound healing (17 %), infection (15 %), hematoma (10 %), seroma (8 %), and total flap loss (4 %). The incidence of pedicled and free-flap complications was not significantly different. The influence of comorbidities on early complications was not significant, except in total flap loss where cardiac disease appeared to have a significant role ($p = 0.012$). From a total of 35 patients who underwent prosthetic material placement, 5 suffered deep infections, and 3 required implant removal. One mesh required removal as a result of deep infection.

Wound healing complications were observed following neoadjuvant chemo- or radiotherapy. Of 14 patients

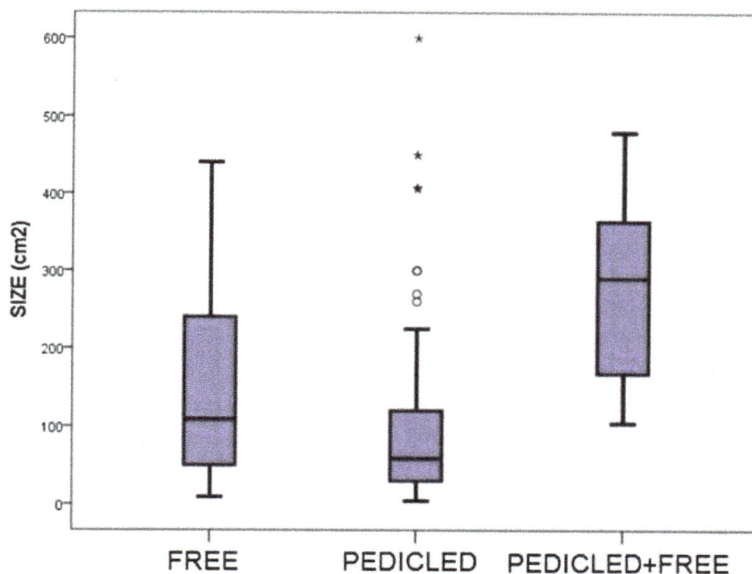

Fig. 1 Sarcoma Defect Size Distribution. Box plot showing the distribution of flap size among the reconstructive groups. Double flap reconstructions were required for larger defect sizes ($p = 0.004$)

Table 4 Flap characteristics: flap type

Flap	Pedicled	Free
Latissimus dorsi	22 (27.1 %)	29 (61.7 %)
ALT	2 (2.4 %)	4 (8.5 %)
ALT + vastus lateralis	2 (2.4 %)	4 (8.5 %)
Vastus lateralis	5 (6.1 %)	1 (2.1 %)
Radial forearm	3 (3.7 %)	2 (4.2 %)
Fibula	1 (1.2 %)	3 (6.3 %)
Rectus abdominis TRAM/VRAM	3 (3.7 %)	1 (2.1 %)
Gracilis neurovascular	-	1 (2.1 %)
Filet Flap	-	2 (4.2 %)
Gluteus	9 (11.1 %)	-
Gastrocnemius	14 (17.2 %)	-
Local fasciocutaneous	11 (13.5 %)	-
Trapezius	1 (1.2 %)	-
Crista iliaca	1 (1.2 %)	-
Tensor fascia lata	2 (2.4 %)	-
Sartorius	1 (1.2 %)	-
Soleus	1 (1.2 %)	-
Biceps femoris	1 (1.2 %)	-
Pectoralis	2 (2.4 %)	-
TOTAL	81 (100 %)	47 (100 %)

[a]Values are expressed as number and percentage. ALT (anterolateral thigh), TRAM/VRAM (transverse/vertical rectus abdominis myocutaneous)

receiving neoadjuvant chemotherapy, 6 reported wound complications such as infections and necrosis that delayed wound healing and required revision surgery ($p = 0.10$). Both patients receiving preoperative radiotherapy presented with complications of recurrent hematoma/seroma formation and infection that required revision surgery ($p = 0.05$).

The revision rates were as follows: 17 % for the pedicled, 13 % for the free, and 4 % for the pedicled + free-flap group. Wound revision for lavage and closure was significantly greater for the pedicled + free-flap group ($p = 0.033$). In the free-flap group, four patients required revisions due to vascular compromise (two required vein and two arterial and venous re-anastomosis); three with reported flap survival. The overall revision differences between the study groups and the number of revisions per patient were not significant ($p = 0.086$ and 0.116).

There was one total flap loss in the free-flap group (97 % survival); 4 total flap losses for the pedicled flap group (94 % survival), and no flap loss in the pedicled + free flap group. The pedicled + free-flap group had significantly more hematomas and wound healing problems than the other groups. The reason for this was the larger defect size in patients receiving both a pedicled and a free-flap reconstruction. When total flap loss was encountered, reconstruction was performed with new free flaps in two cases, with pedicled flaps in two cases, and with negative wound pressure therapy and multiple revision surgery followed by skin grafting in one case. The latter patient required fat grafting for volume replacement. Systemic complications were distributed equally among the groups and included pulmonary, cardiac, thromboembolic events, sepsis, and renal failure.

Local recurrence was 19.3 % and overall survival was 83.5 % (mean [standard deviation] follow-up time 3(2) years, range 0.1-7.7 years). Analysis of the correlation between surgical resection and recurrence revealed that 16/73 (22 %) of the patients with wide resections, 3/24 (18 %) with marginal resections, 2/4 (50 %) with intralesional resections, and 1/10 (10 %) with radical resections had a recurrence. The recurrence rate did not differ significantly among the study groups. Using the American Joint Committee on Cancer TNM clinical-pathologic staging for sarcomas, 28 % were stage I (9 % IA, 19 % IB), 29 % were stage II (15 % IIA, 14 % IIB), and 21 % stage III, for tumors that could be staged; [1] 24 patients (22 %) were considered stage IV. The common sites for tumor metastasis were lung (70 %), bone (15 %), liver (7 %), groin (7 %), and pelvis (4 %). One of the patients had disease progression that led to extremity amputation. Two early deaths were reported (within the first month of surgery). Survival ratios are provided in Fig. 2, and no significant differences were detected in the reconstruction groups. Sarcoma tumor recurrences significantly affected survival, with an 89 % risk of death.

The value of plastic surgery reconstruction was demonstrated in our series. Twelve patients would have been considered inoperable if flap reconstruction was not available. Similarly, without flap reconstruction, 19 patients would have been considered candidates for amputation. Distal limb tumors, tumors resected after whoops procedures, and axial tumors that required flap coverage due to defect size and vital organ exposure benefited the most from reconstructive surgery.

In our series, 96 % of the lower limb and trunk patients were able to ambulate after sarcoma resection and reconstruction, 41 % of these with assisted ambulation or with minor gait disorder. Considering that 27 % of the tumors involved the spine, sacrum, or pelvis axis, and that 39 % involved a lower extremity, functionality was considered adequate Figures 3 and 4 include examples fo hard and soft tissue sarcomas treated in our Department.

Discussion

The goal of primary tissue reconstruction after sarcoma resection is to reconstruct the excised tissue and secure wound healing by filling the dead space. The possibility of primary tissue reconstruction allows the orthopedic oncologist to proceed freely with complete tumor ablation without worrying about wound closure. The SSG guidelines have gradually shifted to accept narrower margins. The patients studied here, however, were operated on at a time when the aim was to achieve wide margin of at least 10 mm of nonfascial tissue. This aim led to

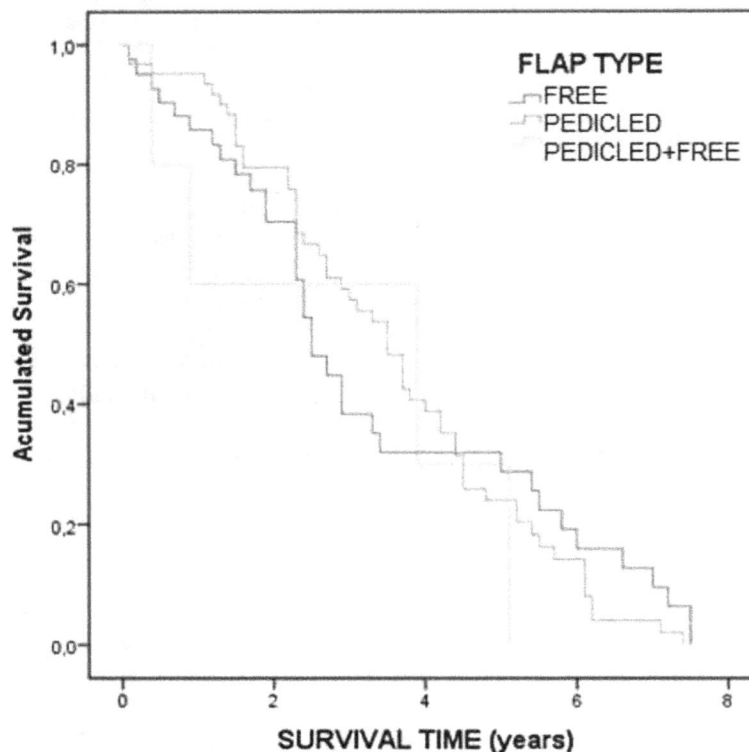

Fig. 2 The Kaplan-Meier survival curve. Survival did not differ significantly among the three reconstructive groups during the study period

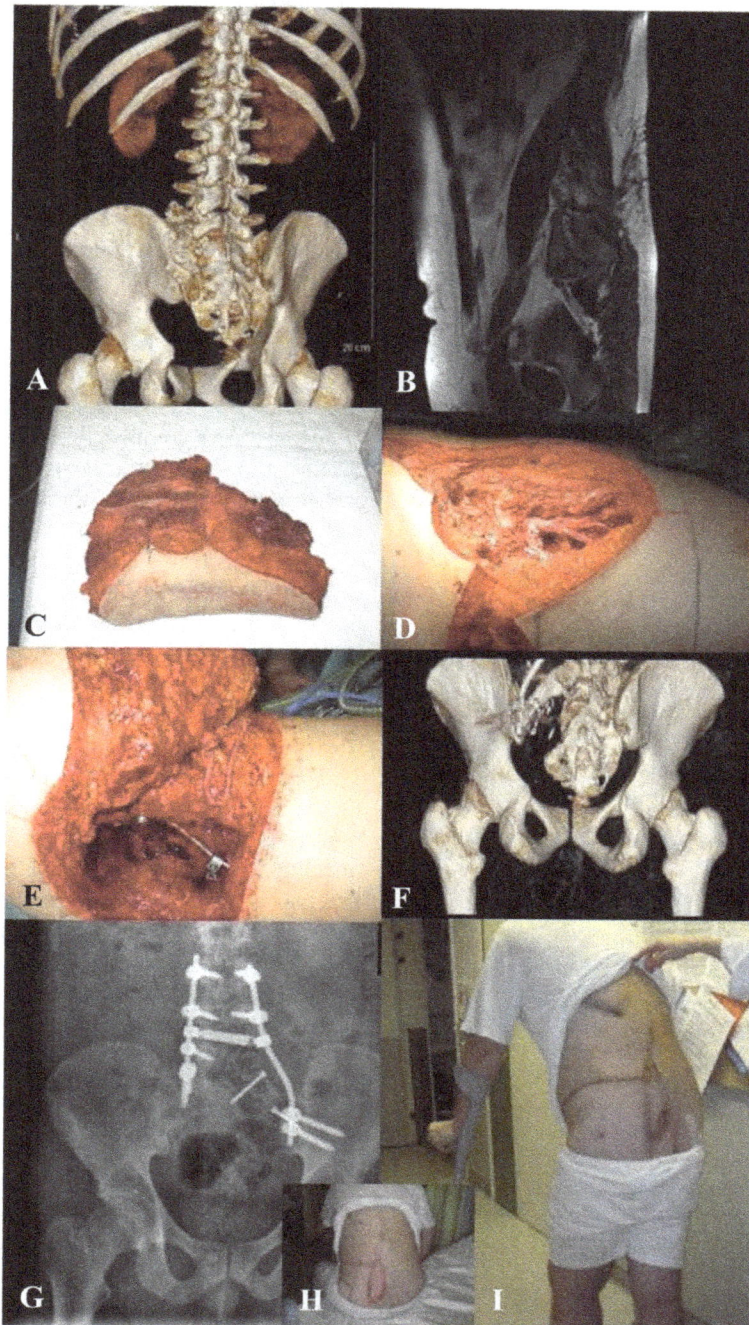

Fig. 3 Patient Photographs. 31 year-old male with left ilium chondrosarcoma, and resection of the medial ilium, partial sacrum, and LV (5th lumbar vertebra) hemicorporectomy, fixation and reconstruction with an osteomyocutaneous latissimus dorsi free-flap and saphenous vein transposition. **a,b** Preoperative images. **c,d** Biopsy specimen and defect. **e** Venous transposition. **f,g** Postoperative images. **h,i** Patient flap progression

extensive resections, as reported here. Although wide margins remain the standard resection for sarcomas, narrower margins have demonstrated comparable outcomes based on longer follow-up and survival numbers [18, 19].

Marginal resections provide similar survival rates compared with wide resections [8, 9, 13, 18, 19]. Intralesional resection yields the highest numbers of recurrence at surgical margins [20]. In our study, the greatest percentage of recurrence was detected in patients undergoing intralesional resections, followed by wide, marginal, and radical, but the differences were not statistically significant. We attribute this result to the remarkably low

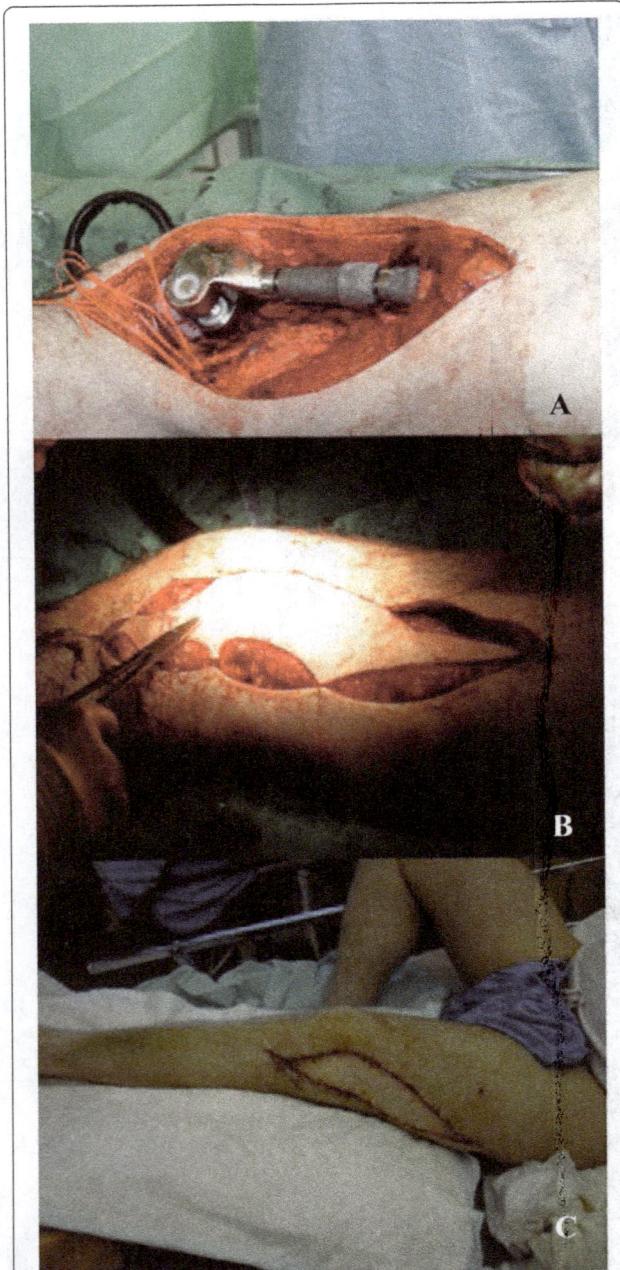

Fig. 4 a,b,c. Patient Photographs. Example of the value of plastic surgery. Patient with megaprosthesis of the knee after sarcoma resection and the resulting defect. Reconstruction with ALT free flap and results

and therefore not commonly used in these patients. Patients with STS are usually older than those with bone sarcoma and chemotherapeutic agents for sarcoma treatment are highly toxic. Therefore, the benefits of chemotherapy are lower than the possible toxic complication rates in this group.

Adequate wound healing is mandatory for postoperative adjuvant therapy [20–22]. In the past, large tumor resections and reconstructions were avoided due to the detrimental effects of adjuvant therapy, patient morbidity, and high recurrence rate. Nonetheless, tissue transfer from unirradiated sites can overcome the detrimental effects of adjuvant therapy on wound healing [20–22]. Sarcoma reconstruction is associated with a high proportion of postoperative complications, likely due to the prolonged surgical time as well as extended postoperative bed rest and immunosuppressive therapies. In the present study, we found that creating two flaps significantly prolonged the operating time. The operating time was significantly shorter for pedicled flaps, compared with free flaps. The main reason for this result, however, is that free-flap surgical time included local options, such as transposition flaps. Cordeiro described major (12 %) and minor complications (7 %) following free-flap reconstruction, reporting flap success in 96 % of cases [12]. In our study, the number of early complications was 17 %, but only 20 % of the patients required revision surgery. Pedicled flaps are commonly considered more reliable and successful for oncologic cases, but we found that the free-flap success rate was equivalent. Our current preference for the use of free flaps in certain cases is due to the advantage of freedom of flap positioning, incorporating healthy vascularized tissue, avoiding kinking or stretching of the vascular pedicle, and quick healing periods. Adding volume and a protective barrier to oncologic defects using reconstructive flaps provides greater tolerance for subsequent adjuvant therapy [23–28].

Recurrences are considered high after flap reconstruction in the setting of advanced and high-grade sarcomas [24]. Initial presentation with recurrent disease and tumor size are important risk factors for subsequent recurrence [20–22, 24, 29, 30]. In our series, planned margins were achieved in over 94 % of the cases, even for large tumors. Overall patient survival was 83.5 % for the study period, which is higher than that reported previously, ranging from 50 % to 80 % [1–3, 31–34]. Sarcoma recurrence is reported to be ~25 % to 60 % [1, 2, 31–34]. In our study, recurrence was 19 %, slightly lower than that in previous reports. Flap reconstruction allows for complete tumor excision, and thus results in a good survival rate.

Proper flap selection is crucial in sarcoma defect reconstruction [29, 30, 35]. In general, free and pedicled flaps were equally effective for defect coverage. The limitations of the current study are the retrospective nature

number of intralesional resections performed compared with the wide or marginal resections.

Although neoadjuvant chemo- and radiotherapy negatively affect wound healing, the effects were not significant. The very low number of patients receiving neoadjuvant therapy may have influenced this result. STS, the most common type of sarcoma, is resistant to chemotherapy of the research and the heterogeneity of the study population. Additionally, the condition of each patient was unique, including tumor type and indication, making their reconstruction almost impossible to compare.

Conclusions

Primary flap reconstructions after sarcoma surgery are often performed in our center for various reasons. The possibility for soft tissue and bone reconstruction allows the oncologic surgeon to perform a complete tumor excision with adequate margins [5]. Primary flap reconstruction also helps to protect orthopedic megaimplants and avoid deep infection. Additionally, an important aim is to maintain maximum patient function without compromising surgical oncologic principles. Enabling a patient to walk and return to daily activities of living after sarcoma resection vastly improves the patient's quality of life. The availability of plastic surgery reconstructions enables surgery to be performed in some patients with complex cases, and can aid in preventing amputations in some cases.

Performing primary flap reconstruction contributes to satisfy the primary goal of sarcoma resection. The choice of the reconstructive method applied is profoundly individualized. Therapeutic planning for sarcoma patients should be accomplished by a multidisciplinary team involving oncologists, radiologists, pathologists, orthopedic oncologists, arthroplastic and spine surgeons, and reconstructive plastic surgeons.

Competing interests
The authors declare that they have no competing interests.

Author' contributions
JL and KH participated in the chart review, data collection, and statistical analysis. JL, IK, and HK designed the study and drafted the manuscript. MK, TK-P, and ML created the study plan and main study points, participated in the study design and coordination, and helped to draft the manuscript. All authors read and approved the final manuscript.

Acknowledgements
We thank Mika Helminen who contributed substantially to the data analysis and interpretation. Source of funding for authors or manuscript preparation: none.

Author details
[1]Department of Plastic Surgery, Unit of Musculoskeletal Diseases, Tampere University Hospital, Pirkanmaa Hospital District, Teiskontie 35, PO BOX 2000, Tampere 33521, Finland. [2]Department of Orthopedics and Trauma, Unit of Musculoskeletal Diseases, Tampere University Hospital, Tampere, Finland.

References
1. American Joint Committee on Cancer. Soft tissues. In: Fleming ID, Cooper JS, Henson DE, editors. AJCC Cancer Staging Manual. 7th ed. Philadelphia: Lippincott-Raven; 2010. p. 149–56.
2. National Cancer Institute 2013. Available at http://www.cancer.gov/cancertopics/pdq/treatment/adult-soft-tissue-sarcoma/HealthProfessional/page1.
3. Finnish Cancer Registry 2011. Available at http://www.cancer.fi/syoparekisteri/en/statistics/cancer-statistics/koko-maa/.
4. Fisher C. Soft tissue sarcomas: Diagnosis, classification and prognostic factors. Br J Plast Surg. 1996;49:27–36.
5. Enneking WF, Spanier SS, Goodman MA. A system for the surgical staging of musculoskeletal sarcoma. Clin Orthop. 1980;153:106–20.
6. Malawer M, Sugarbaker PH. Musculoskeletal Cancer Surgery. Treatment of Sarcomas and Allied Diseases. Netherlands: Springer; 2005. p. 3.
7. Angervall L, Lindblom LG. Principles of pathologic anatomic diagnosis and classification of soft tissue sarcomas. Clin Orthop. 1993;289:9–18.
8. Trovik CS, Bauer HC, Alvegard TA. Surgical margins, local recurrence and metastasis in soft tissue sarcomas: 559 surgically treated patients from the Scandinavian sarcoma group register. Eur J Cancer. 2000;36:710–6.
9. Clement S. Trovik, Sigmund Skjeldal, Henrik Bauer, Anders Rydholm, and Nina Jebsen. Reliability of Margin Assessment after Surgery for Extremity Soft Tissue Sarcoma: The SSG Experience, Sarcoma, vol. 2012, Article ID 290698, 5 pages. doi:10.1155/2012/290698.
10. Zook EG, Russell RC, Asaadi M. A comparative study of free and pedicle flaps for lower extremity wounds. Ann Plast Surg. 1977;59:492–9.
11. Serafin D, Geordiage NG, Smith DH. Comparison of free flaps with pedicle flaps for lower extremity wounds. Plast Reconstr Surg. 1998;102:711–21.
12. Cordeiro PG, Neves RI, Hidalgo DA. The role of free tissue transfer following oncologic resection in the lower extremity. Ann Plast Surg. 1994;33:9–16.
13. O'Donnell PW, Griffin AM, Eward WC, Sternheim A, Catton CN, Chung PW, et al. The effect of the setting of a positive surgical margin in soft tissue sarcoma. Cancer. 2014;120:2866–75.
14. Sukru Y, Chih-Hung L, Yu-Te L, Ali Engin U, Wei F-CMD. Outcome Comparison between Free Muscle and Free Fasciocutaneous Flaps for Reconstruction of Distal Third and Ankle Traumatic Open Tibial Fractures. Plast Reconstr Surg. 2006;117(7):2468–75.
15. Shibata D, Hyland W, Busse P, Kim K, Sentovich SM, Steele G, et al. Immediate Reconstruction of the Perineal Wound With Gracilis Muscle Flaps Following Abdominoperineal Resection and Intraoperative Radiation Therapy for Recurrent Carcinoma of the Rectum. Ann Surg Oncol. 1999;6(1):33–7.
16. Hallock GG. Utility of Both Muscle and Fascia Flaps in Severe Lower Extremity Trauma. J Trauma. 2000;48(5):913–7.
17. Arnold PG, Yugueros P, Hanssen A. Muscle Flaps in Osteomyelitis of the Lower Extremity: A 20-Year Account. Plast Reconstr Surg. 1999;104(1):107–10.
18. Liu CY, Yen CC, Chen WM. Soft tissue sarcoma of extremities: the prognostic significance of adequate surgical margins in primary operation and reoperation after recurrence. Ann Surg Oncol. 2010;17:2102–11.
19. King DM, Hackbarth DA, Kirkpatrick A. Extremity soft tissue sarcoma resections: how wide do you need to be? Clin Orthop Relat Res. 2012;470:692–9.
20. Sawamura C, Springfield DS, Marcus KJ, Perez-Atayde AR, Gerhardt MC. Factors predicting local recurrence, metastasis and survival in pediatric soft tissue sarcoma in extremities. Clin Orthop Relat Res. 2010;468:3019–27.
21. Kane JM, Gibbs JF, McGrath BE, Loree TR, Kraybill WG. Large, deep high-grade extremity sarcomas: When is a myocutaneous flap reconstruction necessary? Surg Oncol. 1999;8:205.
22. Chao AH, Chang DW, Shuaib SW, Hanasono MM. The Effect of Neoadjuvant versus Adjuvant Irradiation on Microvascular Free Flap Reconstruction in Sarcoma Patients. Plast Reconstr Surg. 2012;129:675–82.
23. Kim JY, Subramanian V, Yousef A, Rogers BA, Robb GL, Chang DW. Upper Extremity Limb Salvage with Microvascular Reconstruction in Patients with Advanced Sarcoma. Plas Reconstr Surg. 2004;114:400–8.
24. Pisters PW, Leung DH, Woodruff J, Shi W, Brennan MF. Analysis of prognostic factors in 1,041 patients with localized soft tissue sarcomas of the extremities. J Clin Oncol. 1996;14:1679.
25. Brennan MF. The surgeon as a leader in cancer care: Lessons learned from the study of soft tissue sarcomas. J Am Coll Surg. 1996;182:520.
26. Spark JI, Charalabidis P, Laws P, Seben R, Clayer M. Vascular reconstruction in lower limb musculoskeletal tumours. ANZ J Surg. 2009;79:619–23.
27. Lohman RF, Nabawi AS, Reece GP, Pollock RE, Evans GR. Soft tissue sarcoma of the upper extremity: A 5-year experience at two institutions emphasizing the role of soft tissue flap reconstruction. Cancer. 2002;94:2256.
28. Momeni A, Kalash Z, Stark GB, Bannasch H. The use of the anterolateral thigh flap for microsurgical reconstruction of distal extremities after oncosurgical resection of soft-tissue sarcomas. J Plas, Reconst Aesth Surg. 2011;64:643–8.
29. Malawer MM, Kellar-Graney K. Soft Tissue Reconstruction After Limb-Sparing Surgery for Tumors of the Upper and Lower Extremities. Oper Tech Orthop. 2005;14:276–87.

30. Winkelmann WW. Type-B-IIIa hip rotationplasty: an alternative operation for the treatment of malignant tumors of the femur in early childhood. J Bone Joint Surg Am. 2000;82:814–28.

31. Lehnardt M, Kuhnen C, Drücke D, Homann HH, Joneidi Jafari H, Steinau HU. Liposarcoma of the extremities: recent developments in surgical therapy/ analysis of 167 patients. Chirurg. 2004;75(12):1182–90.

32. Lehnardt M, Hirche A, Daigeler O, Goertz A, Ring TH, Drücke D, et al. Weichgewebssarkome der oberen Extremität. Chirurg. 2012;83(2):143.

33. Steinau HU, Daigeler A, Langer S, et al. Limb Salvage in Malignant Tumors. Seminars in Plastic Surgery. 2010;24(1):18–33.

34. Lehnhardt M, Daigeler A, Homann HH, Schwaiberger V, Goertz O, Kuhnen C, et al. MFH revisited: outcome after surgical treatment of undifferentiated pleomorphic or not otherwise specified (NOS) sarcomas of the extremities – an analysis of 140 patients. Langenbecks Arch Surg. 2009;394(2):313–20.

35. Heller L, Levin LS. Lower extremity microsurgical reconstruction. Plas Reconstr Surg. 2001;108(4):1029–41.

8

Treatment of the diabetic foot – to amputate or not?

Elroy P Weledji[*] and Pius Fokam

Abstract

Background: Diabetic foot infections are a frequent clinical problem. About 50% of patients with diabetic foot infections who have foot amputations die within five years. Properly managed most can be cured, but many patients needlessly undergo amputations because of improper diagnostic and therapeutic approaches.

Discussion: The article debates the pros and cons of amputation of the diabetic foot. The thesis is that if the guidelines on the management of the diabetic foot are followed primary amputation is only necessary for the unsalvageable diabetic foot. This approach would reduce the incidence of lower limb amputations in diabetic patients.

Summary: We favour the argument that a structured clinical and vascular assessment would help clinical decision- making as to which patients to hospitalize, which to send for imaging, or for whom to recommend surgical interventions. Endovascular procedures are the future in the treatment of diabetic arterial disease and hence the diabetic foot.

Keywords: Diabetic foot, Infection, Neuropathy, Ischaemia, Treatment, Amputation

Background

Foot ulcers affect one in ten diabetics during their lifetime [1]. Patients with diabetes have increased risk of lower-extremity amputations and the main cause is diabetic peripheral arterial disease accelerated by the direct damage to the nerves and blood vessels by high blood glucose levels. Wound healing is also impaired from affected collagen synthesis [2,3]. Diabetic vascular disease has three main components: arteritis and small vessel thrombosis; neuropathy (possibly ischaemic in cause); and large vessel atherosclerosis. In combination these are almost bound to cause problems in the weight- bearing areas. The diabetic foot ulcers are often deeper and more frequently infected than other leg ulcers reflecting the severe end vessel ischaemia and opportunistic infection which is the common experience of the diabetic [1-4]. Factors, such as age and the duration of the disease will increase its incidence and risk of death from uncontrolled infection [4,5]. Once tissue damage has occurred in the form of ulceration or gangrene, the aim is preservation of viable tissue, but the two main threats are infection and ischaemia [3]. Ulcers should not be automatically treated with antibiotics since although as open chronic wounds there may be many commensal organisms, about half are not infected [3-5]. Several foot-ulcer classification methods have been proposed in order to organize the proposed appropriate treatment plan but none have been universally accepted. The Wagner- Meggitt classification is based mainly on wound depth and consists of 6 wound grades (Table 1) [6]. The University of Texas system grades the ulcers by depth, then stages them by the presence or absence of infection and ischaemia [6,7]. As there is the need for rapid and more appropriate therapy to facilitate healing, the international working group on the diabetic foot proposed the PEDIS classification which grades the wound on a 5- feature basis: perfusion (arterial supply), extent (area), depth, infection and sensation [1]. They also classified diabetic foot infections into four grades: Grade 1 (no infection; Grade 2 (mild) in subcutaneous tissue only; Grade 3 (moderate) with extensive erythema and infection of deeper tissue and Grade 4 (severe) with systemic inflammatory response indicating severe infection (Table 2) [1-4,7]. Most diabetic foot infections require some surgical intervention, ranging from minor (debridement) to major interventions including amputation. The main emphasis of the current international guidelines on the management of the diabetic foot is prevention, early recognition and

* Correspondence: elroypat@yahoo.co.uk
Department of Surgery, Faculty of Health Sciences, University of Buea, PO Box 126, Limbe, S W Region, Cameroon

Table 1 The Wagner-Meggitt classification

Grade 0	Grade 1	Grade 2	Grade 3	Grade 4	Grade 5
Intact skin	*superficial ulcer*	*deep ulcer to tendon, bone, or joint*	*deep ulcer with abscess or osteomyelitis*	*forefoot gangrene*	*whole foot gangrene*

treatment. Prevention of the diabetic foot entails controlling diabetes, smoking, obesity; daily foot checks, removing callosity (neuropathic foot), daily moisturizing, regular toenail cutting, and well fitted footwear [8].

The thesis is that if the guidelines on the management of the diabetic foot are followed primary amputation is only necessary for the unsalvageable diabetic foot (Table 3). Endovascular procedures are the future in the treatment of diabetic arterial disease and hence the diabetic foot.

Discussion
Arguments for primary amputation

1. Natural history of disease

The aim of primary amputation is to relieve pain and achieve rapid and successful mobility with an artificial limb [9]. Peripheral arterial disease is an independent baseline predictor of the non-healing foot ulcer and along with progressing infection continue to be the main reason for lower extremity amputation (Figure 1) [2,10]. Although the intact foot may withstand markedly reduced skin perfusion, an ulcerated lesion requires a greatly enhanced blood flow to heal; therefore, many ulcers fail to heal where critical ischaemia exists. The progressive development of an abscess in the presence of ischaemia is an ominous sign as it leads to irreparable tissue damage and amputation [4,5].

2. Assessment and treatment

As pre-operative arteriographic studies and ankle-brachial pressure index (ABPI) are usually unhelpful in the diabetic foot, transcutaneous oxygen measurements have been found useful in some units but the apparatus is expensive and the results are not infallible [10,11]. The patient's symptoms, clinical and radiological (duplex ultrasound scanning) findings would dictate the need and level of amputation, including the poorly- controlled diabetic patient with chronic ischaemia who had a failed

Table 2 Classification of diabetic foot infection [1]

Grade 1	Grade 2	Grade 3	Grade 4
No infection	**Mild**	**Moderate**	**Severe**
No signs or symptoms of infection	*Superficial, limited in size and depth*	*Deeper or more extensive*	*Systemic signs or metabolic pertubation*

Table 3 Summary of indications for conservative surgical approach or primary amputation

Debridement/minor amputation	Primary amputation
Good blood supply to foot but infected	*wet gangrene (infection + ischaemia)*
Small vessel disease and gangrenous toes	*life-threatening sepsis*
Successful surgical bypass	*extensive muscle necrosis*
Neuropathic foot with little arterial disease	*revascularisation technically impossible, bed-ridden patients/functionally useless limb*
Osteomyelitis with little arterial disease	

angioplasty to improve the circulation to the lower limb [10,12]. Although bowel gas makes duplex ultrasound scanning less useful in the abdomen, the images obtained are often sufficient to plan intervention without the need to resort to invasive imaging [13]. Digital (conservative) amputations are still rarely successful and secondary amputations are common because of disease progression or a preliminary wrong assessment [14]. In practice, most surgeons inspect and palpate the ischaemic limb pre-operatively and observe the intraoperative bleeding from the severed blood vessels at the time of surgery. Major amputations usually below knee is the gold standard, and should be attempted if there is a reasonable chance that it will succeed. Up to 80% of patients become independently mobile because the knee joint is preserved and also a lighter prosthesis is used [9,12]. The posterior reconstructive transtibial flap (Burgess) method described in 1968 is frequently used but its disadvantage over the equilateral (skew) flap operation described by

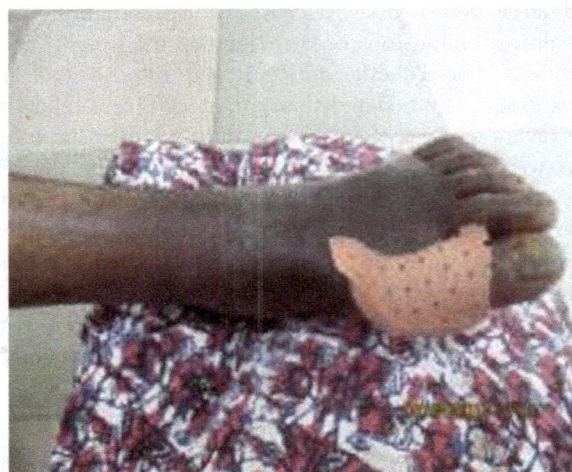

Figure 1 'Wet' gangrene in diabetic patient with peripheral vascular disease (with permission).

Kingsley Robinson in 1982 is the risk of ischaemia in the longer posterior flap and the suture line lying over the end of the tibia [9]. There is no difference in the two amputation methods between the rate of primary healing or the need for higher amputation [12]. More distal amputations in patients with distal small vessel disease or those who have had a successful proximal reconstruction, include the Syme's (forefoot) amputation, a ray amputation of the metatarsal, a transmetatarsal amputation and amputation of the toe [15].

3. Failed revascularization

The greatest immediate danger to these patients after successful revascularization is the 'reperfusion syndrome' caused by the release of toxic metabolites and oxygen free radicals into the systemic circulation from the ischaemic limb [16,17]. This can cause a profound cardiovascular collapse and with renal and sometimes respiratory failure. For this reason revascularisation should not be used in patients with signs of muscle necrosis. Primary amputation is better. A graft should if possible prevent limb loss for at least 2 years if it is to be considered a success. The 2 year patency rate of distal vascular grafts for experienced vascular units should be in the region of 75% [16,17]. There is evidence that failed bypasses result in a higher level of amputations and the combined mortality rate of a failed reconstruction followed by amputation may be higher than a primary amputation [17].

Arguments against primary amputation:

1. Natural history of disease

The 5-year mortality in patients with diabetes and critical limb ischaemia is 30% and about 50% of patients with diabetic foot infections who have foot amputations die within five years [1,3]. The mortality rate is similar to some of the most deadly cancers [18]. Poor treatment can lead to lower extremity amputations. About half of these amputations can be prevented by proper care [19-23]. It is vital that the diabetic condition in patients with infection is urgently controlled, otherwise the vicious cycle of infection leading to the instability of the diabetes and ketosis allows the spread of infection [3]. Patients with a severe infection should be hospitalized immediately as these are often imminently limb-threatening and, in some cases life-threatening [3,18]. When all or part of a foot has dry gangrene, it may be preferable especially for a patient who is a poor surgical candidate to let the necrotic portions auto-amputate. It may also be best to leave adherent eschar in place, especially on the heel, until it softens enough to be more easily removed, provided that there is no underlying focus of infection [12]. Wet gangrene develops if infection supervenes and this spreads rapidly leading to a severely compromised limb, systemic sepsis and death if there is no intervention [21]. However, the required emergency amputation still carries a high mortality of up to 50% because of severe sepsis and the effects of tissue necrosis [24].

2. Assessment and treatment

The diabetic patient presenting with a foot wound should be assessed at three levels- the patient as a whole, the affected limb and foot and the infected wound [1-4]. The affected limb and foot should be assessed for arterial ischaemia, venous insufficiency, presence of protective sensation, and biomechanical problems. There may be an obvious large wound or ulcer associated with erythema and pyrexia. The presence of any exposed bone and ulcer larger than 2 cm [2] increase the likelihood of osteomyelitis [1,3]. It is suspected in a patient with an adequate blood supply to the affected foot that has a deep ulcer which would not heal after 6 weeks of appropriate wound care and off-loading [25]. Some diabetic patients who develop neuropathies or osteomyelitis but with little arterial disease may often benefit from surgical debridement or excision and/or prolonged antibiotic therapy for at least 4 weeks, based on the culture and sensitivity of biopsied bone tissue or the curettage of deep tissues [3,4,26]. Swab specimens, especially of incompletely debrided wounds provide less accurate results [1,27].

It is important to distinguish between the ischaemic and the neuropathic foot with respect to management although these factors may co-exist [28]. The neuropathic foot is characterized by warm, dry, bounding pulses as a result of peripheral vasodilatation, callosities, painless penetrating ulcers at pressure points and sites of minor injury, painless necrosis of toes, spreading infection along plantar spaces, general loss of pain and thermal sensation, decrease ankle jerk reflex, tone and power [29,30]. The ischaemic foot is characterized by cold, absent pulses, dependent rubor, trophic changes, absent callosities, painful ulcers around heels and toes, claudication and rest pain [31].

3. Diabetic foot infection

Diabetic foot infections typically begin in a neuropathic ulceration. An infected diabetic foot with good blood supply would respond to debridement [32]. In neuropathic foot, severe infection is treated with intra-venous antibiotics in hospital and, antiseptics and dressings for ulcers. Necrotic tissue is removed and conservative digital amputations or filleting is sufficient. The surgical approach would optimize the likelihood for healing while attempting to preserve the integrity of the walking surface of the foot [30]. Specialised footwear is used to reduce weight bearing

[1,4]. In ischaemic foot infection is treated by debridement (cleaning the wound, removing pus, dead necrotic tissue and infected bone) [1,31].

While all wounds are colonized with microorganisms, the presence of infection is defined by findings of inflammation or purulence [1,3]. There are usually complex polymicrobial infections, but aerobic gram positive cocci is a vital part of diabetic foot infection. A broad-spectrum intra- venous antibiotic and metronidazole for anaerobes are recommended. Antibiotics can usually be discontinued once the clinical signs and symptoms of infection have resolved usually 1–2 weeks for mild infection and 2–3 weeks for moderate to severe infection, and not until the wound has healed. This is to avoid resistance [4]. If the wound is not easily debrided varidase dressing is used, and inadine or granuflex dressing would promote granulation [33,34]. The use of topical antimicrobials for most clinically uninfected wounds is not advocated for lack of evidence substantiating the benefit over conventional wound care therapy [1,4,35]. Several recent systematic reviews have suggested that silver-containing dressings and topical silver were neither better nor worse than control dressings in preventing wound infection and prolong healing [36]. New techniques for wound debridement include low frequency ultrasound therapy, hydrosurgery, monofilament polyester fibre pad and plasma-mediated bipolar radiofrequency ablation [37]. Skin grafting when no infection is present may be required [24].

The diabetic foot infection classification system (Table 2), along with a vascular assessment, would help determine which patients should be hospitalized, which may require special imaging procedures or surgical interventions including amputation [1,3]. Vascular assessment that reveals small vessel disease with associated gangrenous toes may be successfully treated with debridement and minor amputation [10].

4. Revascularisation

As diabetes is chronic and progressive, it makes sense to have a conservative surgical approach that include surgical revascularization [10]. A successful surgical bypass of larger vessel disease may enable more conservative treatment of the diabetic foot. Revascularisation is, however, considered inappropriate in bedridden patients, in a functionally useless limb, in patients with life threatening sepsis, extensive muscle necrosis and where it is technically impossible. Primary amputation is better in these cases [3,17].

A percutaneous transluminal angioplasty (PTA) and luminal stenting or arterial reconstruction to improve blood flow would aid healing [13]. Because in most cases ischaemia is secondary to larger vessel artherosclerosis rather than to 'small vessel disease', vessels above the

knee and below the ankle tend to be relatively spared. Thus lower extremity artherosclerosis can be amenable to angioplasty or vascular bypass [16]. The indications for a PTA in diabetic peripheral arterial disease are classically for disabling claudication and critical limb ischaemia, Patients with non-critical ischaemia (ankle/brachial pressure index (ABPI- 0.4-0.9) can in some cases be successfully treated without a vascular procedure [17]. Although the prevalence of ABI <0.9 in individuals with normal glucose tolerance was 7% and increased to 20.9% with diabetes, care should be taken when interpreting ABPI in diabetics [11]. Arterial calcification of the vessel media renders the vessels incompressible and causes false 'high' readings. Toe pressure measurements may be of value. Revascularization by percutaneous transluminal angioplasty (PTA) of short segment disease was feasible in more than 96% of diabetics with critical limb ischaemia (ankle systolic pressure of less than 50 mmHg or the toe pressure of less than 30 mmHg) [13]. Many centres have reported successful use of both aggressive endovascular interventions and distal bypass procedures for more severe vascular disease of the foot. The short-term effects are satisfactory with healing of the foot ulcers and thus diminishing the risk of amputation. However, follow-up is required to ascertain the long-term effects [10,17,38]. The feasibility with bypass prosthetic grafting (BPG) is lower but consistent [16]. Studies strongly suggest that early recognition and aggressive surgical drainage of pedal sepsis followed by surgical revascularization is critical to achieving maximal limb salvage of 74% at 5 years in the high risk population [17]. The risks of unsuccessful revascularization leading to limb loss must be weighed against the benefits and the patient informed. However, careful debridement of necrotic, infected diabetic foot wound should not be delayed while awaiting revascularization [3,10].

Aggressive attempts at foot salvage are justified in diabetic patients with advanced forefoot tissue loss/infection. After procuring adequate arterial tissue perfusion, a less conservative transtarsal (mid-foot) amputations salvaged over half of non-healing transmetatarsal amputations with excellent functional results [39].

5. Postoperative sepsis

Smokers, older patients with longer history of uncontrolled diabetes, and those with gangrenous infections and large ulcers have poorer outcome with amputations [4,5,10]. Many patients are elderly with impaired continence and poor hygiene and as a number carry *Clostridium perfringens* in their stools post operative mortality from gas gangrene is high [9]. The major problem is stump infection, which is always caused by the same organisms found in the gangrenous tissues. A swab should therefore be taken from infected lesions in the foot so that appropriate antibiotics can be administered [1]. Normally these are given with the premedication prophylactically unless there is marked infection and cellulitis which require urgent treatment [3].

6. Postoperative amputation pain and rehabilitation

Post-operative amputation pain is mostly due to phantom limb pain (54%) and phantom limb sensation (90-98%) [40]. Phantom limb pain usually continues for more than six months whereas phantom limb sensation (except pain) usually disappears or decreases with time. The true mechanism is not known but many theories overlap a peripheral, spinal and central mechanism. The successful treatment of phantom limb pain is thus difficult and treatment is usually combined and multiple based on the person's level of pain. These include biofeedback to relieve muscle tension, physical therapy, surgery to remove scar tissue entangling a nerve, transcutaneous electrical nerve stimulation (TENS) of the stump, neurostimulation techniques, medications such as analgesics, neuroleptics, anticonvulsants, antidepressants, beta -blockers and sodium channel blockers [41]. The patient must therefore be properly prepared for surgery psychologically with time being spent on assessment by the physiotherapist and reassurance and encouragement being provided by the surgeons, ward nurses or a successful amputee. The patient should be encouraged to spend periods lying prone to help keep the knee straight post-operatively and avoid fixed flexion deformity. The level of amputation may have to be high enough to ensure adequate healing of the stump [42]. Above Knee amputation (AKA) or 'transfemoral amputation' is associated with a much poorer outcome because these patients are more often unwell than those needing a below knee or 'transtibial amputation' (BKA). Although AKA is more likely to heal, rehabilitation is less successful [9]. Most elderly patients are not psychologically prepared and rehabilitation is an up-hill task.

Summary

Many diabetic foot problems are avoidable. Good glycaemic control and patient's education are essential. The main determinant of which patients with a diabetic foot infection need to be hospitalized is the clinical severity of the infection. With minimal surgical trauma and certain curative effect endovascular procedures is the future in the treatment of diabetic peripheral arterial disease and thence the diabetic foot. It is desirable that a vascular surgeon should assess the diabetic foot as the possibility of revascularization must always be considered and the correct sub-group selected for amputation. Guideline-based care for diabetic foot infections and the employment of multi-disciplinary teams would help improve outcome and minimize amputations.

Competing interests
The authors declare that they have no competing interests.

Authors' contributions
EPW carried out the study. PF participated in the literature search and gave relevant advice. Both authors read and approved the final manuscript.

Acknowledgements
We confirm that informed consent for the publication of the image of the diabetic foot was obtained from the patient. Our gratitude to the diabetic foot patients at the Regional hospital Buea, Cameroon who rendered me the impetus to write about this major diabetic complication that incessantly appeared on the surgical ward.

References
1. Lipsky BA, Berendt AR, Cornia PB, Pile JC, Peters EJ, Armstrong DG, Deery HG, Embil JM, Joseph WS, Karchmer AW, Pinzur MS, Senneville E: **Infectious diseases society of America. Clinical practice guidelines for the diagnosis and treatment of diabetic foot infections.** *Clin Infect Dis* 2012, **54**:132–73.
2. Becks PJ, Mackaay AJ, de Neeling JN, de Vries H, Bouter LM, Heine RJ: **Peripheral arterial disease in relation to glycaemic level in an elderly Caucacianpopulation : the Hoorn study.** *Diabetologia* 1995, **38**(1):163–166.
3. Schaper NC, Apelqvist J, Bakker K: **The international consensus and practical guidelines on the management and prevention of the diabetic foot.** *Curr Diab Rep* 2003, **3**:475–9.
4. Lipsky BA, Berendt AR, Deery HG, Embil JM, Joseph WS, Karchmer AW, LeFrock JL, Lew DP, Mader JT, Norden C, Tan JS: **Diagnosis and treatment of diabetic foot infections.** *Clin Infect Dis* 2004, **39**:885–910.
5. Prompers L, Huijberts M, Apelqvist J, Jude E, Piaggesi A, Bakker K, Edmonds M, Holstein P, Jirkovska A, Mauricio D, Ragnarson Tennvall G, Reike H, Spraul M, Uccioli L, Urbancic V, Van Acker K, van Baal J, van Merode F, Schape N: **High prevalence of ischaemia, infection and serious comorbidity in patients with diabetic foot disease in Europe. Baseline results from the Eurodiale study.** *Diabetologia* 2007, **50**:18–25.
6. Oyibo SO, Jude EB, Tarawinch I, Tarawneh I, Nguyen HC, Harkless LB, Boulton AJ: **A comparison of two diabetic foot ulcer classification systems: the Wagner and the University of Texas wound classification systems.** *Diabetes Care* 2001, **24**(1):84–88.
7. Schaper NC: **Diabetic foot ulcer classification system for research purposes; a progress report on criteria for including patients in research studies.** *Diabetes Metab Res Rev* 2004, **20**(Supp1):390–5.
8. Singh N, Armstrong DG, Lipsky B: **Preventing foot ulcers in patients with diabetes.** *JAMA* 2005, **293**:217–28.
9. Callum KG: **Below knee amputation.** *Curr Pract Surg* 1992, **4**:20–24.
10. Hirsh AT, Haskal ZJ, Hertzer NR, Bakal CW, Creager MA, Halperin JL, Hiratzka LF, William RC, Murphy WR, Jeffrey W, Olin JW, Puschett JB, Kenneth A, Rosenfield KA, Sacks D, Stanley JC, Taylor LM, White CJ, John White J, White RA: **ACC/AHA practice guidelines for the management of patients with peripheral arterial disease.** *Circulation* 2006, **113**:e463–6.
11. Bargellini I, Piaggesi A, Cicorelli A, Rizzo L, Cervilli R, Iacopi E, Lunardi A, Cioni R: **Predictive value of angiographic scores for the integrated management of the ischaemic diabetic foot.** *J Vasc Surg* 2013, **57**:1204–12.
12. Pinzur MS, Pinto MA, Schon LC, Smith DG: **Controversies in amputation surgery.** *Instr Course Lect* 2004, **52**:445–51. 39(Suppl 2):S123-8.
13. Sumpio BE, Lee T, Blummet A: **Vascular evaluation and arterial reconstruction of the diabetic foot.** *Clin Podiatr Med Surg* 2003, **20**:689–708.
14. Khan NA, Rahim SA, Anand SS, Simel DL, Panju A: **Does the clinical examination predict lower extremity peripheral arterial disease?** *JAMA* 2006, **295**:536–46.
15. van Battum P, Schaper N, Prompers L, Apelqvist J, Jude E, Piaggesi A, Bakker K, Edmonds M, Holstein P, Jirkovska A, Mauricio D, Ragnarson Tennvall G, Reike H, Spraul M, Uccioli L, Urbancic V, van Acker K, van Baal J, Ferreira I, Huijberts M: **Differences in minor amputation rate in diabetic foot disease throughout Europe are in part explained by differences in disease severity at presentation.** *Diabet Med* 2011, **28**:199–205.
16. Gibbons GW: **Lower extremity bypass in patients with diabetic foot ulcers.** *Surg Clin North Am* 2003, **83**:659–69.

17. Faglia E, Clerici G, Losa S, Tavano D, Cammiti M, Miramonti M, Somalvico F, Airoldi F: **Limb revascularization feasibility in diabetic patients with critical ischaemia: results from a cohort of 344 consecutive unselected diabetic patients evaluated in 2009.** *Diabetes Res Clin Pract* 2012, **95**:364–71.

18. Armstrong DG, Wrobel J, Robbins JM: **Guest editorial: are diabetes-related wounds and amputations worse than cancer?** *Int Wound J* 2007, **4**:286–7.

19. Tan T, Shaw EJ, Siddiqui F, Kandaswamy P, Barry PW, Baker M: **Inpatient management of diabetic foot problems: summary of NICE guidance.** *BMJ* 2011, **342**:1280.

20. Richard JL, Lavigne JP, Got I, Hartemann A, Malgrange D, Tsirtsikolou D, Baleydier A, Senneville E: **Management of patients hospitalized for diabetic foot infection: results of the French OPIDIA study.** *Diabetes Metab* 2010, **37**:208–15.

21. Pecorano RE, Reiber GE, Burgess EM: **Pathways to diabetic limb amputation. Basis for prevention.** *Diabetic Care* 1990, **13**(5):513–521.

22. Trautner C, Haastert B, Mauckner P, Gatcke LM, Giani G: **Reduced incidence of lower-limb amputations in the diabetic population of a German city, 1990–2005: results of the Leverkusen Amputation Reduction Study (LARS).** *Diabetes Care* 2007, **30**:2633–7.

23. Krishnan S, Nash F, Baker N, Fowler D, Rayman G: **Reduction in diabetic amputations over 11 years in a defined U.K. population: benefits of multidisciplinary team work and continuous prospective audit.** *Diabetes Care* 2008, **31**:99–101.

24. Chaytor ER: **Surgical treatment of the diabetic foot.** *Diabetes Metab Res Rev* 2000, **16**(Suppl 1):S66–9.

25. Lavery LA, Peters EJ, Armstrong DG, Wendel CS, Murdoch DP, Lipsky BA: **Risk factors for developing osteomyelitis in patients with diabetic foot wounds.** *Diabetes Res Clin Pract* 2009, **83**:347–52.

26. Goven MF, Karibiber A, Kaynak G, Oyet T: **Conservative and surgical treatment of the chronic Charcot foot and ankle.** *Diabetic Foot Ankle* 2013, In press.

27. Bridges RM Jr, Deitch EA: **Diabetic foot infections. Pathophysiology and treatment.** *Surg Clin North Am* 1994, **7**(4):537–55.

28. Prompers L, Schaper N, Apelqvist J, Edmonds F, Jude E, Mauricio D, Uccoli L, Urbanci V, Bakker K, Holstein B, Jirkovska A, Piaggesi A, Jirkovska A, Ragnaeson-Tennrall G, Reike H, Spraul M, VanAcker K, Van Baal J, Van Merode F, Ferriera I, Huijbets M: **Prediction of outcome in individuals with diabetic foot ulcers: focus on the differences between individuals with and without peripheral arterial disease. The EURODIALE Study.** *Diabetologia* 2008, **51**:747–55.

29. Cheo JJ, Tan SB, Sivathasan C, Pavanni R, Tan SK: **Vascular assessment in the neuropathic diabetic foot.** *Cln Orthop Relat Res* 1995, **320**:95–100.

30. Piaggesi A, Schipani E, Campi F, Romanelli M, Baccetti F, Arvia C, Navalesi R: **Conservative surgical approach versus non-surgical management for diabetic neuropathic foot ulcers: a randomized trial.** *Diabet Med* 1998, **15**:412–7.

31. Shogalefard A, Khorgami Z, Mologen-Tehrain MR, Langam B: **Large and deep diabetic heel ulcers need not lead to amputation.** *Foot Ankle Int* 2013, **34**:215–21.

32. Lipsky BA, Sheehan P, Armstrong DG, Tice AD, Polis AB, Abramson MA: **Clinical predictors of treatment failure for diabetic foot infections: data from a prospective trial.** *Int Wound J* 2007, **4**:30–8.

33. Vermeulen H, Ubbink D, Goossens A, de Vos R, Legemate D: **Dressings and topical agents for surgical wounds healing by secondary intention.** *Cochrane Database Syst Rev* 2004, **2**:CD003554.

34. Weledji EP, Kamga HLF, Assob JC, Nsagha DS: **A critical review of HIV/AIDS and wound care.** *Afr J Cln Exper Microbiol* 2012, **13**(2):66–73.

35. Nelson EA, O'Meara S, Golder S, Dalton J, Craig D, Iglesias C, DASIDU Steering Group: **Systematic review of antimicrobial treatments for diabetic foot ulcers.** *Diabetic Med* 2006, **23**(4):348–359.

36. Storm-Versloot MN, Vos CG, Ubbink DT, Vermeulen H: **Topical silver for preventing wound infection. Cochrane database.** *Syst Rev* 2010, **17**(3):CD066478.

37. Madhok BM, Vowden K, Vowden P: **New techniques for wound debridement.** *Int Wound J* 2013, **10**(3):247–51.

38. Nian- Feng S, Ai-Ling T, Yu-Ling T, San-yuan H, Li X: **The interventional therapy for diabetic peripheral artery disease.** *BMC Surg* 2013, **13**:32.

39. Stone PA, Back MR, Armstrong PA, Flaherty SK, Keeling WB, Johnson BL, Shames ML, Bandyk DF: **Midfoot amputations expand limb salvage rates for diabetic foot infections.** *Ann Vasc Surg* 2005, **19**(6):805–11.

40. Giummarra MJ, Gibson SJ, Georgion-Karistinis N, Bridshaw JC: **Central mechanisms in phantom limb perception: the past, present and furure.** *Brain Res Rev* 2007, **54**:219–23.

41. Ramachandran VS, Hirstein W: **The perception of phantom limbs. 'The D.O.Hebb Lecture".** *Brain: J Neurol* 1998, **121**(9):1603–1630.

42. Wrobel JS, Robbins J, Armstrong DG: **The high-low amputation ratio: a deeper insight into diabetic foot care.** *J Foot Ankle Surg* 2006, **45**:375–9.

9

Randomized control trial to evaluate the effects of acute testosterone administration in men on muscle mass, strength, and physical function following ACL reconstructive surgery: rationale, design, methods

Brian W Wu[1,2]*, Max Berger[1], Jonathan C Sum[2], George F Hatch III[1] and E Todd Schroeder[1,2]

Abstract

Background: The anterior cruciate ligament (ACL) is one of four major ligaments in the knee that provide stability during physical activity. A tear in the ACL is characterized by joint instability that leads to decreased activity, knee dysfunction, reduced quality of life and a loss of muscle mass and strength. While rehabilitation is the standard-of-care for return to daily function, additional surgical reconstruction can provide individuals with an opportunity to return to sports and strenuous physical activity. Over 200,000 ACL reconstructions are performed in the United States each year, and rehabilitation following surgery is slow and expensive. One possible method to improve the recovery process is the use of intramuscular testosterone, which has been shown to increase muscle mass and strength independent of exercise. With short-term use of supraphysiologic doses of testosterone, we hope to reduce loss of muscle mass and strength and minimize loss of physical function following ACL reconstruction compared to standard-of-care alone.

Methods/design: This study is a double-blinded randomized control trial. Men 18–50 years of age, scheduled for ACL reconstruction are randomized into two groups. Participants randomized to the testosterone group receive intramuscular testosterone administration once per week for 8 weeks starting 2 weeks prior to surgery. Participants randomized to the control group receive a saline placebo intramuscularly instead of testosterone. Lean mass, muscle strength and physical function are measured at 5 time points: 2 weeks pre-surgery, 1 day pre-surgery, and 6, 12, 24 weeks post-surgery. Both groups follow standard-of-care rehabilitation protocol.

Discussion: We believe that testosterone therapy will help reduce the loss of muscle mass and strength experienced after ACL injury and reconstruction. Hopefully this will provide a way to shorten the rehabilitation necessary following ACL reconstruction. If successful, testosterone therapy may also be used for other injuries involving trauma and muscle atrophy.

Trial registration: NCT01595581, Registration: May 8, 2012

Keywords: Anterior cruciate ligament, Rehabilitation, Testosterone, Orthopedic surgery

* Correspondence: brianwlwu@gmail.com
[1]Keck School of Medicine, University of Southern California, Los Angeles, CA, USA
[2]Biokinesiology and Physical Therapy, University of Southern California, Los Angeles, CA, USA

Background

The anterior cruciate ligament is one of four major ligaments in the knee and provides stability during physical activity. A tear in the ligament is characterized by joint instability that leads to decreased activity, knee dysfunction, and reduced quality of life [1]. The initial knee injury is associated with rapid loss of muscle mass and strength, which can be regained with structured rehabilitation [1]. While rehabilitation is the standard-of-care for return to daily function, additional surgical reconstruction can provide individuals with an opportunity to return to sports and strenuous physical activity [2]. However, surgery will initially add more trauma to the knee and prolong rehabilitation. Together, these components can lead to a slow and expensive recovery [3]. Because there are at least 200,000 anterior cruciate ligament (ACL) reconstructions performed each year in the United States [1], it will be beneficial to improve the recovery process. One possible method may be the use of intramuscular testosterone, which has been shown to increase muscle mass and strength independent of exercise [4,5]. Inducing an anabolic environment with a short course of testosterone may be an efficient method to improve recovery.

Muscle mass is dependent on the ratio of muscle protein synthesis (anabolism) to muscle protein breakdown (catabolism). Trauma from surgery and limited movement of the knee result in atrophy and breakdown due to a catabolic state and reduced anabolism of skeletal muscle proteins. Furthermore, ACL injuries can result in weeks of immobilization of the knee, and animal studies have shown that anabolism decreases after as few as 6 hours of cast immobilization [6]. The combination of surgery, the initial knee injury, and the associated limited movement contribute to the delayed and intensive rehabilitative process.

Testosterone increases myofibrillar protein synthesis and promotes anabolism of muscle tissue. It also modulates the activity of immune, fibroblast, and myogenic precursor cells, which are all involved in muscle regeneration. Furthermore, testosterone administration increases lean tissue and maximal voluntary strength in a dose-dependent manner [5]. Animal models have shown that exogenous testosterone aids in muscle regeneration following several types of injury, such as crush injuries, venom-induced muscle injury, muscle disuse atrophy, and injury following muscle graft surgery [7]. With testosterone, successful regeneration of healthy mouse muscle can occur within 2–3 weeks of injury where muscle strength can return to pre-injured values [7].

Testosterone may also induce muscle growth via growth hormone (GH) and insulin-like growth factor 1 (IGF-1) [7,8]. IGF-1 can stimulate muscle protein synthesis and satellite cell activity and anabolic steroids increase both circulating IGF-1 and muscle mRNA expression of *IGF-1*. Akt (protein kinase B) is a signaling mediator of IGF-1

that can regulate muscle mass. However, it is also known that testosterone can work outside of the Akt signaling pathway in order to maintain skeletal muscle hypertrophy [7,9]. We are studying key regulatory proteins such as Akt1, mTOR, and FOXO3a, which have not been studied in concurrent states of muscle trauma and testosterone administration.

There is evidence that the Akt pathway regulates gene transcription through the inactivation of a group of transcription factors (FOXOs) located in the nucleus [10,11]. FOXO3a increases the transcription of atrophy related genes (atrogens), decreases protein degradation, and results in muscle atrophy. Phosphorylation of FOXO3a by phosphorylated Akt1 inactivates the transcription factor, releasing it from DNA and resulting in translocation of the inactive FOXO3a to the cytosol [11]. Phosphorylated Akt1 will also activate the mTOR pathway to stimulate protein synthesis and result in hypertrophy [11]. Therefore, the Akt pathway may regulate both skeletal muscle protein synthesis and degradation by different but complimentary mechanisms in response to testosterone (Figure 1). By analyzing muscle tissue following an ACL rupture with or without testosterone administration, we can learn more about the mechanism through which muscle adapts to trauma and how testosterone affects this process. Therefore, we may learn more about testosterone's mechanism of action in skeletal muscle during the catabolic stimulus of bedrest and surgery.

In addition to understanding the possible mechanisms of testosterone, there may be improved recovery time as measured by questionnaires and function tests. In a study using the Tegner Activity Scale [12], a questionnaire developed to describe a patient's physical activity, 60% of participants who received ACL reconstruction did not return to pre-injury activity level within 2 years [1]. In another study where supraphysiologic doses of testosterone were given to older men undergoing knee replacement, the physical function as measured by the Functional Independence Measure ability to stand was significantly higher by 30% in patients who received testosterone. Similarly, we hope to improve recovery following ACL reconstruction using supraphysiologic doses of testosterone. Specifically, we hope to reduce the loss of muscle mass and strength and minimize loss of physical function. Should acute testosterone improve rehabilitation following ACL surgery, it may be possible to apply the same concept to other injuries that involve muscle atrophy.

Objectives

The overall objective of this study is to determine if 8 weeks of testosterone first administered 2 weeks prior to surgery, can improve the outcome of ACL reconstruction. Specifically, we will evaluate the effect of testosterone administration on lean muscle mass and strength, physical

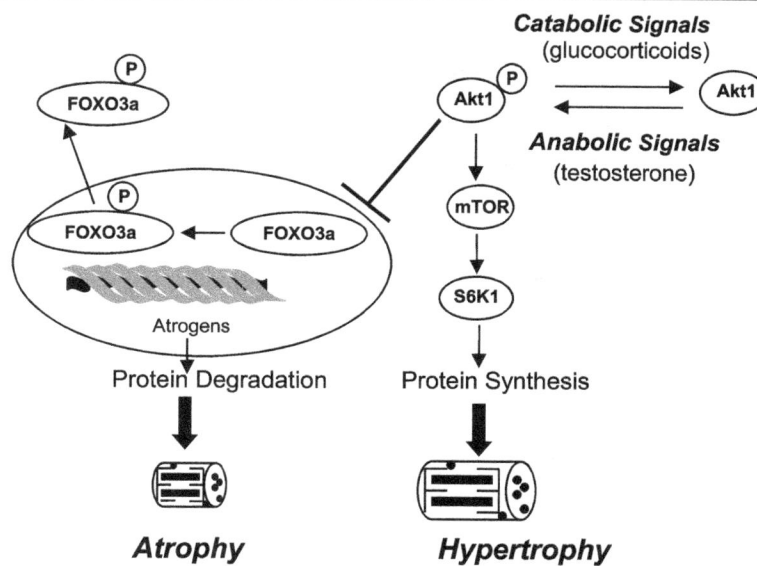

Figure 1 Akt1 signaling and control of skeletal muscle hypertrophy and atrophy. Anabolic signals (e.g. testosterone) initiate phosphorylation (P) of Akt1, which activates protein synthesis via the mTOR pathway. At the same time, Akt1(P) inactivates FOXO3a by phosphorylation and facilitates translocation of FOXO3a out of the nucleus, resulting in inhibition of the atrophy-related genes (atrogens), and thereby decreasing protein degradation. On the other hand, catabolic stimuli (e.g. glucocorticoids) dephosphorylate and thereby inactivate the Akt1 protein. Inactivation of the Akt1 protein allows expression of *FOXO3a* in the nucleus and subsequent activation of the atrogens, resulting in protein degradation. (Figure adapted from G.A. Nader) [10].

function, clinical outcomes, and skeletal muscle myogenic regulators following ACL reconstructive surgery. We hypothesize that testosterone will minimize the reductions or potentially increase muscle mass and strength following surgery and may hasten a patient's return to physical activity. If testosterone improves recovery after ACL surgery, the same treatment may be used for other injuries that involve trauma and muscle atrophy. Furthermore, this study will examine the effect of trauma with or without testosterone on myogenic regulators in muscle tissue taken during ACL surgery—providing possible mechanistic insights for the clinical outcomes.

Methods
Study design
Men, 18–50 years of age, scheduled for ACL reconstructive surgery will be randomized to one of two groups. Although most ACL tears occur in women [2], this study will be limited to men due to the gender-related side effects of testosterone. According to our power analysis, we aim to have at least 7 patients in each group after recruiting and screening approximately 70 patients. The dosing is based on a previous study using supraphysiological dose of testosterone for knee replacement surgery [13]. Intramuscular testosterone cypionate will be used because it has been more widely studied and is less expensive than the gel or patch forms of testosterone. Group 1 will receive testosterone administration, one weekly 200 mg dose intramuscularly of testosterone in sesame oil, for 8 continuous weeks beginning

2 weeks prior to surgery and standard-of-care rehabilitation following surgery. Group 2 will follow the same dosing and rehabilitation schedule but receive a saline placebo instead of testosterone. The dose will be given intramuscularly to minimize systemic side effects; however, we expect the total systemic levels of testosterone to increase to an average of 1200 ng/dl. Lean mass, muscle strength, and physical function will be measured 2 weeks prior to surgery, 1 day prior to surgery, and 6, 12, and 24 weeks following surgery. By administering the dose 2 weeks prior to surgery, there will be sufficient time to develop an anabolic state before the catabolic stimulus of surgery. The dose will continue for 8 weeks to try to maintain muscle mass when there is limited movement and endogenous anabolic stimulus. After 6 weeks from the surgery, testosterone will no longer be administered because KOOS function and sports score appear to stabilize after this time [1]. The study will be a double-blinded experiment.

Patients will follow a standard rehabilitation protocol [14] customized by an orthopedic physician. Rehabilitation will begin shortly after surgery and will be supervised by a licensed physical therapist. The protocol includes goals for range of motion, muscle function, and functional performance at different post-operative stages. The goals for each stage must be met before patient progresses to the next stage and the amount of exercises will be closely monitored by physical therapists and the graduate student. A quicker progression is expected in patients assigned to standard-of-care rehabilitation with testosterone. If any pain or swelling slows progression, the patient will see the treating clinician.

The study will be conducted at the University of Southern California (USC), Keck School of Medicine in Los Angeles, California and was approved by the Institutional Review Board of the University of California (HS-11-00649).

Selection and randomization of subjects

Male participants, 18–50 years of age, who present to the orthopedic surgeon with recent knee trauma will be screened for eligibility. Eligible patients will have had rotational trauma to a previously uninjured knee within the preceding 8 months, ACL insufficiency as determined by clinical examination (positive pivot shift and/or positive Lachmann test), and a score of 5 to 9 on the Tegner Activity Scale (TAS) [12] before the injury (scores range from 1 to 10, with a score of 5 indicating participation in recreation sports, and a score of 9 indicating participation in competitive sports on a nonprofessional level).

All eligible participants (see Table 1) will receive information about the trial orally and in writing. After signing a written informed consent, they will be randomly assigned to undergo either standard-of-care structured rehabilitation with testosterone administration or standard-of-care structured rehabilitation with placebo. An investigator not involved in the randomization procedure will prepare sequentially numbered, opaque, sealed envelopes containing the assigned interventions to ensure randomness which will then be provided to the research pharmacist. The study is a double blind study. Only the research pharmacist will know which patient is receiving study drug or placebo. The surgeon, PI, study team, and physical therapist will not know which study arm the patient was randomized. The protocol for rehabilitation will remain the same for all patients.

Study agent administration and safety

Although the study involves a very short course of testosterone, it may still have side effects on the endocrine systems; and therefore, common markers of endocrine function are monitored. Blood analysis will be performed at USC. Pituitary hormones (LH and FSH), prostate-specific antigen (PSA), liver enzymes, hematocrit, and blood pressure are measured at two weeks preoperatively, 1 day preoperatively, and 2, 3, 6, 12, and 24 weeks postoperatively.

Orthopedic surgery

Surgery will be performed for all eligible patients within 8 months after the injury by a licensed orthopedic surgeon. Surgery will be performed while the patient is under general anesthesia. Meniscal surgery will be carried out as

Table 1 Inclusion and exclusion criteria

Inclusion criteria	Exclusion criteria
Eligible participants will have had:	• Previous major knee injury or knee surgery
• A complete ACL tear as visualized on MRI	• Associated posterior cruciate ligament (PCL) or medical collateral ligament (MCL) injury grade III
° The ACL injury can be either "isolated" or combined with one or several of the following injuries visualized on MRI and/or arthroscopy:	• Concomitant severe injury to contra-lateral knee
▪ A meniscus tear that is either left untreated or treated with a partial resection	• Injury to the lateral/posterolateral ligament complex with significantly increased laxity
▪ A small, stable meniscus tear treated with fixation, but with the fixation not interfering with the rehabilitation protocol	• Unstable longitudinal meniscus tear that requires repair and where the following postoperative treatment (e.g. bracing and limited range of motion) interferes with the rehabilitation protocol
▪ Cartilage changes verified on MRI with an arthroscopically determined intact surface.	• Bi-compartmental extensive meniscus resections
• A radiographic examination with normal joint status or combined with either one of the following findings:	• Cartilage injury representing a full thickness loss down to bone
° A small-avulsed fragment located laterally, usually described as a Segond fracture, JSN grade 1 or osteophytes grade 1 as determined by the OARSI atlas[15]	• Total rupture of MCL/LCL as visualized on MRI.
	• History of deep vein thrombosis (DVT) or a disorder of the coagulative system
	• Claustrophobia
	• Prior or current use of anabolic steroids
	• General systemic disease affecting physical function
	• Chromosomal disorders
	• Medications that interfere with testosterone production or function, including but not limited to 5α-reductase inhibitors
	• Any other condition or treatment interfering with the completion of the trial

needed, followed by ACL reconstruction. All surgeons have similar success rates for ACL reconstruction.

Rehabilitation

Rehabilitation will follow a standard guideline [16] under the supervision of a licensed physical therapist and the participant's doctor.

Muscle biopsies

During surgery, vastus lateralis muscle tissue will be obtained. The tissue will then be examined by q-PCR for changes in the gene expression of *Akt-1*, *mTOR*, and *FOXO3a* [17-21]. In tissues that have received 2 weeks of testosterone, we expect to see up-regulated expression of *Akt-1* and *mTOR*, and down-regulated expression of *FOXO3a*. Akt-1 phosphorylation will also be detected by western blotting, and should be higher in patients receiving testosterone.

Clinical and laboratory evaluations

The patient will be tested on multiple occasions. All testing takes place at the USC Clinical Exercise Research Center (CERC). Information will be collected 2 weeks prior to surgery, followed by measurements 1 day prior to surgery, and 2, 6, 12, and 24 weeks after surgery. Surgery will be performed on an arranged date with the orthopedic surgeon. Physical therapy will follow a pre-defined protocol with a physical therapist.

Table 2 outlines the timeline used for the study including the dates of each visit and what takes place on each visit.

Drug delivery

Either testosterone or placebo will be injected intramuscularly once per week for 8 weeks, starting 2 weeks prior to surgery and ending 5 weeks post-surgery.

Blood draw

Blood will be collected to monitor any adverse effects on the participant's health.

Body composition testing by bioelectrical impedance

The Biospace InBody 520 [22] device measures body composition as the participant stands on a scale-like device while grasping two handles; one in each hand. The device works by sending a very low-voltage electrical signal through the body to determine water content, body fat percentage, and lean (muscle) mass.

Body composition testing by DXA

We will also measure the participant's lean mass and body fat percentage by whole-body dual-energy x-ray absorptiometry [22-24] (DXA), which is more sensitive to small changes in body composition than bioelectrical impedance. The subject will have DXA scans throughout the study. The DXA works by passing low energy x-rays through the subject's body. The x-ray is absorbed differently by muscle tissue than fat tissue which allows the device to differentiate the amount of lean mass and fat mass in the participant's body.

Physical function tests

At 2 weeks prior to surgery, 1 day prior to surgery, and 6, 12, and 24 weeks after surgery, tests of maximal muscle strength using a Cybex dynamometer [25-27] will be performed on the subject's unaffected and affected leg. In addition, knee stability and flexibility tests of the affected leg are typically performed during rehabilitation. During later stages of rehabilitation, tests may include the single leg squat, single leg hop, X-hop, triple hop, and timed hop tests [19,28-31].

Questionnaires

The subject will be asked to complete the Knee Injury and Osteoarthritis Outcome Score [32,33] (KOOS), a commonly used test to measure progression after ACL reconstruction, and the Tegner Activity Scale [12,34-37] to determine physical activity level.

Statistical data analysis

Descriptive statistics will be performed for participant characteristics as well as baseline testosterone, strength, and body composition. Comparisons across groups will be

Table 2 Study calendar

Timeline	Drug delivery	Blood collection	BC testing	PF testing	Questionnaires
2 weeks prior to surgery	X	X	X	X	X
1 week prior to surgery	X				
1 day prior to surgery	X	X	X	X	X
1 week post-surgery	X				
2 weeks post-surgery	X	X			
3 weeks post-surgery	X				
4 weeks post-surgery	X				
5 weeks post-surgery	X				
6 weeks post-surgery		X	X	X	X
12 weeks post-surgery		X	X	X	X
24 weeks post-surgery		X	X	X	X

BC = Body Composition, PF = Physical function.

made for each measurement (t-test) to determine if bias exists between the randomized groups. If bias does exist, these variables will be included as covariates in the primary analysis. The raw data (pre- and post-test) will be plotted to determine if outliers exist. Because the sample size is small if outliers are found, transformations of the data (e.g. log transformation) will be attempted. If this is not feasible, results will be compared using non-parametric analogs to the parametric tests listed below. Intent to treat analyses for specific hypotheses are listed below. In addition, effect sizes will be computed with Cohen's D to determine the clinical relevance of the results and assist in powering further research. Analyses will be performed using SPSS for all analyses with $\alpha = 0.05$. If there is any missing data, the analyses can be performed with the SPSS multiple imputation procedure.

Intent to treat will be tested by comparing changes in lean mass and strength using ANCOVA models, with group adjusting for baseline values. KOOS and TAS scores will be analyzed by ANCOVA models. Physical function tests scores on the Lachman and pivot shift tests will be analyzed by χ^2 test. The changes in gene expression of *Akt1*, *mTOR*, and *FOXO3a* will be compared by ANCOVA models.

Power analysis

Sample size estimates were computed with Nquery (v4) for $\alpha = 0.05$ and $1\text{-}\beta = 0.80$. Preliminary data was taken from a study that provided 12 weeks of oxandrolone/day in 32 healthy 60–87 year old men [24]. Effects sizes between changes in means from baseline to 12 weeks for lean body mass and maximal voluntary strength were used to estimate the changes in mass and strength for Aim 1. The effect size was 2.0 for mass and 2.03 for strength. For similar effects, a minimum of 6 men would be needed for each group. Assuming a 20% attrition rate [1] and similarly very large effect, our sample of 7 per group should be sufficient to see statistically significant effects.

Discussion

In this study, we are testing the hypothesis that standard-of-care rehabilitation with the addition of supraphysiologic doses of testosterone for 8 weeks will augment muscle mass, strength, and physical function following ACL reconstructive surgery compared to standard rehabilitation alone.

Use of testosterone

Testosterone is the principal male sex hormone and an anabolic steroid. It is essential for healthy males. In men, testosterone plays a key role in the development of male reproductive tissues and promotes secondary sexual characteristics such as increased muscle, bone mass, and

the growth of body hair. In young healthy male subjects similar to those used in our study, supraphysiologic doses of testosterone have been shown to increase fat-free mass, muscle size and strength independent of exercise [4]. This effect was even greater when testosterone was used in conjunction with strength training. Additionally, testosterone likely causes some of its effects, such as muscle strength, in a dose dependent manner [38].

While few studies have used supraphysiologic doses of testosterone, the ideal dosing for adjunctive therapy with ACL surgery is not known. Because our patients will not necessarily be hypogonadal, as is typical for testosterone replacement studies, there is a risk that our dose may not be large enough to have a significant influence on muscle mass and strength. Alternatively, a dose that is too high (>600 mg/wk) [38] or given for long duration (6 months) [39] may have deleterious effects by increasing risk of cardiovascular disease. However, we believe that our chosen dose regimen will be safe and successful as it is based on the current literature and the expertise of our study team [5,13].

The potential detrimental cardiovascular side effects of testosterone have recently been featured in both the literature and the media [40]. However, these studies focus primarily on testosterone replacement therapy for an extended duration and are mainly in hypogonadal men and therefore are not as applicable to our current study. We do not anticipate any negative side effects of the testosterone treatment, but will be monitoring all patients closely for any potential complications.

Study participants

In our study, we will use young healthy males aged 18–50 with recent acute ACL tears. This demographic will be used in an attempt to isolate the effect of testosterone and minimize any confounding factors such as age, comorbidities and sex. Women will not be used in this initial study due to the gender related side effects of testosterone. Additionally, the results showing the ability of supraphysiologic doses of testosterone to augment muscle size and strength were reported for young healthy males [38]. However, we do not believe that the benefits of testosterone on rehabilitation are isolated to this demographic alone. If this study shows significant results, the next step would be to expand our age range and conduct studies with other atrophy-related surgeries such as total knee arthoplasty.

Limitations

Testosterone therapy is currently a controversial topic but previous studies have shown positive results [8,41-48]. It may have been ideal to personalize the supraphysiologic doses according to baseline for each participant. However, for ease of administration and future research viability, we attempted to standardize this value. It may be interesting to note variability of the peak testosterone values and results for those participants. Similarly, there is a large age range of participants and studies have shown differences in testosterone level as early as 40 years of age [44,48-52]. However, additional studies show that the effects in males will still exist with supraphysiologic doses [48,53,54] and we expect an effect to be measured independent of age or race.

Recruitment of participants who meet all inclusion criteria will be challenging. Although we are working with multiple orthopedic surgeons, there are a number of challenges in recruiting patients with ACL injury into randomized clinical trials [55]. It will likely be necessary to recruit and screen approximately 70 participants – 5 times as many potential participants as our power analysis indicates to demonstrate significant differences.

Additionally, while we aim to work with as few physical therapists as possible and are following a standardized protocol, there are differences in the techniques and progression of individual therapists. We intend to monitor progress of individual participants as standardized as possible and to also focus on the 24 week result as the primary outcome time point.

Relevance for investigating the effects of testosterone on rehabilitation

The present study will contribute to the field of rehabilitation following invasive surgery with respect to understanding an innovative approach towards treating injury induced muscle atrophy. By examining the effects of testosterone following surgery as an adjunct therapy, we can observe the effects on multiple translational levels including clinical outcomes, quality of life, and mechanisms. The results of the study will help provide the framework for additional large scale and multi-centered investigations to optimize rehabilitation in surgeries that affect many persons and injuries.

Because many patients do not return to pre-surgical levels of activity and strength [1,29,56], continued research is necessary to study muscle atrophy, a critical component of this poor return. Furthermore, these effects are often compounded in elite athletes [28,57] and although this present study does not focus on these patients, they are a crucial group that may benefit from such research. Ideally, such methods for targeting muscle atrophy should be applicable across gender, age, and injury type. Future and vigorous research will be required to test such hypotheses, as testosterone levels play a critical role in overall health.

Testosterone has never been studied in the age range of our patients for therapy following injuries associated with muscle atrophy. We believe that testosterone will improve the outcome of ACL reconstruction and augment muscle mass, strength, and physical function compared to standard-of-care alone. If our study demonstrates that acute testosterone improves rehabilitation following ACL

reconstruction, it may be possible to apply the same concept to other injuries that involve muscle atrophy. With almost every orthopedic injury and accompanying surgery, there is a disuse muscle atrophy that occurs that will ultimately lengthen the period of rehabilitation needed to get back to full strength [6]. We believe that testosterone therapy will help prevent this loss of muscle mass and can shorten the length of rehabilitation needed in these patients. In addition, by analyzing muscle tissue following an ACL rupture with or without testosterone administration, we can learn more about the mechanism through which muscle adapts to trauma and how testosterone affects this process. Therefore, we may learn more about testosterone's mechanism of action in skeletal muscle during the catabolic stimulus of bedrest and surgery.

A unique aspect of our proposed adjunct therapy to ACL reconstruction is its clinical feasibility. Testosterone therapy is easily added to the standard-of-care rehabilitation with little additional time or effort required by the patient. The testosterone injections can be administered at routine preoperative and postoperative visits, with few extra office visits necessary. This would allow many additional patients to have access to the therapy regardless of time constraints.

Conclusion

This study will contribute to the understanding of skeletal muscle adaptations to trauma and surgery, and how testosterone can affect this process. We believe that testosterone will augment muscle mass and improve rehabilitation times following ACL reconstructive surgery and quality of life for patients with this injury. In the future, we hope that the principles of testosterone therapy following injury and disuse atrophy can be expanded to a larger cohort of patients and a more diverse range of injuries and surgeries. The results from this study will allow for larger scale studies investigating the optimization of testosterone therapy in rehabilitation for various types of injuries.

Abbreviations
ACL: Anterior cruciate ligament; GH: Growth hormone; IGF-1: Insulin-like growth factor 1; KOOS: Knee Injury and Osteoarthritis Outcome Score; TAS: Tegner Activity Score; PCL: Posterior cruciate ligament; MCL: Medial collateral ligament; LH: Luteinizing hormone; FSH: Follicle stimulating hormone; PSA: Prostate specific antigen; CERM: USC Clinical Exercise Research Center; BC: Body composition; PF: Physical function; DXA: Dual Energy X-ray Absorptiometry; SPSS: Statistical Package for the Social Sciences; ANCOVA: Analysis of covariance.

Competing interests
The authors declare that they have no competing interests.

Authors' contributions
BW, JS, RH, TS provided conception, design, trial protocol and initiation of the project; BW is the study coordinator, providing supervision of physical function testing and specimen collection; MB and BW patient recruitment, data collection and entry, drafted and finalized the manuscript. All authors have read and approved the final manuscript.

Authors' information
BW, JS, RH, TS provided conception, design, trial protocol and initiation of the project; BW is the study coordinator, providing supervision of physical function testing and specimen collection; MB and BW patient recruitment, data collection and entry, drafted and finalized the manuscript. All authors have read and approved the final manuscript.

Acknowledgements
We would like to thank the USC Intradepartmental Award for Interdisciplinary Work, Division of Biokinesiology and Physical Therapy, Southern California Clinical and Translational Science Institute (SC CTSI) Funding Program and American Orthopaedic Soc. for Sports Medicine (AOSSM) Sandy Kirkley Clinical Outcome Research Grant for funding of this project. We would also like to thank the administration and clinical staff that aided in the project.

References
1. Frobell RB, Roos EM, Roos HP, Ranstam J, Lohmander LS: A randomized trial of treatment for acute anterior cruciate ligament tears. N Engl J Med 2010, 363(4):331–342.
2. Spindler KP, Wright RW: Anterior Cruciate Ligament Tear. N Eng J Med 2008, 359(20):2135–2142.
3. Arangio GA, Chen C, Kalady M, Reed JF 3rd: Thigh muscle size and strength after anterior cruciate ligament reconstruction and rehabilitation. J Orthop Sports Phys Ther 1997, 26(5):238–243.
4. Bhasin S, Storer TW, Berman N, Callegari C, Clevenger B, Phillips J, Bunnell TJ, Tricker R, Shirazi A, Casaburi R: The effects of supraphysiologic doses of testosterone on muscle size and strength in normal men. N Engl J Med 1996, 335(1):1–7.
5. Schroeder ET, Terk M, Sattler FR: Androgen therapy improves muscle mass and strength but not muscle quality: results from two studies. Am J Physiol Endocrinol Metab 2003, 285(1):E16–E24.
6. Marimuthu K, Murton AJ, Greenhaff PL: Mechanisms regulating muscle mass during disuse atrophy and rehabilitation in humans. J Appl Physiol (Bethesda, Md : 1985) 2011, 110(2):555–560.
7. White JP, Baltgalvis K, Sato S, Wilson LB, Carson JA: Effect of nandrolone decanoate administration on recovery from bupivacaine-induced muscle injury. J Appl Physiol (Bethesda, Md: 1985) 2009, 107(5):1420–1430.
8. Serra C, Bhasin S, Tangherlini F, Barton ER, Ganno M, Zhang A, Shansky J, Vandenburgh HH, Travison TG, Jasuja R, Morris C: The role of GH and IGF-I in mediating anabolic effects of testosterone on androgen-responsive muscle. Endocrinology 2011, 152(1):193–206.
9. Hourdé C, Jagerschmidt C, Clément-Lacroix P, Vignaud A, Ammann P, Butler-Browne GS, Ferry A: Androgen replacement therapy improves function in male rat muscles independently of hypertrophy and activation of the Akt/mTOR pathway. Acta Physiologica (Oxford, England) 2009, 195(4):471–482.
10. Nader GA: Molecular determinants of skeletal muscle mass: getting the "AKT" together. Int J Biochem Cell Biol 2005, 37(10):1985–1996.
11. Sandri M, Sandri C, Gilbert A, Skurk C, Calabria E, Picard A, Walsh K, Schiaffino S, Lecker SH, Goldberg AL: Foxo transcription factors induce the atrophy-related ubiquitin ligase atrogin-1 and cause skeletal muscle atrophy. Cell 2004, 117(3):399–412.
12. Tegner Y, Lysholm J: Rating systems in the evaluation of knee ligament injuries. Clin Orthop Relat Res 1985, 198:43–49.
13. Amory JK, Chansky HA, Chansky KL, Camuso MR, Hoey CT, Anawalt BD, Matsumoto AM, Bremner WJ: Preoperative supraphysiological testosterone in older men undergoing knee replacement surgery. J Am Geriatr Soc 2002, 50(10):1698–1701.
14. Oiestad BE, Engebretsen L, Storheim K, Risberg MA: Knee osteoarthritis after anterior cruciate ligament injury: a systematic review. Am J Sports Med 2009, 37(7):1434–1443.
15. Hochberg MC, Altman RD, Brandt KD, Clark BM, Dieppe PA, Griffin MR, Moskowitz RW, Schnitzer TJ: Guidelines for the medical management of osteoarthritis. Part I Osteoarthritis of the hip American College of Rheumatology. Arthritis Rheum 1995, 38(11):1535–1540.
16. Wilk KE, Macrina LC, Cain EL, Dugas JR, Andrews JR: Recent advances in the rehabilitation of anterior cruciate ligament injuries. J Orthop Sports Phys Ther 2012, 42(3):153–171.
17. Jorge MLMP, de Oliveira VN, Resende NM, Paraiso LF, Calixto A, Diniz ALD, Resende ES, Ropelle ER, Carvalheira JB, Espindola FS, Jorge PT, Geloneze B: The effects of aerobic, resistance, and combined exercise on metabolic control, inflammatory markers, adipocytokines, and muscle insulin signaling in patients with type 2 diabetes mellitus. Metab Clin Exp 2011, 1–9.
18. Wolsk E, Mygind H, Grøndahl TS, Pedersen BK, van Hall G: IL-6 selectively stimulates fat metabolism in human skeletal muscle. Am J Physiol Endocrinol Metab 2010, 299(5):E832–E840.
19. Barker T, Leonard SW, Hansen J, Trawick RH, Ingram R, Burdett G, Lebold KM, Walker JA, Traber MG: Vitamin E and C supplementation does not ameliorate muscle dysfunction after anterior cruciate ligament surgery. Free Radic Biol Med 2009, 47(11):1611–1618.
20. Wilborn CD, Taylor LW, Greenwood M, Kreider RB, Willoughby DS: Effects of different intensities of resistance exercise on regulators of myogenesis. J Strength Cond Res 2009, 23(8):2179–2187.
21. Chen YW, Zhao P, Borup R, Hoffman EP: Expression profiling in the muscular dystrophies: identification of novel aspects of molecular pathophysiology. J Cell Biol 2000, 151(6):1321–1336.
22. Jensky-Squires NE, Dieli-Conwright CM, Rossuello A, Erceg DN, McCauley S, Schroeder ET: Validity and reliability of body composition analysers in children and adults. Br J Nutr 2008, 100(4):859–865.
23. Schroeder ET, He J, Yarasheski KE, Binder EF, Castaneda-Sceppa C, Bhasin S, Dieli-Conwright CM, Kawakubo M, Roubenoff R, Azen SP, Sattler FR: Value of measuring muscle performance to assess changes in lean mass with testosterone and growth hormone supplementation. Eur J Appl Physiol 2011, 112(3):1123–1131.
24. Schroeder ET, Zheng L, Yarasheski KE, Qian D, Stewart Y, Flores C, Martinez C, Terk M, Sattler FR: Treatment with oxandrolone and the durability of effects in older men. J Appl Physiol 2004, 96(3):1055–1062.
25. Brown K, Swank AM, Quesada PM, Nyland J, Malkani A, Topp R: Prehabilitation versus usual care before total knee arthroplasty: A case report comparing outcomes within the same individual. Physiother Theory Pract 2010, 26(6):399–407.
26. Meier WA, Marcus RL, Dibble LE, Foreman KB, Peters CL, Mizner RL, LaStayo PC: The long-term contribution of muscle activation and muscle size to quadriceps weakness following total knee arthroplasty. J Geriatr Phys Ther 2009, 32(2):79–82.
27. Heijne A, Werner S: Early versus late start of open kinetic chain quadriceps exercises after ACL reconstruction with patellar tendon or hamstring grafts: a prospective randomized outcome study. Knee Surg, Sports Traumatol, Arthroscopy : Off J ESSKA 2007, 15(4):402–414.
28. Myer GD: Utilization of Modified NFL Combine Testing to Identify Functional Deficits in Athletes Following ACL Reconstruction. J Orthopaedic Sports Physical Therapy 2011.
29. Cimino F, Volk BS, Setter D: Anterior cruciate ligament injury: diagnosis, management, and prevention. Am Fam Physician 2010, 82(8):917–922.
30. Hohmann E, Tetsworth K, Hohmann S, Bryant AL: Anabolic steroids after total knee arthroplasty. A double blinded prospective pilot study. J Orthop Surg Res 2010, 5:93.
31. Samuelsson K, Andersson D, Karlsson J: Treatment of anterior cruciate ligament injuries with special reference to graft type and surgical technique: an assessment of randomized controlled trials. Arthroscopy: J Arthrosc Relat Surg: Off Publ Arthrosc Assoc N Am Int Arthrosc Assoc 2009, 25(10):1139–1174.
32. Hambly K, Griva K: IKDC or KOOS: which one captures symptoms and disabilities most important to patients who have undergone initial anterior cruciate ligament reconstruction? Am J Sports Med 2010, 38(7):1395–1404.
33. Roos EM, Roos HP, Lohmander LS, Ekdahl C, Beynnon BD: Knee Injury and Osteoarthritis Outcome Score (KOOS)–development of a self-administered outcome measure. J Orthop Sports Phys Ther 1998, 28(2):88–96.
34. Lind M, Menhert F, Pedersen AB: The first results from the Danish ACL reconstruction registry: epidemiologic and 2 year follow-up results from 5,818 knee ligament reconstructions. Knee Surg Sports Traumatol Arthrosc 2009, 17(2):117–124.
35. Kessler MA, Behrend H, Henz S, Stutz G, Rukavina A, Kuster MS: Function, osteoarthritis and activity after ACL-rupture: 11 years follow-up results of conservative versus reconstructive treatment. Knee Surg Sports Traumatol Arthrosc 2008, 16(5):442–448.

Randomized control trial to evaluate the effects of acute testosterone administration in men on muscle...

63

36. Maletis GB, Cameron SL, Tengan JJ, Burchette RJ: A prospective randomized study of anterior cruciate ligament reconstruction: a comparison of patellar tendon and quadruple-strand semitendinosus/gracilis tendons fixed with bioabsorbable interference screws. *Am J Sports Med* 2007, 35(3):384–394.

37. Spindler KP, Kuhn JE, Freedman KB, Matthews CE, Dittus RS, Harrell FE Jr: Anterior cruciate ligament reconstruction autograft choice: bone-tendon-bone versus hamstring: does it really matter? A systematic review. *Am J Sports Med* 2004, 32(8):1986–1995.

38. Bhasin S, Woodhouse L, Casaburi R, Singh AB, Bhasin D, Berman N, Chen X, Yarasheski KE, Magliano L, Dzekov C, Dzekov J, Bross R, Phillips J, Sinha-Hikim I, Shen R, Storer TW: Testosterone dose–response relationships in healthy young men. *Am J Physiol Endocrinol Metab* 2001, 281(6):E1172–E1181.

39. Basaria S, Coviello AD, Travison TG, Storer TW, Farwell WR, Jette AM, Eder R, Tennstedt S, Ulloor J, Zhang A, Choong K, Lakshman KM, Mazer NA, Miciek R, Krasnoff J, Elmi A, Knapp PE, Brooks B, Appleman E, Aggarwal S, Bhasin G, Hede-Brierley L, Bhatia A, Collins L, LeBrasseur N, Fiore LD, Bhasin S: Adverse events associated with testosterone administration. *N Engl J Med* 2010, 363(2):109–122.

40. Finkle WD, Greenland S, Ridgeway GK, Adams JL, Frasco MA, Cook MB, Fraumeni JF Jr, Hoover RN: Increased risk of non-fatal myocardial infarction following testosterone therapy prescription in men. *PLoS One* 2014, 9(1):e85805.

41. Fu R, Liu J, Fan J, Li R, Li D, Yin J, Cui S: Novel evidence that testosterone promotes cell proliferation and differentiation via G protein-coupled receptors in the rat L6 skeletal muscle myoblast cell line. *J Cell Physiol* 2010, 2011:1–27.

42. O'Connell MDL, Roberts SA, Srinivas-Shankar U, Tajar A, Connolly MJ, Adams JE, Oldham JA, Wu FCW: Do the effects of testosterone on muscle strength, physical function, body composition, and quality of life persist six months after treatment in intermediate-frail and frail elderly men? *J Clin Endocrinol Metab* 2011, 96(2):454–458.

43. Saad F, Gooren LJ: The role of testosterone in the etiology and treatment of obesity, the metabolic syndrome, and diabetes mellitus type 2. *J Obes* 2011, 2011.

44. Sattler FR, Bhasin S, He J, Yarasheski K, Binder E, Todd Schroeder E, Castaneda-Sceppa C, Kawakubo M, Roubenoff R, Dunn M, Hanh C, Stewart Y, Martinez C, Azen SP: Durability of the Effects of Testosterone and Growth Hormone Supplementation in Older Community Dwelling Men: The HORMA Trial. *Clin Endocrinol* 2011, 103–111.

45. Travison TG, Basaria S, Storer TW, Jette AM, Miciek R, Farwell WR, Choong K, Lakshman K, Mazer NA, Coviello AD, Knapp PE, Ulloor J, Zhang A, Brooks B, Nguyen AH, Eder R, LeBrasseur N, Elmi A, Appleman E, Hede-Brierly L, Bhasin G, Bhatia A, Lazzari A, Davis S, Ni P, Collins L, Bhasin S: Clinical Meaningfulness of the Changes in Muscle Performance and Physical Function Associated With Testosterone Administration in Older Men With Mobility Limitation. *J Gerontol Series A, Biol Sci Med Sci* 2011, 66(10):1090–1099.

46. Wang C, Ilani N, Arver S, McLachlan RI, Soulis T, Watkinson A: Efficacy and safety of the 2% formulation of testosterone topical solution applied to the axillae in androgen-deficient men. *Clin endocrinol* 2011, 75(6):836–843.

47. Bhasin S, Cunningham GR, Hayes FJ, Matsumoto AM, Snyder PJ, Swerdloff RS, Montori VM: Testosterone therapy in men with androgen deficiency syndromes: an Endocrine Society clinical practice guideline. *J Clin Endocrinol Metab* 2010, 95(6):2536–2559.

48. Bhasin S, Woodhouse L, Casaburi R, Singh AB, Mac RP, Lee M, Yarasheski KE, Sinha-Hikim I, Dzekov C, Dzekov J, Magliano L, Storer TW: Older men are as responsive as young men to the anabolic effects of graded doses of testosterone on the skeletal muscle. *J Clin Endocrinol Metab* 2005, 90(2):678–688.

49. Hyde Z, Flicker L, Almeida OP, Hankey GJ, McCaul KA, Chubb SAP, Yeap BB: Low free testosterone predicts frailty in older men: the health in men study. *J Clin Endocrinol Metab* 2010, 95(7):3165–3172.

50. Krasnoff JB, Basaria S, Pencina MJ, Jasuja GK, Vasan RS, Ulloor J, Zhang A, Coviello A, Kelly-Hayes M, D'Agostino RB, Wolf PA, Bhasin S, Murabito JM: Free testosterone levels are associated with mobility limitation and physical performance in community-dwelling men: the Framingham Offspring Study. *J Clin Endocrinol Metab* 2010, 95(6):2790–2799.

51. Srinivas-Shankar U, Roberts SA, Connolly MJ, O'Connell MDL, Adams JE, Oldham JA, Wu FCW: Effects of testosterone on muscle strength, physical function, body composition, and quality of life in intermediate-frail and frail elderly men: a randomized, double-blind, placebo-controlled study. *J Clin Endocrinol Metab* 2010, 95(2):639–650.

52. Sattler FR, Castaneda-Sceppa C, Binder EF, Schroeder ET, Wang Y, Bhasin S, Kawakubo M, Stewart Y, Yarasheski KE, Ulloor J, Colletti P, Roubenof R, Azen SP: Testosterone and growth hormone improve body composition and muscle performance in older men. *J Clin Endocrinol Metab* 2009, 94(6):1991–2001.

53. Auyeung TW, Lee JSW, Kwok T, Leung J, Ohlsson C, Vandenput L, Leung PC, Woo J: Testosterone but not estradiol level is positively related to muscle strength and physical performance independent of muscle mass: a cross-sectional study in 1489 older men. *Eur J Endocrinol/Eur Fed Endocr Soc* 2011, 164(5):811–817.

54. Chen F, Lam R, Shaywitz D, Hendrickson RC, Opiteck GJ, Wishengrad D, Liaw A, Song Q, Stewart AJ, Cummings CE, Beals C, Yarasheshki KE, Reicin A, Ruddy M, Hu X, Yates NA, Menteski J, Herman GA: Evaluation of early biomarkers of muscle anabolic response to testosterone. *J Cachex Sarcopenia Muscle* 2011, 2(1):45–56.

55. Frobell RB, Lohmander LS, Roos EM: The challenge of recruiting patients with anterior cruciate ligament injury of the knee into a randomized clinical trial comparing surgical and non-surgical treatment. *Contemp Clin Trials* 2007, 28(3):295–302.

56. Comins J, Brodersen J, Krogsgaard M: Treatment for acute anterior cruciate ligament tear. *N Engl J Med* 2010, 363(19):1871. author reply 1872–1873.

57. Shah VM, Andrews JR, Fleisig GS, McMichael CS, Lemak LJ: Return to play after anterior cruciate ligament reconstruction in National Football League athletes. *Am J Sports Med* 2010, 38(11):2233–2239.

10

Deltopectoral flap revisited for reconstruction surgery in patients with advanced thyroid cancer

Taro Mikami[1*], Shintaro Kagimoto[1], Yuichiro Yabuki[1], Kazunori Yasumura[1], Toshinori Iwai[2], Jiro Maegawa[1], Nobuyasu Suganuma[3], Shohei Hirakawa[3] and Katsuhiko Masudo[3]

Abstract

Background: We present the cases of 2 patients with invasive thyroid cancer, who underwent reconstructive surgery using a deltopectoral flap. Although the overall rate of extrathyroidal extension in patients with thyroid cancer is quite low, skin invasion is the most common pattern observed. Reconstructive surgery, involving local skin flaps, is required in these patients. The deltopectoral flap relies on the blood supply from intercostal perforators of the internal thoracic artery and usually requires skin grafting to the donor site. The internal thoracic artery is rarely sacrificed in these cases, even in an advanced surgery such as in patients with invasive thyroid cancer.

Case presentation: A 55-year-old man with a distended thyroid gland presented to our hospital. He underwent advanced surgery, including skin excision, because we suspected that his tumor was thyroid cancer. The defect was covered with an ipsilateral deltopectoral flap via transposition of the flap, without skin grafting. In the second case, a 67-year-old woman with thyroid cancer that metastasized to her neck lymph nodes presented to our institution. Although the ipsilateral internal thoracic artery was sacrificed near its origin during tumor resection, the deltopectoral flap was raised in the usual manner without any complications. The skin defect caused by the tumor resection was covered with the flap. The patient had an uneventful clinical course for more than 2 years of follow-up.
These 2 cases show the effectiveness of using the deltopectoral flap as a reconstructive option for patients with thyroid cancer who underwent radical surgery, resulting in a skin defect. The first case shows that this flap does not always require skin grafting to the donor site. To our knowledge, the second case may be the first report of a deltopectoral flap that was safely raised and applied with resection of the bifurcation of the ipsilateral internal thoracic artery.

Conclusions: Although thyroid cancer surgery with surrounding skin excision is a rare procedure, we found that the deltopectoral flap was useful and should be the first choice for patients undergoing reconstructive surgery, whether the bifurcation of the ipsilateral internal thoracic artery is sacrificed.

Keywords: Thyroid cancer, Deltopectoral flap, Reconstruction, Neck dissection, Advanced stage

Background

The incidence of thyroid cancer is relatively low in Japan—13 per 10 million individuals—however, it is of particular interest now because of the recent accidents involving nuclear power plants, including those in Fukushima, not only in this country, but also in other countries [1–3].

Although skin invasion is the most common pattern of extrathyroidal extension in patients with thyroid cancer, the overall rate of invasion is only 4%, even in well-differentiated adenocarcinoma [4]. Therefore, there are only a few reports of reconstruction in advanced thyroid cancer cases.

In the past 10 years, only 2 of approximately 600 cases of thyroid cancer surgery performed at our institution included reconstructive surgery; both cases involved invasion of the skin from the neck. A deltopectoral (DP) flap, a well-known flap used in reconstructive surgery, was applied in both cases using the standard technique. One

* Correspondence: zeong3@mac.com
[1]Department of Plastic and Reconstructive Surgery, Yokohama City University Hospital, 236-0004 Kanazawa-ku, Yokohama city, Kanagawa prefecture, Japan
Full list of author information is available at the end of the article

case provided new information concerning blood flow of the DP flap, and the second one, an example of irregular treatment of the donor site.

Case presentation
Patient 1
A 55-year-old man presented to our hospital with suspected carcinoma of the thyroid gland. The tumor in the center of the neck was large enough for us to suspect that the skin invasion had been present for many years, although the patient had no remarkable symptoms. Based on needle biopsy findings, the tumor was diagnosed as papillary carcinoma. In addition to total thyroidectomy, we planned for an optional skin excision with bilateral neck dissection based on the CT findings (Fig. 1). We originally planned to use a local flap of the neck to cover the skin defect, but the size of the defect was too large and we had to make an extended skin incision (Fig. 2a). A DP flap was designed with substantial undermining to the pectoral region, followed by direct closure of the surgical wound and donor site, using suction drains and without a skin graft (Fig. 2b-d). No adverse events occurred during hospitalization. The patient initially

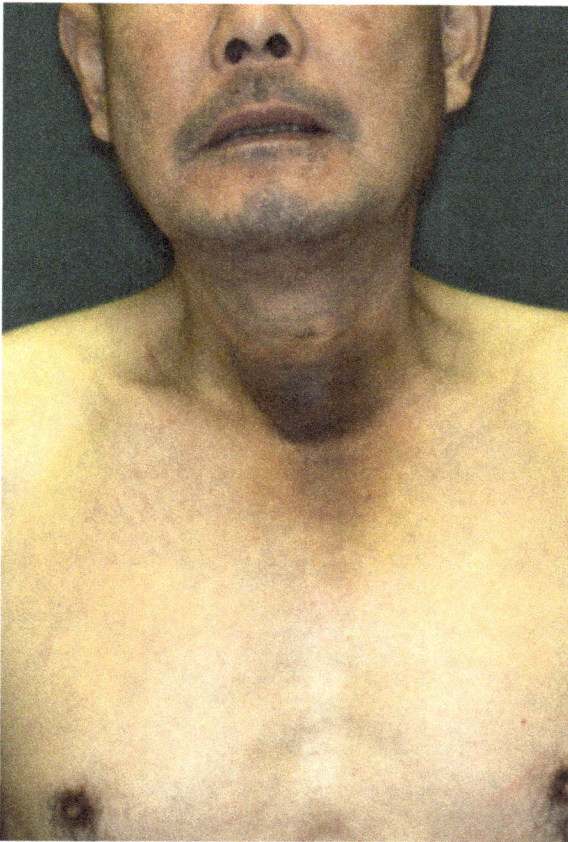

Fig. 1 Preoperative findings of case 1. The lower neck shows obvious swelling. The skin is pigmented, presumably due to inflammation caused by thyroid cancer

declined multiple z-plasty 6 months after the initial surgery to treat the scar contracture around his neck, but later accepted our recommendation (Fig. 3 and Additional file 1: Figure S1).

Patient 2
A 67-year-old woman presented to our hospital with undifferentiated carcinoma of the thyroid gland with local metastasis to neck lymph nodes that was diagnosed based on needle biopsy outside our hospital. The patient presented with no other remarkable symptoms while she had few past medical histories. The tumor size was large enough to raise suspicion of skin involvement during her evaluation at the referring hospital. She was then referred to our hospital due to skin involvement and the need to sacrifice the surrounding large vessels, such as the right common carotid artery and right subclavian artery and vein, during tumor resection and total thyroidectomy (Fig. 4). At first, various flaps such as the DP flap, the pectoralis major myocutaneous flap, the latissimus dorsi flap, and free flaps were considered as candidates for reconstruction of the skin defect. We decided against using a pectoralis major myocutaneous flap because a portion of the right subclavian vein, brachiocephalic vein, and proximal portion of the right internal thoracic artery and vein would have to be sacrificed with dissection of the right neck and paratracheal lymph nodes, while salvaging the right common carotid artery (Fig. 5 a, b). The right DP flap was likely to be excluded as an option before pulsation of the second intercostal perforator artery was confirmed using a Doppler stethoscope. Ultimately, the DP flap was designed and elevated in the usual manner because the 2nd and 3rd intercostal perforator arteries were detected by the Doppler stethoscope. Bleeding from the distal edge of the flap was enough to confirm blood supply of the flap, even after sacrificing the branch of the thoracoacromial artery, and the flap was elevated completely. A portion of the skin on the right side of the neck was undermined and used as a skin flap, followed by setting of the DP flap, which allowed for the airtight closure of the skin defect (Fig. 5 c-e). A portion of the donor site of the DP flap was covered by a meshed skin graft taken from the lower left abdomen. The postoperative clinical course was uneventful to hospital discharge. Because the pathological diagnosis was undifferentiated carcinoma of the thyroid gland, chemoradiotherapy was administered, with no adverse effects. There were no signs of recurrence or metastasis 2 years postoperatively, while the range of motion of the right shoulder improved and no scar contracture developed around the skin graft (Fig. 6, Additional file 2: Figure S2 and Additional file 3: Figure S3).

Discussion and conclusions
In cases of small sized defects in the neck, direct closure or a small local flap is the first choice for reconstruction,

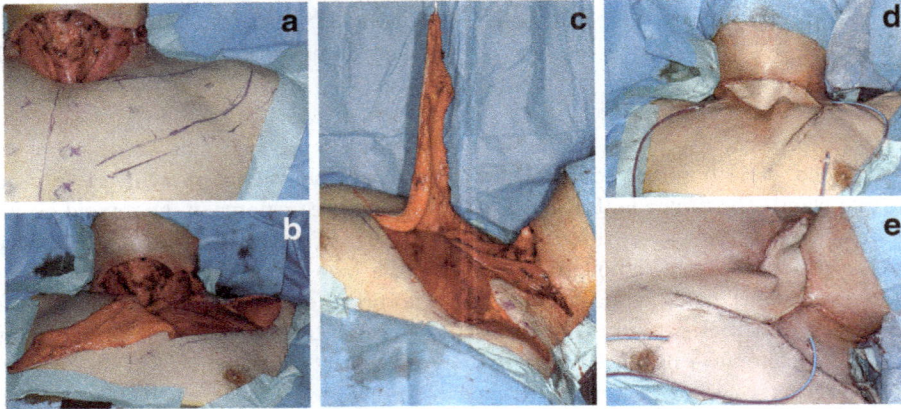

Fig. 2 The DP flap design and dimensions of case 1. **a** The design and landmarks were drawn on the patient's skin, using gentian violet. Previously, the thyroid gland was entirely removed, followed by bilateral neck dissection. The DP flap included the 2nd and 3rd intercostal perforator vessels, as per the usual technique, which was thought to provide adequate blood supply for the flap in this case. **b, c** Dimensions of the flap. As the surface of the pectoralis major and the deltoid muscle can be seen, the DP flap is confirmed as a fascio-cutaneous flap, as is usually found. **d, e** Final patient outcome. The donor site of the flap was closed directly by undermining the wound edges of the incision for left neck dissection. Suction drains were fixed without air leak

because the skin of the neck is thin and has good extensibility. In patients with thyroid cancer and skin invasion, however, the thyroid gland has to be completely resected with some amount of adjacent skin and paratracheal nodes, because the lesion is classified as stage T4, according to the Unio Internationalis Contra Cancrum. In these cases, additional skin incisions are often made that lead to difficulty in design and elevation of local flaps.

The DP flap was first described by Aymard in 1917 as a method for nasal reconstruction [5]. The history of the DP flap is so old that this flap was regarded a useful candidate for head and neck reconstruction in the 1960s; myocutaneous flaps and vascularized flaps have replaced it in recent years [6]. However, the DP flap is the first choice for closure of neck skin defects because it is thin, pliant, and provides a

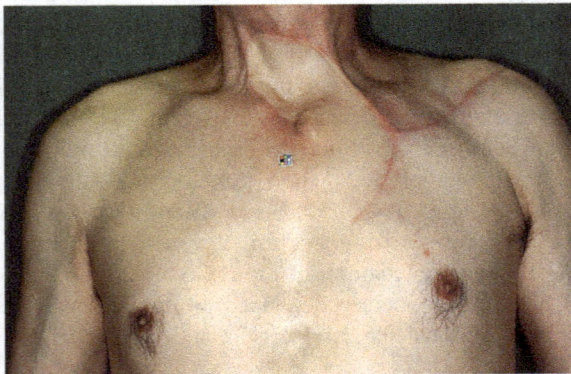

Fig. 3 Local findings of case 1 at postoperative 6 months. There is no obvious deformity, except for upper deviation of the left nipple. A mild scar contracture is observed around the left clavicle, which was revised 15 months after primary surgery by performing multiple z-plasty

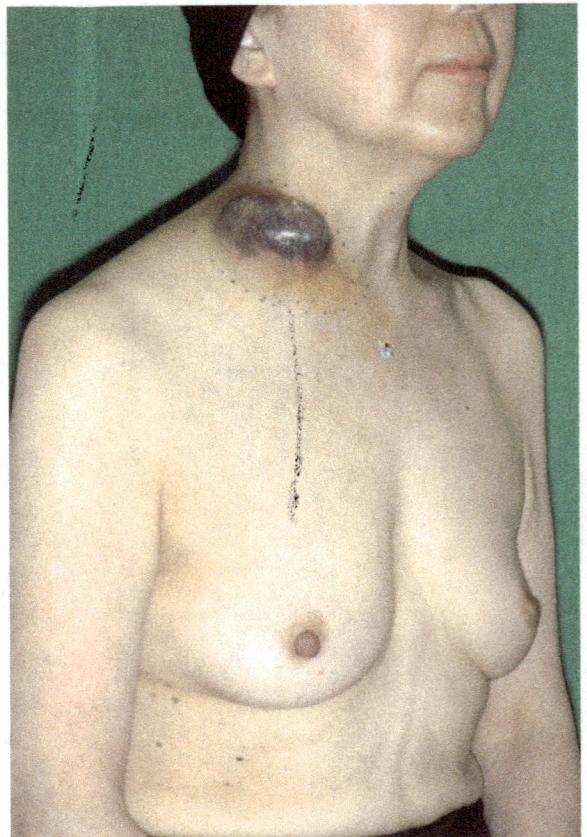

Fig. 4 Preoperative status of case 2. A large tumor was observed in the right neck. The size was approximately 10 × 8 cm, based on the marker on the sternal notch

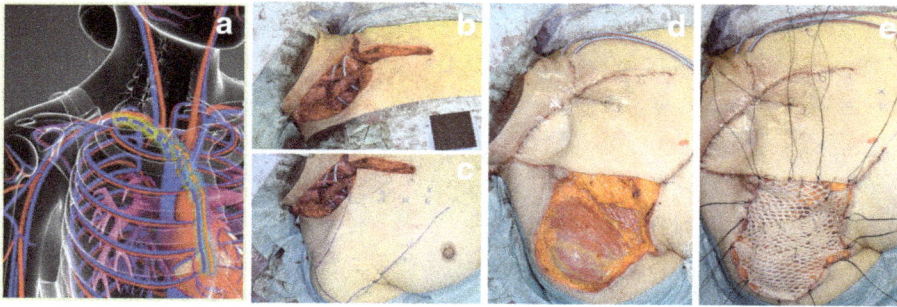

Fig. 5 Intraoperative findings in case 2. **a** The schema shows the arteries and veins of the operative site. The interrupted lines show the sacrificed vessels, including the internal thoracic artery and vein, subclavian vein, and brachiocephalic vein. **b** Right anterior oblique view of the operation. The anterior surface of the trachea can be seen, as the thyroid gland had been entirely removed. The right sternocleidomastoid muscle was reconstructed to cover the arteries and veins of the neck while two suction drains were placed under the muscle. **c** The design of the DP flap was drawn in the usual manner. The distal edge was extended to the mid-lateral line of the shoulder. **d** The deltoid muscle and the pectoralis major muscle are observed after DP flap setting. Airtight conditions were ensured to maintain efficacy of the suction drains. **e** Split thickness skin grafting was performed to the donor site of the DP flap. The skin graft had been processed using a mesh dermatome to fit the uneven surface of the muscle and fatty tissue

color and texture match. Moreover, this flap is easy and safe to raise. Its only disadvantage seems to be the need to process the pedicle 2 or 3 weeks after the primary surgery [7, 8]. Skin grafting to the donor site is usually required, but is not always necessary in few cases, as in case 1 reported here.

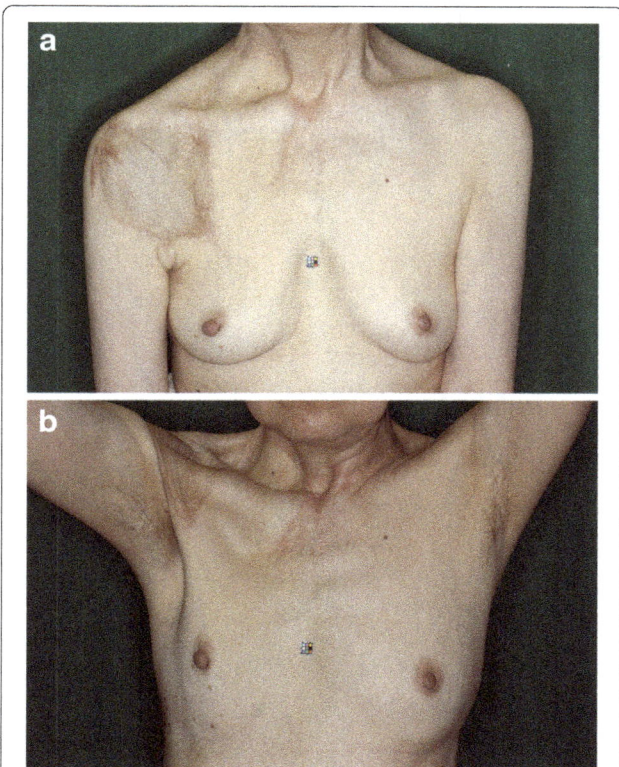

Fig. 6 Outcome of case 2 at postoperative 2 years. **a** The flap and the skin graft fit well with the surrounding skin. No obvious scars were observed. **b** The patient can raise her right arm as well as the left arm. There is no derangement of the right shoulder

In cases of neck skin defects caused by radical surgery for the treatment of patients with thyroid cancers, there is little need to perform pedicle treatment as a secondary surgery if DP flaps are applied. Therefore, the DP flap is considered the first choice in most cases of advanced surgery for thyroid cancer, unless the defect is too large [9].

However, blood supply to the flap needs to be taken into consideration. The blood supply of a DP flap is usually provided primarily by the 2nd, 3rd, and 4th intercostal perforating vessels, which arise from the ipsilateral superior costal artery and internal thoracic artery. The internal thoracic artery provides the anterior intercostal arteries in each intercostal space, which connect to the posterior intercostal arteries, the branches of the thoracic aorta, or the supreme intercostal artery. In cases that require sacrificing the proximal ipsilateral internal thoracic artery, arterial blood flow to the DP flap is provided theoretically via bypass of the thoracic aorta. According to some reports, using this flap is contraindicated when the internal thoracic artery has been previously compromised (Fig. 6) [6]. However, if a bypass vessel can supply sufficient blood flow in a short time, the DP flap can be raised safely in the usual manner, namely without the so-called "delay" technique. Based on the clinical course of case 2, our data support this hypothesis, despite the limited number of similar cases in the literature.

In case of radical surgery for late stage thyroid cancer as in case 2, the usual size of the DP flap can be applied to the skin defect even if the ipsilateral internal thoracic artery is sacrificed at its origin. However, it is necessary to confirm survival of the second intercostal perforator artery, which is regarded as the most important nutrient vessel of the DP flap, by Doppler stethoscope. With extreme caution, it is best to confirm bleeding from the distal edge of the flap even after dividing the flap from the branch of the thoracoacromial artery.

The DP flap is still an important reconstructive tool for neck skin defects and has reliable blood supply even after radical surgery for advanced thyroid cancer and other malignant neoplasms of the neck.

Additional files

> **Additional file 1: Figure S1.** Touch-up surgery for the scar contracture. a: Multiple z-plasty was designed for the scar contracture on the left neck. b: The scar contracture was released after removal of the scar and incisions of the flaps. Each small flap was elevated over the superficial fascia. c: The wound was closed with some trimming of the flap edges. d: Local finding 1 year after multiple z-plasty. The scar contracture was released almost completely although hypertrophic scar was formed again. (ZIP 12226 kb)
>
> **Additional file 2: Figure S2.** Preoperative reconstructed 3D–CT angiography. a: The left anterior oblique view shows the origin of the left internal thoracic artery (ITA) while the right ITA is observed clearly in the picture. b: In the right anterior oblique view, the arising portion of the right ITA can be seen just behind the yellowish shadow of the tumor in the right neck. The right ITA is clearly seen in this view. (ZIP 1109 kb)
>
> **Additional file 3: Figure S3.** Postoperative reconstructed 3D–CT angiography. a: The left ITA is located just in front of the aortic arch in this left anterior oblique view. The disconnected portion of the left subclavian artery is due to artifact from the clavicle. The right ITA is quite shallow compared with the left, whereas the arising portion is difficult to visualize. b: In the right anterior oblique view, the right ITA is totally obscured while the left ITA can be seen clearly. (ZIP 512 kb)

Abbreviations
DP flap: Deltopectoral flap

Acknowledgments
We would like to thank Editage (www.editage.jp) for English language editing.

Funding
There is no funding obtained for this study.

Authors' contributions
TM, KY, TI and NS were involved in data collection, case analysis and writing the manuscript. SK, YY, and JM assisted in drafting the manuscript and reviewed this article. SH, KM, TM and NS performed the surgeries as main operators. All authors read and approved the final manuscript.

Competing interests
The authors declare that they have no competing interests.

Author details
[1]Department of Plastic and Reconstructive Surgery, Yokohama City University Hospital, 236-0004 Kanazawa-ku, Yokohama city, Kanagawa prefecture, Japan. [2]Department of Oral and Maxillofacial Surgery, Yokohama City University Graduate School of Medicine, Yokohama, Japan. [3]Department of General Surgery, Yokohama City University Hospital, Yokohama, Japan.

References
1. Ohira T, Takahashi H, Yasumura S, Ohtsuru A, Midorikawa S, Suzuki S, Fukushima T, Shimura H, Ishikawa T, Sakai A, et al. Comparison of childhood thyroid cancer prevalence among 3 areas based on external radiation dose after the Fukushima Daiichi nuclear power plant accident: the Fukushima health management survey. Medicine (Baltimore). 2016;95(35):e4472.
2. Ojino M, Yoshida S, Nagata T, Ishii M, Akashi M. First successful pre-distribution of stable iodine tablets under Japan's new policy after the Fukushima Daiichi nuclear accident. Disaster Med Public Health Prep. 2016:1–5.
3. Michel LA, Donckier J, Rosiere A, Fervaille C, Lemaire J, Bertrand C. Post-Chernobyl incidence of papillary thyroid cancer among Belgian children less than 15 years of age in April 1986: a 30-year surgical experience. Acta Chir Belg. 2016;116(2):101–13.
4. Cody HS 3rd, Shah JP. Locally invasive, well-differentiated thyroid cancer. 22 years' Experience at Memorial Sloan-Kettering Cancer Center. Am J Surg. 1981;142(4):480–3.
5. Aymard JL. Some new points on the anatomy of the nasal septum, and their surgical significance. J Anat. 1917;51(Pt 3):293–303.
6. Chan RC, Chan JY. Deltopectoral flap in the era of microsurgery. Surg Res Pract. 2014;2014:420892.
7. Lash H, Maser MR, Apfelberg DB. Deltopectoral flap with a segmental dermal pedicle in head and neck reconstruction. Plast Reconstr Surg. 1977;59(2):235–40.
8. Mortensen M, Genden EM. Role of the island deltopectoral flap in contemporary head and neck reconstruction. Ann Otol Rhinol Laryngol. 2006;115(5):361–4.
9. Mebed AH. Aggressive surgical therapy for locally invasive differentiated thyroid carcinoma: an experience of nineteen (19) cases. J Egypt Natl Canc Inst. 2007;19(4):282–91.

11

Combined anterior lumbar interbody fusion and instrumented posterolateral fusion for degenerative lumbar scoliosis: indication and surgical outcomes

Ming-Kai Hsieh, Lih-Huei Chen, Chi-Chien Niu, Tsai-Sheng Fu, Po-Liang Lai and Wen-Jer Chen[*]

Abstract

Background: Traditional approaches to deformity correction of degenerative lumbar scoliosis include anterior-posterior approaches and posterior-only approaches. Most patients are treated with posterior-only approaches because the high complication rate of anterior approach. Our purpose is to compare and assess outcomes of combined anterior lumbar interbody fusion and instrumented posterolateral fusion with posterior alone approach for degenerative lumbar scoliosis with spinal stenosis.

Methods: Between November 2002 and November 2011, a total of 110 patients with degenerative spinal deformity and curves measuring over 30°were included. Of the 110 patients who underwent surgery, 56 underwent the combined anterior and posterior approach and 54 underwent posterior surgery at our institution. The following were the indications of anterior lumbar interbody fusion: (1) rigid or frank lumbar kyphosis, (2) anterior or lateral bridged traction osteophytes, (3) gross coronal and sagittal deformity or imbalance, and (4) severe disc space narrowing that is not identifiable when performing posterior or transforaminal lumbar interbody fusion. The clinical outcomes were evaluated using the Oswestry disability index and the visual analog scale. The status of fusion were assessed according to the radiographic findings.

Results: All patients received clinical and radiographic follow-up for a minimum of 24 months, with an average follow-up of 53 months (range, 26–96 months). At the final follow-up, the mean ODI score improved from 28.8 to 6.4, and the mean back/leg VAS, from 8.2/5.5 to 2.1/0.9 in AP group and the mean ODI score improved from 29.1 to 6.2, and the mean back/leg VAS, from 9.0/6.5 to 2.3/0.5 in P group. The mean scoliotic angle changed from 41.3° preoperatively to 9.3°, and the lumbar lordotic angle, from 3.1° preoperatively to 35.7°in AP group and the mean scoliotic angle from 38.5 to 21.4 and the lumbar lordotic angle from 6 to 15.8 in P group. There were significant differences in sagittal (P = 0.009) and coronal (P = 0.02) plane correction between the two groups.

Conclusions: Our results demonstrate that combined anterior lumbar interbody fusion and instrumented posterolateral fusion for adult degenerative lumbar scoliosis effectively improves sagittal and coronal plane alignment than posterior group and both group were effectively improves clinical scores.

Keywords: Degenerative lumbar scoliosis, De novo scoliosis, Anterior lumbar interbody fusion, Instrumented fusion

* Correspondence: chenwenj@adm.cgmh.org.tw
Department of Orthopedic Surgery, Chang Gung Memorial Hospital and
Chang Gung University, 5, Fu-Hsin Street, Kweishan Shiang, Taoyuan 333,
Taiwan

Background

Degenerative lumbar scoliosis is believed to develop secondary to asymmetric collapse of the intervertebral disc spaces [1-5]. This leads to poor body posture, back pain, and neurological deterioration owing to decreased foraminal height with nerve root compression on the concave side of the deformity, and nerve stretching on the convex side [1,2,6]. The commonly presenting symptoms include chronic back pain and neurogenic claudication caused by concurrent stenosis with a structural degenerative deformity [7]. Traditional approaches to deformity correction of degenerative lumbar scoliosis include anterior-posterior approaches and, more commonly, posterior-only approaches. Most patients are treated with posterior-only approaches because the anterior approach has been shown to be associated with complications such as vascular injury, ileus, and retrograde ejaculation and involves performing 2 large surgical procedures and, hence, increases the operating time [8,9]. The use of posterior decompression with posterior spinal instrumentation and fusion may obviate the need for extensive abdominal surgery by enabling significant correction through a posterior-only approach. However, degenerative lumbar scoliosis secondary to an idiopathic curve tends to become rigid anteriorly, which gets more difficult to be corrected via a posterior-only approach [10]. Combined anterior lumbar interbody fusion and instrumented posterolateral fusion provides several benefits over the posterior-only approach, in terms of improved stability, decreased stress on screws, improved fusion rates, and better lumbar lordosis [11-13]. To our knowledge, no study has yet mentioned the indications of combined anterior lumbar interbody fusion and instrumented posterolateral fusion for degenerative lumbar scoliosis with spinal stenosis and compare and assess outcomes with posterior alone approach.

The goals of adult deformity surgery are to obtain sagittal and coronal balance, symptom relief, and solid fusion [14,15]. Various techniques have been reported for correcting degenerative lumbar deformities with instrumentation and fusion using pedicle screw systems and various types of interbody cages. Interbody cages allow for the correction of the deformity, anterior column support, increased foraminal height, circumferential arthrodesis, and restoration of the anterior column height as well as lumbar lordosis. Interbody cages can be placed via either a posterior approach, as for the posterior lumbar interbody fusion (PLIF) and transforaminal lumbar interbody fusion (TLIF), or an anterior approach, as for the anterior lumbar interbody fusion (ALIF), by using either an autograft or allograft, metal cages, or poly-ether-ether-ketone (PEEK) cages [11,16-18]. Herein, we describe our experience as well as indications for performing combined anterior lumbar interbody fusion and instrumented posterolateral fusion for degenerative lumbar scoliosis with spinal stenosis.

Methods

Patients

From November 2002 to November 2011, 1834 patients with degenerative lumbar scoliosis underwent surgery in our institution. The Chang Gung Medical Foundation Institutional Review Board approved this study (99-0771B) and waived the requirement for informed consent due to the retrospective nature of the study. All patients presented with neurological claudication with mechanical back pain that was refractory to at least 6 months of conservative management such as physical therapy, activity modification, chiropractic manipulation, administration of oral analgesics and nonsteroidal anti-inflammatory drugs, epidural steroids, and facet injections. The inclusion criteria of combined anterior and posterior approach were (1) rigid or frank lumbar kyphosis, (2) anterior or lateral bridged traction vertebral osteophytes, (3) gross coronal and sagittal deformity or imbalance, and (4) severe disc space narrowing that is not identifiable when performing PLIF or TLIF (Figure 1) and exclusion criteria were previous abdominal or retroperitoneal surgery.

A total of 110 patients with degenerative spinal deformity and curves measuring over 30°who underwent reconstructive spinal fusion surgery from 2002 to 2011 were included. Of the 110 patients who underwent surgery, 56 underwent the combined anterior and posterior approach and 54 underwent posterior surgery at our institution. This posterior (P) group included 34 females and 20 males with an average age of 62 years. 56 patients underwent combined anterior release and fusion of multiple lumbar levels followed by posterior instrumented fusion (AP group) included 35 females and 21 males with an average age of 61 years. Eighteen patients underwent ALIF followed by simultaneous instrumented posterolateral fusion. The remaining 38 patients underwent staged operations between 1 and 2 weeks.

Clinical assessment

The clinical outcome was evaluated using the Oswestry disability index (ODI) and the visual analog scale (VAS) preoperatively and at the final follow-up. All patients were scheduled for follow-up at 3 months, 6 months, and 1 year after the surgery and then annually. The following comorbidities were preoperatively diagnosed in AP and P groups : diabetes mellitus (n = 6;8); hypertension (n = 8;8); corticosteroid usage (n = 3;4); and valvular heart disease (n = 2;1).

Surgical technique

Anterior surgery in the combined anterior-posterior group, the patient was placed in the lateral decubitus

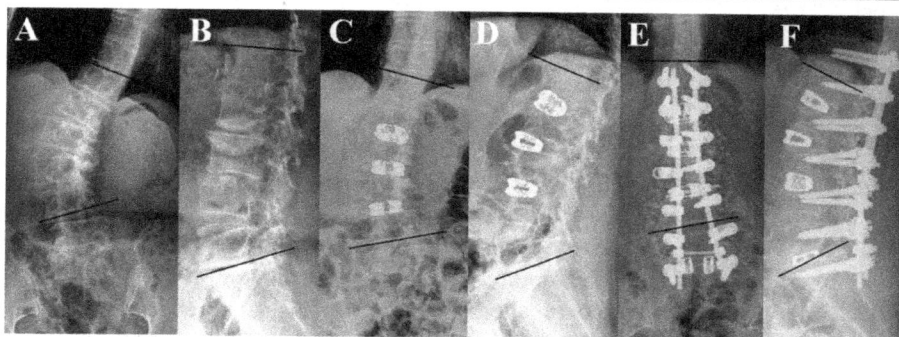

Figure 1 A 64-year-old woman complained low back pain with bilateral sciatica and claudication for several years. Radiographs of anteroposterior view **(A)** and lateral view **(B)** showing degenerative lumbar scoliosis from T12 to L5 with lateral bridged traction vertebral osteophytes over L2-3,L3-4 associated with severe disc space narrowing over L1-2 ,L2-3. After anterior lumbar interbody fusion with three SynCages over L1-2, L2-3, and L3-4, the scoliotic angle (T12-L4) was improved from 37° to 17° **(C)** and the lumbar lordotic curve was improved from 4° to 29° **(D)**. One week later, posterior instrumentation of T12-S1 with posterior interbody fusion of L5-S1 was performed. The scoliotic angle was improved from 17° to 6° **(E)** and the lumbar lordotic curve was improved from 29° to 36° **(F)**.

position with the concave side up, with the intention to directly correct the scoliosis. ALIF was performed using the flank retroperitoneal approach. After exposure of the anterior part of the disc, the anterior longitudinal ligament was transversely incised, and the disc was completely removed. Next, the vertebral endplates were cleared of cartilage using sharp curettes, taking care that damage to the subchondral bone of the endplates is avoided. Maximum distraction of disc space was achieved by manual lordotic force. After a satisfactory trial implantation, the SynCage (Synthes Spine, West Chester, PA, USA), which was filled with a morselized cancellous allograft, was implanted.

Posterior surgery in the combined anterior-posterior group and the posterior group ,all posterior instrumentation was placed via an open posterior approach. After subperiosteal exposure of the dorsal spine using a standard midline approach, an autologous bone graft was harvested via a subcutaneous access to the posterior iliac crest. After adequate decompression, pedicle screw instrumentation with TriFix G (Aspine, Oakland, CA, USA), with or without PLIF or TLIF was performed. Finally, rod derotation maneuver and compression on the convex side with the rod carefully contoured to the lordosis was performed to restore lumbar lordosis and correct lumbar scoliosis.

Radiographic evaluation
Plain radiographs in the standing posteroanterior (PA), lateral, and flexion-extension views were obtained for all patients preoperatively, postoperatively, 1 year after the surgery, and at the final follow-up. Preoperative and postoperative radiographs were compared to determine the degree of correction achieved following surgery. The coronal Cobb angle was determined from the standing PA radiograph by drawing a line parallel to the superior endplate of the most superior vertebra and a second line

parallel to the inferior endplate of the most inferior vertebra of the scoliotic curve. Lumbar lordosis was measured using the Cobb method [18] between the superior endplate of L-1 and S-1. Hyperlordosis was defined as any Cobb angle >60°, and hypolordosis was defined as any angle <20°. We also measure the lordotic angle correction for each level and SynCage position. End-plate fractures, cage malpositioning, and the status of the anterior and posterolateral fusion were also recorded. Anterior fusion was classified as solid, probable, or pseudoarthrosis. Solid fusion was defined as visible, continuous trabeculae of bridging fusion masses across the disc space and lack of instability in the flexion-extension radiographs. Probable fusion was defined as unclear bony trabecular continuity with no radiolucent interruption or motion seen in the stress radiographs. Pseudoarthrosis was defined as radiolucent interruption of the cage, and as motion, in stress radiographs. Posterolateral fusion was also classified as solid, probable, and pseudoarthrosis. Solid fusion was defined as visible, continuous trabeculae of bridging fusion masses over the bilateral transverse processes and no motion in the flexion and extension stress radiographs. Probable fusion was defined as unclear bony trabecular continuity with no radiolucent interruption or motion in stress radiographs. Radiolucent interruption of the fusion mass was labeled as pseudoarthrosis [19]. The fusion status was decided by the senior surgeons (W-J,Chen).

Statistical analysis
Data were analyzed using the SPSS statistical software package (SPSS, Inc, Chicago, IL, USA). Means were calculated for different variables including the ODI score, VAS, and angles of lumbar lordosis and scoliosis. Preoperative and postoperative measurements and values between the different subgroups were compared using the paired t-test with statistical significance set at a

P value of <0.05. The position of SynCage and the lordotic angle correction was compared using the Student's *t*-test with statistical significance set at a P value of <0.05.

Results

All patients received clinical and radiographic follow-up for a minimum of 24 months, with an average follow-up of 53 months (range, 26–96 months). The operation time of anterior lumbar interbody fusion is 172.5 minutes (range,115-301 minutes) and instrumented posterolateral fusion is 262.5 minutes (range, 195–375 minutes) in AP group and 350.5 minutes (range, 210–452 minutes) in P group, estimated blood loss of anterior lumbar interbody fusion is 250 ml (range,150-1750 ml) and instrumented posterolateral fusion is 1650 ml (range,1000-4850 ml) in AP group and 3250 ml (range,2000-6500 ml) in P group, transfusion amount of anterior lumbar interbody fusion is 700 ml (range,500-2000 ml) and instrumented posterolateral fusion is 1500 ml (range,1000-5000 ml) in AP group and 4000 ml (range,2000-8000 ml) in P group, and length of stay is 16 days (range ,10-21 days) in AP group and 10 days (range ,7-14 days) in P group.

Clinical outcomes

The VAS and ODI scores were evaluated preoperatively and at the final follow-up (Table 1). At final follow-up, the average ODI score was significantly lower than that determined preoperatively in both groups. The mean back and leg VAS scores also improved significantly in both groups.

Radiographic outcomes

Preoperative and postoperative coronal Cobb angles and lumbar lordosis angles were compared (Table 1). The average preoperative coronal Cobb angle was 41.3° (range, 32°–85°), which decreased to 9.3° post-operatively in AP group, demonstrating a significant mean scoliosis correction of 78% (P = 0.042). The mean preoperative lumbar lordosis angle increased from 3.1° (range, kyphosis 30° to lordosis 33°) to 35.7° (range, lordosis 9° to 60°), demonstrating a mean improvement of 32.6° (P = 0.009).In P group , the average preoperative coronal Cobb angle was 38.5° (range, 32°–55°), which decreased to 21.4° post-operatively, demonstrating a significant mean scoliosis correction of 44%. The mean preoperative lumbar lordosis angle increased from 6° (range, kyphosis 25° to lordosis 25°) to 15.8° (range, lordosis 10° to 40°), demonstrating a mean improvement of 9.8°. Both in coronal and sagittal plane ,angle improvement were better in AP group than P group.As shown in Table 2, ALIF was performed for a total of 171 disc levels in the 56 patients as follows: 1-level procedure (n = 3), 2-level (n = 15), 3-level (n = 18), 4-level (n = 16), and 5-level (n = 4). As seen in Figure 2, the ALIF procedures were correlated with a higher rate of scoliosis and lordosis correction. In Figure 3 and Table 3, an ALIF cage placed in the posterior half provides more lordosis at the instrumented level, whereas a cage placed in the anterior half may not provide better sagittal plane correction. (10.9° to 6.1°; P = 0.0058). Two patients exhibited asymptomatic SynCage subsidence, and 1 patient had asymptomatic S1 screw loosening. The fusion status was decided by the senior surgeons (W-J,Chen). At the final follow-up, 36 of the 56 patients (64.3%) exhibited solid anterior

Table 1 Clinical and radiographic outcomes

	AP[#] group	P[##] group	P value
Pre-op mean back VAS[+]	8.2	9.0	0.54
2-year post-op mean back VAS	2.1	2.3	0.23
Pre-op mean leg VAS	5.5	6.5	0.45
2-year post-op mean leg VAS	0.9	0.5	0.22
Pre-op ODI[++] score	28.8	29.1	0.15
2-year post-op ODI[#] score	6.4	6.2	0.45
Pre-op mean scoliotic angle(°)	41.3	38.5	0.48
2-year post-op mean scoliotic angle(°)	9.3	21.4	0.02*
Scoliosis correction(%)	78	44	0.02*
Pre-op mean lumbar lordotic angle(°)	3.1	6	0.21
2-year post–op mean lumbar lordotic angle(°)	35.7	15.8	0.009*

[+]: VAS, Visual analog scale.
[++]: ODI, Oswestry Disability Index.
#AP, Combined anterior and posterior approach.
##:P, Posterior approach.
*:P value < 0.05.

Table 2 ALIF levels and angle correction

ALIF*	Patients	Scoliotic angle (°)			Lumbar lordotic angle (°)		
		Pre-op	2-year F/U+	Correction	Pre-op	2-year F/U	Correction
1	3	22	2	20	2	20	18
2	15	39	6.8	32.2	4.1	32	27.9
3	18	41	9	32	2	33.7	31.7
4	16	44	11	33	7.8	46	38.2
5	4	62	22	40	0.5	56	55.5

*ALIF: Anterior lumbar interbody fusion levels.
+F/U: Follow up.

fusion; 40 (71.4%), solid posterolateral fusion; 20 (35.7%), probable anterior fusion; and 16 (28.6%), probable posterolateral fusion in AP group and 39 of the 54 patients (72.2%) exhibited solid posterolateral fusion; 15 (27.8%), probable posterolateral fusion in P group. No anterior or posterolateral pseudoarthrosis was noted.

Complications

There were no major complications such as intraoperative cerebrospinal fluid (CSF) leak, postoperative weakness, deep venous thrombosis, ureteral trauma, or injury to the peritoneal or retroperitoneal structures. Perioperative complications, which presented as postoperative superficial wound infections, occurred in 5 patients in the AP group and 7 in P group, but the symptoms subsided after debridement and antibiotic treatment. Six patients experienced transient postoperative anterior thigh numbness in the AP group, ipsilateral to the approach, in the distribution of the anterior femoral cutaneous nerve.

Discussion

Adult degenerative scoliosis is believed to develop as a result of asymmetrical degeneration of the spine. It most commonly occurs in the lumbar spine and typically presents as pain, which is the primary complaint in 90% of the patients [7]. This axial back pain occurs most commonly due to a combination of muscle fatigue, trunk imbalance, facet arthropathy, and degenerative disc disease [20,21]. The flat-back deformity and forward sagittal imbalance have been shown to be a significant source of pain and disability in patients [22,23]. Several studies showed that radiographic parameters were correlated with clinical symptoms in adults [24-27]. Many radiographic parameters may affect functional scores in degenerative lumbar

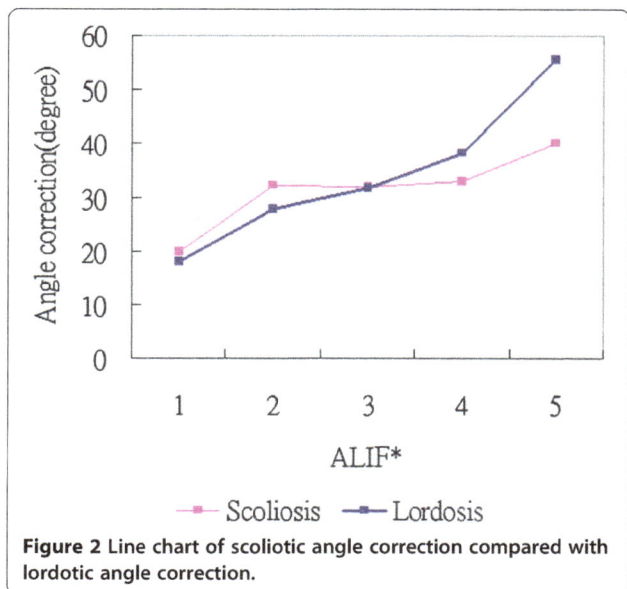

Figure 2 Line chart of scoliotic angle correction compared with lordotic angle correction.

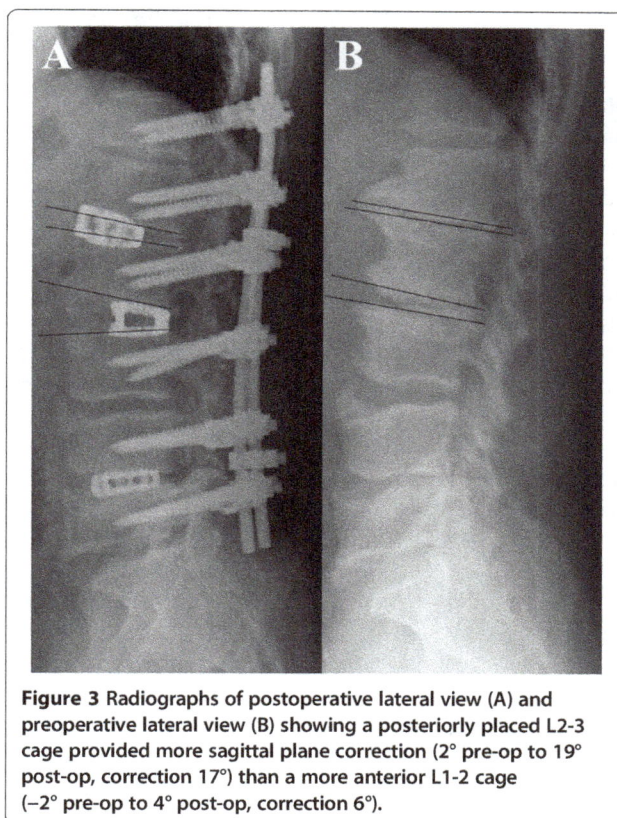

Figure 3 Radiographs of postoperative lateral view (A) and preoperative lateral view (B) showing a posteriorly placed L2-3 cage provided more sagittal plane correction (2° pre-op to 19° post-op, correction 17°) than a more anterior L1-2 cage (−2° pre-op to 4° post-op, correction 6°).

Table 3 Position of SynCages and lordotic angle correction

SynCage position	Number	Mean lordotic angle correction	P value
Anterior half	78 cages	6.1° (1°–12°)	
Posterior half	93 cages	10.9° (6°–24°)	0.0058

scoliosis, including the Cobb scoliosis angle in all major thoracolumbar or lumbar and lumbosacral curves, maximal intervertebral lateral olisthesis, thoracic kyphosis, thoracolumbar kyphosis, lumbar lordosis, plumbline offset from C7 to the posterosuperior corner of the S1 vertebral body, and maximal intervertebral anteroposterior olisthesis. Avraam et al. [26] reported that a loss of normal lordosis could affect health outcomes even when the sagittal balance is preserved in patients with degenerative lumbar scoliosis. Decreased lumbar lordosis and an increased lumbosacral hemicurve have led to poorer results of health status. The average curve correction in our series was 78% of maximal Cobb angle with maintenance of the correction seen at the 2-year follow-up. The mean scoliotic and lumbar lordotic angle were improved from 41.3° and 3.1° pre-operatively to 9.3° and 35.7° at the 2-year follow-up in our combined group. However , the mean scoliotic and lumbar lordotic angle were improved from 38.5° and 6° pre-operatively to 21.4° and 15.8° in our posterior approach. There were significant differences in sagittal (P = 0.009) and coronal (P = 0.02) plane correction between the combined anterior-posterior group and the posterior group. The radiographic outcome in our combined approach was superior to that via a posterior approach (Table 1).

Degenerative lumbar scoliosis with spinal stenosis has been traditionally treated with posterior decompression along with posterior spinal instrumentation and fusion. From 2002 to 2011, 1834 patients with degenerative lumbar scoliosis underwent surgery in our institution and 1778 patients were treated via a posterior-only approach. Only 56 patients received combined anterior lumbar interbody fusion and instrumented posterolateral fusion. The obvious disadvantages of using an anterior approach to the lumbar spine include retroperitoneal dissection with associated vascular manipulation, 2 major surgical procedures required, and increased operating time [8,9]. In our experience, the following are the indications for ALIF in addition to instrumented posterolateral fusion: (1) rigid or frank lumbar kyphosis; (2) anterior or lateral bridged traction vertebral osteophytes; (3) gross coronal and sagittal deformity or imbalance; and (4) severe disc space narrowing that is not identifiable when performing PLIF or TLIF. In de novo degenerative lumbar scoliosis, the curves tend to be more rigid posteriorly and, therefore, are amenable to correction via a posterior-only approach [10]. In our result ,rigid or frank lumbar kyphoscoliotic

deformity secondary to idiopathic curves were difficult to correct via a posterior-only approach with scoliosis correction only 44% and lordotic angle correction only 9.8°, and better scoliosis and lordosis correction were achieved through the combined anterior and posterior approach with statistically significant. Anterior or lateral bridged traction vertebral osteophytes restrict not only graft placement but also lordosis restoration and can only be removed via an anterior approach. When performing PLIF or TLIF in osteoporotic endplate or severe disc narrowing cases, violation of the endplate always results in cage subsidence and poor angle correction.

The use of interbody grafts associated with posterior instrumentation in deformity correction surgery has gained popularity for providing anterior column structural stability, increased fusion rates, as well as enable restoration and preservation of lumbar lordosis [11-13,28]. Graft placement has traditionally been achieved through either an anterior (ALIF) or a posterior (PLIF or TLIF) approach.

Anterior lumbar interbody fusion is superior to posterior lumbar fusion because of the larger surface area available between the vertebral bodies, which facilitates the use of wider cages that can rest on a strong peripheral cortical bone on either side, thus minimizing the risk of cage subsidence, which is especially important in elderly patients with osteoporotic bones [11,17,29,30].

We found that the ALIF approach using the anterior-posterior wedge cages was effective for correcting sagittal plane deformities. An ALIF cage placed in the posterior half provides more lordosis at the instrumented level, whereas a cage placed in the anterior half may not provide better sagittal plane correction. (10.9° to 6.1°; P = 0.0058) (Figure 3, Table 3).

We have observed that the transpsoas approach leads to a high frequency of thigh numbness, pain, weakness, and dysesthesias, which are likely the result of retraction proximal to the lumbosacral plexus, and have been well described in previous anatomical studies [31]. Prior reports of lateral retroperitoneal approaches including mobilization of the psoas muscle from the lumbar spine have demonstrated high incidence (30%) of paresthesias in the thigh/groin region [32]. Knight et al. [33] reported 10% incidence of lateral femoral cutaneous nerve deficit and 3% incidence of L4 motor deficit using the lateral retroperitoneal transpsoas approach. In our study, we identified 6 patients (10.7%) with transient postoperative ipsilateral sensory deficits that had resolved before the last follow-up visit. Because these deficits were transient, we believe they were stretch or neuropraxic injuries.

Conclusions

ALIF with SynCages and supplemental instrumented posterolateral fusion resulted in better coronal and sagittal plane correction than posterior approach in all patients and was maintained in the 2-year follow-up. The VAS and ODI scores significantly improved after the operation, and no major complications occurred.

Competing interests
The authors declare that they have no competing interests.

Authors' contributions
Each author has made substantive intellectual contributions to this multicentre study: M–K H and W-J C participated in the study design, in collecting the data, the statistically analyses ,drafting and contributed equally to the manuscript. C-C N, T-S F , P-L L ,and L–H C, participated in the study design. W-J C advised and assisted drafting of the manuscript. All authors read and approved the final manuscript.

Acknowledgements
We thank the Department of Orthopaedic Surgery for their contribution to the study.

References
1. Ploumis A, Transfledt EE, Denis F. Degenerative lumbar scoliosis associated with spinal stenosis. Spine J. 2007;7:428–36.
2. Aebi M. The adult scoliosis. Eur Spine J. 2005;14:925–48.
3. Berven SH, Deviren V, Mitchell B, Wahba G, Hu SS, Bradford DS. Operative management of degenerative scoliosis:an evidence-based approach to surgical strategies based on clinical and radiographic outcomes. Neurosurg Clin N Am. 2007;18:261–72.
4. Oskouian Jr RJ, Shaffrey CI. Degenerative lumbar scoliosis. Neurosurg Clin N Am. 2006;17:299–315.
5. Daffner SD, Vaccaro AR. Adult degenerative lumbar scoliosis. Am J Orthop. 2003;32:77–82.
6. Anand N, Baron EM, Thaiyananthan G, Khalsa K, Goldstein TB. Minimally invasive multilevel percutaneous correction and fusion for adult lumbar degenerative scoliosis: a technique and feasibility study. J Spinal Disord Tech. 2008;21:459–67.
7. Winter RB, Lonstein JE, Denis F. Pain patterns in adult scoliosis. Orthop Clin North Am. 1988;19:339–45.
8. Crandall DG, Revella J. Transforaminal lumbar interbody fusion versus anterior lumbar interbody fusion as an adjunct to posterior instrumented correction of degenerative lumbar scoliosis: three year clinical and radiographic outcomes. Spine (Phila Pa 1976). 2009;34:2126–33.
9. Rajaraman V, Vingan R, Roth P, Heary RF, Conklin L, Jacobs GB. Visceral and vascular complications resulting from anterior lumbar interbody fusion. J Neurosurg. 1999;91(1 Suppl):60–4.
10. Pateder DB, Kebaish KM, Cascio BM, Neubaeur P, Matusz DM, Kostuik JP. Posterior Only Versus Combined Anterior and Posterior Approaches to Lumbar Scoliosis in Adults. A Radiographic Analysis. Spine. 2007;32:1551–4.
11. Hsieh PC, Koski TR, O'Shaughnessy BA, Sugrue P, Salehi S, Ondra S, et al. Anterior lumbar interbody fusion in comparison with transforaminal lumbar interbody fusion: implications for the restoration of foraminal height, local disc angle, lumbar lordosis, and sagittal balance. J Neurosurg Spine. 2007;7:379–86.
12. Ploumis A, Wu C, Fischer G, Mehbod AA, Wu W, Faundez A, et al. Biomechanical comparison of anterior lumbar interbody fusion and transforaminal lumbar interbody fusion. J Spinal Disord Tech. 2008;21:120–5.
13. Potter BK, Freedman BA, Verwiebe EG, Hall JM, Polly Jr DW, Kuklo TR. Transforaminal lumbar interbody fusion: clinical and radiographic results and complications in 100 consecutive patients. J Spinal Disord Tech. 2005;18:337–46.
14. Birknes JK, White AP, Albert TJ, Shaffrey CI, Harrop JS. Adult degenerative scoliosis: a review. Neurosurgery. 2008;63(3 Suppl):94–103.
15. Heary RF, Kumar S, Bono CM. Decision making in adult deformity. Neurosurgery. 2008;63(3 Suppl):69–77.
16. Blumenthal SL, Ohnmeiss DD. Intervertebral cages for degenerative spinal diseases. Spine J. 2003;3:301–9.
17. Janssen ME, Lam C, Beckham R. Outcomes of allogenic cages in anterior and posterior lumbar interbody fusion. Eur Spine J. 2001;10(2 suppl):S158–68.
18. Groth AT, Kuklo TR, Klemme WR, Polly DW, Schroeder TM. Comparison of sagittal contour and posterior disc height following interbody fusion: threaded cylindrical cages versus structural allograft versus vertical cages. J Spinal Disord Tech. 2005;18:332–6.
19. Wu CH, Wong CB, Chen LH, Niu CC, Tsai TT, Chen WJ. Instrumented Posterior Lumbar Interbody Fusion for Patients With Degenerative Lumbar Scoliosis. J Spinal Disord Tech. 2008;21:310–5.
20. Cobb JR. Outline for the study of scoliosis. Instructional course lectures. In: Bechtol CA, editor. American Academy of Orthopedic Surgeons, vol. 5. Edwards: Ann Arbor, MI; 1948. p. 261–75.
21. Bradford DS, Tay BK, Hu SS. Adult scoliosis: surgical indications, operative management, complications, and outcomes. Spine (Phila Pa 1976). 1999;24:2617–29.
22. Jang JS, Lee SH, Min JH, Maeng DH. Changes in sagittal alignment after restoration of lower lumbar lordosis in patients with degenerative flat back syndrome. J Neurosurg Spine. 2007;7:387–92.
23. Wiggins GC, Ondra SL, Shaffrey CI. Management of iatrogenic flat-back syndrome. Neurosurg Focus. 2003;15:E8.
24. Glassman SD, Berven S, Bridwell K, Horton W, Dimar JR. Correlation of radiographic parameters and clinical symptoms in adult scoliosis. Spine. 2005;30:682–8.
25. Jackson RP, Simmons EH, Stripinis D. Coronal and sagittal plane spinal deformities correlating with back pain and pulmonary function in adult idiopathic scoliosis. Spine. 1989;14:1391–7.
26. Ploumis A, Liu H, Mehbod AA, Transfeldt EE, Winter RB. A correlation of radiographic and functional measurements in adult degenerative scoliosis. Spine. 2009;34:1581–4.
27. Schwab FJ, Smith VA, Biserni M, Gamez L, Farcy JP, Pagala M. Adult scoliosis: a quantitative radiographic and clinical analysis. Spine. 2002;27:387–92.
28. Jagannathan J, Sansur CA, Oskouian Jr RJ, Fu KM, Shaffrey CI. Radiographic restoration of lumbar alignment after transforaminal lumbar interbody fusion. Neurosurgery. 2009;64:955–64.
29. Gödde S, Fritsch E, Dienst M, Kohn D. Influence of cage geometry on sagittal alignment in instrumented posterior lumbar interbody fusion. Spine (Phila Pa 1976). 2003;28:1693–9.
30. Hart RA, Prendergast MA. Spine surgery for lumbar degenerative disease in elderly and osteoporotic patients. Instr Course Lect. 2007;56:257–72.
31. Benglis DM, Vanni S, Levi AD. An anatomical study of the lumbosacral plexus as related to the minimally invasive transpsoas approach to the lumbar spine. J Neurosurg Spine. 2009;10:139–44.
32. Bergey DL, Villavicencio AT, Goldstein T, Regan JJ. Endoscopic lateral transpsoas approach to the lumbar spine. Spine (Phila Pa 1976). 2004;29:1681–8.
33. Knight RQ, Schwaegler P, Hanscom D, Roh J. Direct lateral lumbar interbody fusion for degenerative conditions: early complication profile. J Spinal Disord Tech. 2009;22:34–7.

12

Choroid vascular occlusion and ischemic optic neuropathy after facial calcium hydroxyapatite injection

Chien-Chih Chou[1], Hsin-Han Chen[2], Yi-Yu Tsai[1], You-Ling Li[1] and Hui-Ju Lin[1,3,4*]

Abstract

Background: We reported a case of sudden monocular vision loss after calcium hydroxyapatite (CaHA) injection into the nasal tip and dorsum with detailed retina images.

Case presentation: A healthy, 35-year-old woman received CaHA filler injection for nose augmentation. Ten minutes after the procedure, she developed nausea, vomiting, headache, ptosis, and left periorbital pain. After 30 minutes, she complained of progressively blurring vision in the left eye. The best-corrected visual acuity (BCVA) in her left eye was 30 cm ahead of hand motion. Left exotropia was noted in primary gaze. Limitations in adduction, supraduction, and infraduction of the left eye were also observed. Slit lamp examination of the left eye revealed a pink conjunctiva, a clear cornea, a mild anterior chamber reaction, a sluggish papillary light reflex, and a semi-dilated pupil. A positive relative afferent pupillary defect was observed in the left eye. Fundus examination revealed optic disc edema and some linear whitish opacity over the superior and temporal sites in the left eye, suggesting multiple CaHA emboli in the choroid vessels.

Conclusions: Although the majority of adverse reactions are mild and transient, surgeons should be alert about extremely rare serious adverse events such as visual loss.

Keywords: Calcium hydroxyapatite, Nose augmentation, Choroid vascular occlusion, Ischemic optic neuropathy, Vision loss, Filler

Background

Facial plastic surgery reverses the signs of aging. Injectable facial fillers are effective in ameliorating certain signs of aging [1], and calcium hydroxyapatite (CaHA) is one of the most commonly used fillers for this purpose [2]. Serious adverse events are rarely observed, and the majority of adverse reactions are mild and transient [3]. Here we report the case of a 35-year-old woman who developed sudden monocular vision loss after CaHA injection into the nasal tip and dorsum.

Case presentation

A healthy, 35-year-old woman without any history of ocular and systemic disease received CaHA filler injections

* Correspondence: irisluu2396@gmail.com
[1]Department of Ophthalmology, China Medical University Hospital, No. 2 Yuh Der Road, Taichung 404, Taiwan
[3]Department of Medical Research, China Medical University Hospital, Taichung, Taiwan
Full list of author information is available at the end of the article

(RADIESSE® 1.5 ml) for cosmetic nose augmentation. Multiple injections along midline of the nasal dorsum from nasal tip to glabella were performed under local anesthesia. Ten minutes after the procedure, she developed nausea, vomiting, headache, ptosis, and left periorbital pain. After 30 minutes, she complained of progressively blurring vision in the left eye. The best-corrected visual acuity (BCVA) in her left eye was 30 cm ahead of hand motion. Skin necrosis developed over the nasal dorsum, glabellar region, and left forehead (Figure 1a). Left exotropia was noted in primary gaze. Limitations in adduction, supraduction, and infraduction of the left eye were also observed (Figure 1b). Slit lamp examination of the left eye revealed a pink conjunctiva, a clear cornea, a mild anterior chamber reaction, a sluggish pupillary light reflex, and a semi-dilated pupil. A positive relative afferent pupillary defect was observed in the left eye. The intraocular pressure was normal in both eyes. Fundus examination revealed optic disc edema and some linear whitish opacities over the

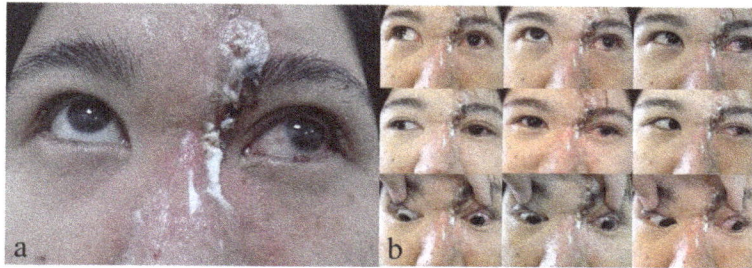

Figure 1 Skin necrosis developed at nasal dorsum, glabellar region, and left forehead (a). Left exotropia was noted in primary gaze, and limitations on adduction, supraduction, and infraduction in left eye were also noted **(b)**.

superior and temporal sites in the left eye, suggesting multiple CaHA emboli in the choroid vessels (Figure 2a,b). Optical coherence tomography (OCT) revealed disc edema without macular edema in the left eye (Figure 2c). Fluorescein angiography revealed neither delayed filling nor hypofluroescence in the left eye. Visual field testing revealed an inferior altitudinal visual field defect in the left eye. Measurement of the visual evoked potential (VEP) showed a decreased amplitude and marked delay in the appearance of peaks. Electroretinography (ERG) showed a normal waveform. All examinations were normal in the right eye. Orbital computed tomography (CT) demonstrated high-density deposits in the nose region and left medial orbital cavity (Figure 3). No evident lesion was noted on brain magnetic resonance imaging (MRI).

Alprostadil and dextran were administered for improving blood supply. Moreover, ten sessions of hyperbaric oxygen therapy were administered. One month later, the visual acuity in her left eye improved to 6/60. A pale disc was observed, with persistent plaque occlusions in the choroid vessels.

Discussion

There are few reports of vision loss following facial injection of autologous fat or hyaluronic acid [4-6]. In a previous study, Lazzeri et al. [7] reported 32 cases of blindness caused by iatrogenic retinal embolism

after cosmetic facial filler injections, while Park et al. [8] reported 12 cases of retinal artery occlusion caused by cosmetic facial filler injections. Furthermore, Park et al. [9] showed the clinical and angiographic features of occlusion of the ophthalmic artery and its branches caused by cosmetic facial filler injections. In these 44 cases, only one was attributed to CaHA, and no CaHA emboli were clearly observed on fundus photography.

Sung et al. [10] postulated that emboli may move in a retrograde fashion to the ophthalmic artery under a high injection pressure. In the present case, multiple emboli localized on the choroidal layer without retinal vessel occlusion, resulting in normal ERG waveform. However, poor vision, a positive RAPD sign, and a pale, swollen disc were present. Visual field testing showed an inferior altitudinal visual field defect. We postulate that the CaHA emboli migrated via the dorsonasal artery back to the main ciliary arteries and occluded the short posterior ciliary arteries, which supply the superior nasal choroid and the optic nerve. Subsequently, ischemic optic neuropathy developed and caused poor vision, a positive RAPD sign, a pale, swollen disc, and an abnormal waveform on VEP. Furthermore, we first postulated that the occluded vessel was Haller's layer because the distribution pattern of affected vessels was consistent with the Haller's layer distribution pattern.

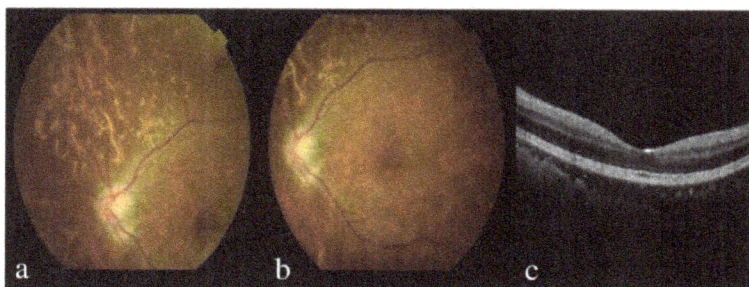

Figure 2 Fundus examination revealed optic disc edema and some linear whitish opacities over the superior and temporal sites in the left eye, suggesting multiple CaHA emboli in the choroid vessels (a). No macular edema in left eye was revealed on fundus examination **(b)**, or OCT **(c)**.

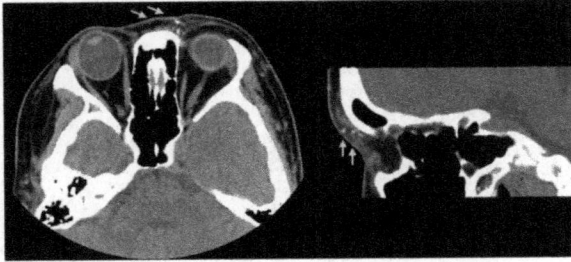

Figure 3 Orbital CT demonstrates multiple radiopaque spots in the subcutaneous layer of medial aspect of left periorbital region, suggesting CaHA deposition.

The emboli moved back to branches supplying the oculomotor nerve, causing blepheroptosis and ophtalmoplegia. This is compatible with the CT findings (Figure 3). The ptosis and limitation in supraduction subsided gradually. We postulate that the superior division of the oculomotor nerve innervating the levator and superior rectus muscles recovered early.

In previously reported cases of CaHA injections and in this case, there was no cerebral infarction, which is more frequently observed after autologous fat injections [9]. This may be related to properties of the filler material, such as molecular weight or size.

To decrease the risk of intravascular injection and retrograde occlusion, Park et al. suggested slow injection in a fractionated dose and the use of a blunt cannula [9]. We suggest the use of a mixture of CaHA and epinephrine because epinephrine leads to vasoconstriction and thus decreases the possibility of intravascular injection. Soft tissue can be dissected to create a subcutaneous space for subsequent filler injection. Furthermore, an injection device with a valve that can relieve excessive injection pressure can be designed for this purpose.

Injectable facial fillers have become increasingly popular these days. Although the majority of adverse reactions are mild and transient, surgeons should be alert about extremely rare serious adverse events such as visual loss. Most cases of blindness are caused by autologous fat and hyaluronic acid injections. To the best of our knowledge, localized choroid vascular occlusion, ischemic optic neuropathy, and cranial nerve III palsy without evidence of compromised retinal or choroidal circulation after CaHA injection have not been reported.

Conclusion

In conclusion, we reported a case of sudden monocular vision loss after CaHA filler injection into the nasal tip and dorsum. CaHA emboli were clearly observed in this case, providing direct evidence to prove the mechanism underlying retrograde occlusion after facial filler injection.

Consent statement
Written informed consent was obtained from the patient for publication of this case report and any accompanying images. A copy of the written consent is available for review by the Editor of this journal.

Competing interests
All authors certify that they have NO affiliations with or involvement in any organization or entity with any financial interest (such as honoraria; educational grants; participation in speakers' bureaus; membership, employment, consultancies, stock ownership, or other equity interest; and expert testimony or patent-licensing arrangements), or non-financial interest (such as personal or professional relationships, affiliations, knowledge or beliefs) in the subject matter or materials discussed in this manuscript.

Authors' contributions
CCC and YLL participated in the drafted the manuscript. HJL, HHC, and YYT, participated in the design of the study and helped to draft the manuscript. All authors read and approved the final manuscript.

Author details
[1]Department of Ophthalmology, China Medical University Hospital, No. 2 Yuh Der Road, Taichung 404, Taiwan. [2]Department of Plastic and Reconstructive Surgery, China Medical University Hospital, Taichung, Taiwan. [3]Department of Medical Research, China Medical University Hospital, Taichung, Taiwan. [4]School of Chinese Medicine, College of Chinese Medicine, China Medical University, Taichung, Taiwan.

References
1. Jacovella PF. Use of calcium hydroxylapatite (Radiesse®) for facial augmentation. Clin Interv Aging. 2008;3(1):161–74.
2. Jurado JR, Lima LF, Olivetti IP, Arroyo HH, de Oliveira IH. Innovations in minimally invasive facial treatments. Facial Plast Surg. 2013;29(3):154–60.
3. Funt D, Pavicic T. Dermal fillers in aesthetics: an overview of adverse events and treatment approaches. Clin Cosmet Investig Dermatol. 2013;6:295–316.
4. Dreizen NG, Framm L. Sudden visual loss after autologous fat injection into the glabellar area. Am J Ophthalmol. 1989;107:85–7.
5. Danesh-Meyer HV, Savino PJ, Sergott RC. Case reports and small case series: ocular and cerebral ischemia following facial injection of autologous fat. Arch Ophthalmol. 2011;119:777–8.
6. Peter S, Mennel S. Retinal branch artery occlusion following injection of hyaluronic acid (Restylane). Clin Experiment Ophthalmol. 2006;34:363–4.
7. Lazzeri D, Agostini T, Figus M, Nardi M, Pantaloni M, Lazzeri S. Blindness following cosmetic injections of the face. Plast Reconstr Surg. 2012;129 (4):995–1012.
8. Park SW, Woo SJ, Park KH, Huh JW, Jung C, Kwon OK. Iatrogenic retinal artery occlusion caused by cosmetic facial filler injections. Am Ophthalmol. 2012;154(4):653–66.
9. Park KH, Kim YK, Woo SJ, Kang SW, Lee WK, Choi KS, et al. Iatrogenic retinal artery occlusion caused by cosmetic facial filler injections: a national survey by the Korean Retina Society. JAMA Ophthalmol. 2014;132(6):714–23.
10. Sung MS, Kim HG, Woo KI, Kim YD. Ocular ischemia and ischemic oculomotor nerve palsy after vascular embolization of injectable calcium hydroxylapatite filler. Ophthal Plast Reconstr Surg. 2010;26:289–91.

13

Recurrence of post burn contractures of the elbow and shoulder joints: experience from a ugandan hospital

Deo Darius Balumuka[1*], George William Galiwango[2] and Rose Alenyo[3]

Abstract

Background: Recurrence of post-burn contractures, following inadequate management of post-burn contractures (PBC), is under reported. It is associated with multiple operations and an increased cost to patients and their families. The purpose of this study was to determine the frequency of recurrence of PBC of the shoulder and the elbow joint three months after surgical intervention and the associated risk- factors.

Methods: This was a prospective cohort study conducted at CoRSU hospital from March 2012 to November 2014. All patients with PBC of the elbow and/or shoulder joint who consented to be in the study and met the inclusion criteria were enrolled. Data was collected using a pretested, coded questionnaire. A goniometer was used to measure the active range of motion of the involved joint. The measurements were recorded in degrees. The data was analysed with STATA version 12.1.

Results: 58 patients were enrolled consecutively in the study. There were 36 females and 22 males, with a female to male ratio of 1.6:1. The age range was 0.75–45 years, with a median age of 5 years. The average age at the time of injury was 3.4 years. The most common cause of initial burn injury was scalding. The average number of joints involved per patient was two. There was a high incidence of recurrence of PBC (52 %) among the participants. The shoulder had the highest frequency of recurrence at 67 %. The elbow joint had a frequency of recurrence of 27 %. All participants with both elbow and shoulder joint involvement had PBC recur. The risk factors for recurrence were flame burn ($p = 0.007$), duration of PBC of more than 1 year ($p = 0.018$), and incomplete release of the contracture ($p = 0.002$). The presence of keloids, hypertrophic scars, ulcers and the occurrence of complications at the contracture site were not associated with recurrence of PBC.

Conclusion: Recurrence of PBC of the elbow and shoulder joint is a common problem. The risk factors should be kept in mind during management of PBC to reduce the recurrence rate.

Keywords: Recurrence, Post Burn Contractures, Elbow joint, Shoulder joint, PBC

Background

Post-burn contractures (PBC) are a distressing problem in both the developed and developing worlds [1–3]. They usually occur following inadequate primary burn injury management [4]. Children are the most affected by PBC, and the elbow and shoulder joints are the most involved regions [1, 5, 6]. Management of PBC of the elbow and

* Correspondence: balumukad@gmail.com
[1]Mbarara University of Science and Technology, PO Box 1410, Mbarara, Uganda
Full list of author information is available at the end of the article

shoulder joints is challenging, primarily because they have a tendency to recur [7–9].

Just as the inappropriate management of burns leads to the occurrence of PBC, inadequate management of PBC leads to their recurrence [1, 9, 10]. Recurrence has been reported in developed and developing countries following both surgical and non-surgical management [7–9]. Shoulder joint PBC have been reported to be more challenging to manage due to the wide range of motion of the joint. Management of these contractures has been reported to have complications which predispose to recurrences [11]. Elbow joint PBC are more likely to recur the longer the contractures have been present [3, 11], however, any joint involved by PBC, if inadequately managed, will have recurrence of the contracture.

There is a dearth of data available on the frequency of recurrence of PBC of the elbow and shoulder joint, especially in low-income countries such as Uganda. This study was carried out to determine the frequency of recurrence of PBC of the shoulder and elbow joint and the associated risk-factors among patients managed at our centre.

Methods

Study design

This was a prospective study involving all patients who had PBC of the elbow and/or shoulder joint who were managed at Comprehensive Rehabilitation Services Uganda (CoRSU) hospital from 2012 to 2014.

Study setting

The study was conducted at the Plastic Surgery department of CoRSU Hospital, a specialised centre offering plastic and reconstructive surgery services in Uganda. It has a capacity of 84 beds and also serves as a training centre for the Mbarara University plastic surgery programme. CoRSU provides services to patients from the neighbouring towns and also the neighbouring countries like South Sudan, Kenya, Tanzania and D.R. Congo.

Study population

The study population included patients of all age groups and sexes who had a PBC of the elbow and/or shoulder joint who were consecutively managed and reassessed at CoRSU hospital during the study period.

Inclusion criteria

All patients with a PBC of the shoulder joint and/or elbow joint operated on at CoRSU hospital.

Exclusion criteria

All patients who had severe disease co-morbidities, including malignancy (Marjolin's ulcer) involving the affected limb, or with infection of the upper affected limb, were excluded from the study. All patients who were not residents of Uganda and were not to be followed up at CoRSU hospital were also excluded.

Study materials

Data was collected using a coded questionnaire. A clear plastic goniometer with a 360 degree head and three scales calibrated to the International Standard of Measurements was used to measure the active range of motion of the affected joints.

Study procedure

After obtaining informed consent, the participant's socio-demographics, history of burn injury, and history of contracture were obtained. Examination of the affected joints for type of PBC, presence of ulcers, hypertrophic scars and/or keloids was done.

The active range of motion at each involved joint was measured using a manual goniometer with a standardized technique. The severity of contractures was recorded in degrees. Multiple planes of motion, i.e. flexion, extension, abduction, and adduction were measured at the involved shoulder joint(s) and recorded before surgery. Extension and flexion planes of motion were recorded before surgery for the elbow joint(s). The extension plane of motion was recorded as negative showing the extension deficit of the involved elbow joint.

After surgery the active range of motion of the operated joint(s) and the type of operative management, STSG, FTSG, Flap or a combination, were recorded. Any post-operative complications were recorded. The patients were seen by a physiotherapist and/or occupational therapist for splinting and mobilisation exercises. The patient was then discharged and given a date for follow-up.

After 1 month post-operation the patient's use of splints, joint mobilisation regimen and supervision of physiotherapy were asked and recorded. The active range of motion of the operated joint(s) was measured using a goniometer. The presence of any complications was sought and recorded.

After 3 months post-operation the use of splints, joint mobilisation regimen and supervision of physiotherapy were again asked and recorded. The range of motion of the affected joint(s) was measured again. The presence of any complications at the operated joints was sought and recorded.

The information was entered in the database using Epidata Version 3.1. The range, consistency and validity checks were built in to minimize errors.

Elbow joint PBC were classified depending on the loss of joint extension as follows;

- Negligible, when there is less than 10 degrees of extension loss;
- Mild, when 11–49 degrees of extension loss
- Moderate, when there is 50–89 degrees of extension loss
- Severe when greater than 90 degrees of extension loss exists [3].

Shoulder joint PBC were classified depending on deficit in abduction as follows;

- Mild type; the arm abduction is above 150 degrees,

- Moderate type; limitation of abduction was from 120–150 degrees and the
- Severe type; limitation of abduction to less than 120 degrees [12].

The active range of motion of the joint measured after three months post operation was subtracted from the active range of motion obtained immediately post operation to get the degree of recurrence of post burn contracture.

Ethical consideration
Clearance was obtained from the Faculty Research Ethics Committee of Mbarara University of Science and Technology (FREC-MUST) prior to commencement of the study and the patients or care givers gave informed consent to partake in the study.

Statistical analysis
Data was exported to STATA version 12.1; stratification and univariate analysis was done. Poisson regression methods were used to estimate the overall incidence, risk and respective confidence intervals. A p value of < 0.05 was considered statistically significant.

Results
During the study period 72 patients met the inclusion criteria, 4 patients were excluded because they were not to be followed up at CoRSU. 10 patients were lost to follow-up. 58 patients were analysed.

There were 36 females and 22 males, with a female-to-male ratio of 1.6:1. The age-range was 0.75–45 years, with a median age of 5 years. The average age at time of the initial burn injury was 3.4 years and the commonest cause of the initial burn injury was hot liquids (57 %). Flame burns affected 43 % of the participants [Table 1].

97 % of the participants had been treated in a hospital for the initial burn injury. 67 % of the participants had multiple-joint involvements, with the average number of joints involved by PBC being two. 10 % had prior treatment for post-burn contracture having already had recurrence, and of these 4 patients had recurrence at the shoulder joint and two at the elbow joint. More than half of the participants had had a contracture duration of over a year [Table 1]. The range of participant follow-up was 3 months to 2 years.

Elbow joint
All the PBC were flexion contractures, with a right to left ratio of 1.2:1. Hypertrophic scars affected 15 % right and 26 % of left elbow joints. Keloids affected 11 % right and 13 % of the left elbow joints. No ulcers at the contracture site were observed. Additional file 1 shows a case of elbow post burn contracture and its managment with a local flap.

Table 1 Participants Characteristics

Characteristic	Participants' distribution	
	Number	Percentage
Age categories in years		
≤5 years	29	51.79
>5 years	27	48.21
Gender		
Female	36	62.07
Male	22	37.93
Age categories at initial burn injury		
<1 year	11	18.97
1–5 years	36	62.07
>5 years	11	18.97
Cause of initial burn injury		
Flame	25	43.10
Hot Liquid	33	56.90
Treatment after initial burn injury		
No	2	3.45
Yes	56	96.55
Contracture duration in years		
≤1 year	28	48.28
>1 year	30	51.72
Number of large joints involved by PBCs		
Single	19	32.76
Multiple	39	67.24
Any previous contracture treatment		
No	52	89.66
Yes	6	10.34
Recurrence of elbow PBCs at initial presentation	50	96.15
No	2	3.85
Yes		
Recurrence of shoulder contracture at initial presentation.	54	93.10
No	4	6.90
Yes		

50 % of the elbow joint PBC were managed by skin grafting, and 50 % by local flaps, the commonest being Z-plasty. Complete release of the PBC was achieved in 57 % of the right elbow and 63 % of the left elbow joints [Table 2].

Shoulder joint
The right shoulder joint was more involved than the left shoulder joint, with a right to left ratio of 1.6:1. In the right shoulder joint the anterior fold (Type 1) was the most affected by the contracture where as in the left shoulder joint both the anterior and posterior folds were

Table 2 Operative management employed and completeness of release

Patient treatment	PBC Shoulder		PBC Elbow	
	Right	Left	Right	Left
	N =14 (%)	N = 9 (%)	N = 28 (%)	N = 24 (%)
Operative management				
SSG	1 (7.14)	2 (22.22)	7 (25.00)	5 (20.83)
FTSG	0	0	7 (25.00)	4 (16.67)
Z-plasty	4 (28.57)	1 (11.11)	6 (21.43)	4 (16.67)
Y-V fap	3 (21.43)	2 (22.22)	2 (7.14)	2 (8.33)
Jumping man flap	5 (35.71)	1 (11.11)	2 (7.14)	4 (16.67)
Transposition flap	1 (7.14)	3 (33.33)	4 (14.29)	4 (16.67)
Bilobed flap	0	0	0	1 (4.17)
Completeness of Release of Pbc	N = 14	N = 9	N = 28	N = 24
No	9 (64.29)	6 (66.67)	12 (42.86)	9 (37.50)
Yes	5 (35.71)	3 (33.33)	16 (57.14)	15 (62.50)

equally involved. Hypertrophic scars were present in over 50 % of both joints affected by PBC (57 % right side and 56 % left side). Keloids affected only 22 % of left shoulder joints and 7 % of the right shoulder joint.

The commonest operative technique employed was local flaps. Only 6 patients were managed by split skin grafting and none by full thickness grafts. Complete release of the contracture at the shoulder joint was achieved in 56 % of the right shoulder joint PBC and 33 % of the left joint contractures [Table 2].

The complications observed included wound dehiscence (14 %), wound infection (14 %), skin graft loss (7 %) and flap tip necrosis (7 %).

Patients managed by flaps had shorter hospital stays, approximately 6 days in total; compared to those managed by skin grafting, approximately 10 days. The difference in hospital stay was statistically significant ($p = 0.009$) [Table 3]. Among the patients managed by flaps, physiotherapy was started within 12 days of surgery compared to those managed by skin grafting where physiotherapy was started within 18 days. This difference was however, not statistically significant [Table 3].

Incidence of recurrence of PBC

Out of 58 participants, 30 patients (52 %) had a recurrence of the PBC. The frequency of recurrence of PBCs of the shoulder joint was 67 %, the elbow joint 27 %, and 100 % among participants who had a combination of elbow and shoulder joint PBC.

Risk factors were: flame as the cause of the initial burn ($p = 0.007$), duration of post burn contracture of more than one year ($p = 0.018$), and incomplete release of post burn contracture ($p = 0.002$).

Discussion

In this study 30 participants (52 %) with PBC had a recurrence after operative management. The shoulder joint had a high frequency of recurrence at 67 %. Despite the frequency, the recurrent PBC of the shoulder joint were mostly of mild-to-moderate severity [Table 4]. The elbow joint had a lower frequency of recurrence (27 %) than the shoulder joint. Although the initial PBC of the elbow joint were mostly mild-to-severe, the recurrent contractures were mostly of a negligible-to-mild severity [Table 4]. This shows a general improvement in the active range of motion after operative management. Patients with a combination of elbow and shoulder joint PBC had 100 % recurrence of contractures.

Recurrence of PBC of the shoulder has been reported mostly following management of the contracture with skin grafting. The uneven axillary area presents a challenge for graft application as well as an increased occurrence of graft loss, flap loss and split-skin graft contraction after healing. This is the purported reason for the high recurrence of axillary contractures [11, 13, 14].

In our study the majority of patients with axillary PBC were managed by local flaps, however, we still observed

Table 3 Length of Hospital Stay and Time prior to start of physiotherapy

	Mean (standard deviation) days			Mean difference	p-value
	Overall	Among graft	Among flap		
Hospital stay	7.49(5.70)	10.35(8.22)	5.97(2.92)	4.38	0.009
Time prior to Start of physiotherapy	14.18(10.68)	18.18(14.99)	12.06(6.89)	6.11	0.055

Table 4 Severity of recurrence of post burn contractures

	Shoulder joint	
	Right (%)	Left (%)
Flexion		
Mild	12 (80.00)	5 (62.50)
Moderate	3 (20.00)	3 (37.50)
Severe	0	0
Extension		
Mild	15 (100)	8 (100)
Moderate	0	0
Severe	0	0
Abduction		
Mild	3 (20.00)	2 (25.00)
Moderate	6 (40.00)	3 (37.50)
Severe	6 (40.00)	3 (37.50)
Adduction		
Mild	15 (100)	8 (100)
Moderate	0	0
Severe	0	0
	Elbow Joint	
Extension		
Negligible	15 (55.56)	18 (75.00)
Mild	7 (25.93)	4 (16.67)
Moderate	3 (11.11)	2 (8.33)
Severe	2 (7.41)	0

post burn contracture recurrence. This finding was also reported by other authors [7]. In our study, the PBC of the axilla tended to be severe [Table 5] and residual contractures persisted after surgery [Table 2]. This was compounded by the limited appropriate use of splints; only 38 % of participants used splints, which may have led to recurrence of these contractures. The splints may have been inappropriately used because they were fashioned from Plaster of Paris. Our patients found these splints cumbersome and abandoned them while playing; this finding has been reported by other authors [14].

The severity of the recurrent elbow joint PBC in our study was either negligible (<10 degrees extension deficit) or mild (between 11–49 degrees of extension loss) [Table 4]. This resulted in very little functional limitation, despite post burn contracture recurrence.

The highest incidence of recurrence was observed among patients who had a combination of both elbow and shoulder joint PBC. In our study, 100 % of participants experienced recurrence. All patients who presented to our centre with both elbow and shoulder joint PBC had the two contractures managed in a single operation. The practice of operating on both the elbow and the shoulder joints when a patient presents with a

combination of PBC affecting these joints may have led to the high recurrence in this group. In our study, operating on both joints made post-operative management more demanding, especially the splinting of the joints in the anti-contracture positions and full mobilisation of these joints during physiotherapy. These challenges were especially salient in children. The practice of operating on as many joints as possible has been supported by other authors [11]. This practice is said to reduce costs for the patients and their families and the duration of anaesthetic exposure. However, other authors, such as Hudson et al. [15], recommend the release of the proximal joint followed by the distal joint, with each joint being released completely and rehabilitated to reduce recurrence of PBC.

The other reason for the high incidence of recurrence among the patients with both elbow and shoulder joint involvement may be due to the compensatory motions that patients with axillary joint PBC develop while performing activities of daily living. Plamieri et al. [17] showed that patients with post burn axillary contractures develop compensatory motions which include increased elbow flexion (to aid raising the hand over the head) and reduced internal rotation of the shoulder (to augment shoulder joint flexion). These compensatory motions, the authors believe, subject the patients to an increased risk of recurrence not only at the shoulder joint but also at the elbow joint.

We do believe the best practice may be to release each joint separately and completely, followed by adequate splinting and physiotherapy for the shoulder joint then the distal elbow joint. This would ensure adequate mobilisation of each operated joint and also prevent the compensatory motions that tend to occur in patients who have both axillary and elbow joint PBC.

Factors associated with recurrence of PBC in our study included: flame as the cause of the initial burn injury ($p = 0.007$), duration of contracture of more than one year ($p = 0.018$) and failure to achieve complete release of the contracture ($p = 0.002$). Patients with PBC following flame burn were twice as likely to have recurrence compared to those who had had scalds. Flame burns are usually deep dermal or mixed thickness compared to scalds [16]. Because of this flame, burns may lead to more severe PBC that, if managed inappropriately, could lead to recurrence of the contracture.

Duration of post burn contracture of more than one year was associated with recurrence of PBC. This is contrary to other studies which advocate for the release of the contracture after one year [10, 11]. The waiting period of one year is supposedly to allow the post-burn scar to mature, which is said to reduce the recurrence rate. PBC of a longer duration lead to severe shortening of the musculotendinous units, the joint capsule and the

Table 5 Post Burn Contracture description before and after Operative management

Range of motion	Contracture descriptions			
	Shoulder joint			
	Right		Left	
	Before Treatment %	After Treatment %	Before Treatment %	After Treatment %
Flexion				
Mild	6 (42.86)	11 (78.57)	1 (11.11)	5 (55.56)
Moderate	7 (50.00)	3 (21.43)	5 (55.55)	4 (44.44)
Severe	1 (7.14)	0	3 (33.33)	0
Extension				
Mild	12 (85.71)	14 (100)	5 (55.56)	8 (88.88)
Moderate	1 (7.14)	0	3 (33.33)	1 (11.11)
Severe	1 (7.14)	0	1 (11.11)	0
Abduction				
Mild	1 (7.14)	4 (28.57)	0	3 (33.33)
Moderate	0	7 (50.00)	0	1 (11.11)
Severe	13 (92.86)	3 (21.43)	9 (100)	5 (55.55)
Adduction				
Mild	11 (78.57)	13 (92.86)	5 (55.56)	9 (100)
Moderate	2 (14.29)	1 (7.14)	4 (44.44)	0
Severe	1 (7.14)	0	0	0
	Elbow joint			
Extension				
Negligible	2 (7.14)	17 (60.71)	0	14 (58.33)
Mild	10 (35.71)	6 (21.43)	9 (37.50)	7 (29.17)
Moderate	10 (35.71)	3 (10.71)	11 (45.83)	3 (12.50)
Severe	6 (21.43)	2 (7.14)	4 (16.67)	0

neurovascular structures, which may predispose the patients to recurrence of contractures and our findings are in agreement. However, Schwarz et al. [11] reported that in children a complete range of motion can be expected in spite of the duration of contracture, as long as the operation is done before the child is 12 years old.

Failure to achieve complete release of the contracture was associated with a high risk of recurrence ($p = 0.002$). The residual contractures were observed in cases of severe contracture of long standing duration, in which there was severe shortening of the underlying structures. This made it challenging to safely release the contracture in a single stage. The residual contractures may also have led to compensatory motions especially at the shoulder joint increasing the tendency of recurrence [17].

Physiotherapy has been reported to reduce the incidence of recurrence by ensuring active range of motion of the affected joint [3, 18, 19]. However, in our study, some of the patients who reported having had physiotherapy had a recurrence of PBC. This may be because following wound healing the physiotherapy was started in-hospital and supervised by a therapist. However, upon

reaching home, there was no longer any supervision by a qualified therapist. This is shown in our study, where patients' attendants were the supervisors of the physiotherapy in 57 % of cases, and a qualified therapist in only 10 %. We believe the physiotherapy at home may not have been performed adequately on a daily basis due in part to inadequate supervision and poor pain management.

Factors which were not associated with an increased risk of recurrence of PBC at a statistically significant level included: Age at initial burn injury ($p = 0.671$), presence of keloids ($p = 0.802$), hypertrophic scars ($p = 0.1644$), ulcers at the contracture site ($p = 0.142$), and presence of complications ($p = 0.103$) (including infection, graft loss, wound dehiscence and flap tip necrosis).

Limitation of the study

The duration of follow-up of may not have been enough to determine the frequency of recurrence in all the participants.

The immediate post-operative range of motion could have been limited by post-operative pain and tissue oedema.

The measurement of active range of motion of a joint by goniometry does not translate into the equivalent limitation of recurrent PBC on the activities of daily living. Some patients may be functioning well even with some limitation in the active range of motion as measured by goniometry.

Burning agents in the study were limited to flame and hot liquid.

Materials that have been shown to reduce recurrence of PBC like Acellular dermal matrix (ADM) and Integra were not used due to their prohibitive cost.

Conclusion

Recurrence of PBC of the elbow and shoulder joint is common. Patients who were initially burnt by flame, have contractures for more than one year, have involvement of both the shoulder and elbow joint, and/or have incomplete release of contracture during surgery, are at an increased risk for recurrence.

Surgeons managing PBC of the elbow and/or shoulder joint should take into consideration the associated risk factors and modify operative and post-operative management accordingly. Appropriate splinting, physiotherapy, supervision of the physiotherapy regimen and splint usage should be done to reduce the recurrence rate of PBC.

Recommendation

PBC should be released within the first 12 months if at all possible.

Shoulder joint PBC should be released with flap coverage followed by appropriate use of splints and physiotherapy.

The presence of keloids, hypertrophic scars or ulcers at the contracture site should not deter or delay management of PBC.

Competing interests
The authors declared that they have no competing interests.

Authors' contributions
DDB designed the study, analysed and interpreted the data; GWG interpreted and critically reviewed the manuscript. RA- critically reviewed the manuscript for the intellectual content. All the authors approved the final copy of the manuscript.

Acknowledgement
The authors would like to thank Dr. Humfrey Wanzira for the statistical Analysis, the entire CoRSU staff specifically Dr. Andrew Hodges, Dr. Martin Tungotyo, and Dr. Otim Henry, violet kyakumanya who helped us during the follow-up of the patients and the surgeries.

Author details
[1]Mbarara University of Science and Technology, PO Box 1410, Mbarara, Uganda. [2]CoRSU hospital, PO Box 46, Kisubi, Uganda. [3]College of Health Sciences School of Medicine, Makerere University, PO Box 7062, Kampala, Uganda.

References
1. Schneider JC, Radha H, Helma P, Richard G, Karen K. Contractures in burn injury: Defining the problem. J Burn Care Res. 2006;27:508–14.
2. Oladele AO, Olabanji JK. Burns in Nigeria. Rev Ann Burns Fire Disaster. 2010;23(3):120–7.
3. Richard SJ. Management of Post Burn Contractures of the upper extremity. J Burn Care Res. 2007;28:212–9.
4. A/Samie AM, Mohamed KM. Outcome of conservative management of Burns: Critical Review. Sudan JMS. 2007;2(1):25–8.
5. Viktor GM. Post burn shoulder medial –adduction contracture: Anatomy and treatment with trapeze-plasty. Burns. 2013;39:341–8.
6. Viktor GM. The post –burn elbow medial flexion scar contracture treatment with trapeze flap plasty. Burns. 2009;35:280–7.
7. Ogawa R, Hyakusoku H, Murakami M, Koike S. Reconstruction of axillary scar contractures –retrospective study of 124 cases over 25 years. Br J Plast Surg. 2003;56(2):100–5.
8. Erdem G, Ete UL, Hocaoglu E, Vash KS, Huseyin E. Treatment of post burn upper extremity, neck and facial contractures report of 77 cases. Turkish J Trauma Emergency Surg. 2010;16(5):401–6.
9. Saaiq M, Zaib S, Ahmad S. The menace of post burn contractures: A developing country's perspective. Ann Burns and fire Disasters. 2012;25(3):152–8.
10. Arun G, Prabhat S. Post- burn scars and scar contractures. Indian J Plast Surg. 2010;43:63–71.
11. Schwarz J, Richard, Joshi K D. Management of post burn contractures. J Nepal Med Assoc. 2004;43:211–7.
12. Basha Hamdy MD, Abdulla Mohamed Hamdy FRCS. Classification of post burn axillary contractures: Reappraisal of its Rational. Egypt J Plastic/ reconstructive Surg. 1999;23(2):203–7.
13. Olaitn P.B., Onah I.I., Oduezue A.O., Duru N.E.2007. Options for Axillary contractures. The internet journal of plastic surgery [online] vol 3(1). www.ispub.com.
14. Obaidullah HU, Aslam M. Figure-of-8 sling for prevention of recurrent axillary contracture after release and skin grafting. Burns. 2005;31:283–9.
15. Donald HA, Anthony R. An algorithm for the release of burn contractures of the extremities. Burn. 2006;32:663–8.
16. Chukwuanukwu TOG, Opara KO, Nnabuko REE. Peadiatric post burn contractures in Enungu Nigeria. Nigeria J Plastic Surg. 2007;3(1):1–4.
17. Palmieri LT, Petuskey K, Bagley A, Takashiba S, Greenhalgh DG, Rab TG. Alteration in functional movement after Axillary burn scar contraction: A motion analysis study. J Burn Care Rehabil. 2003;24(2):104–8.
18. Ankur PN. Principles of treatment of burn contractures: Repair and Reconstruction. A J Injury, Deformity Dis. 2001;2(2):12–3.
19. Proctor F. Rehabilitation of a Burn Patient. Indian J Plast Surg. 2010;43(suppl):S101–3.

14

Failed pneumoperitoneum for laparoscopic surgery following autologous Deep Inferior Epigastric Perforator (DIEP) flap breast reconstruction

Daniel M Balkin[1], Quan-Yang Duh[2], Gabriel M Kind[3], David S Chang[3] and Mary H McGrath[1*]

Abstract

Background: Laparoscopic abdominal surgery may prove difficult in patients who have undergone previous abdominal procedures. No reports in the medical literature have presented an aborted laparoscopic procedure for failed pneumoperitoneum following autologous flap-based breast reconstruction.

Case presentation: A 55-year-old woman presented with recurrent invasive lobular carcinoma of the right breast as well as a history of ductal carcinoma in situ of the left breast. The patient desired to proceed with bilateral skin- and nipple-sparing mastectomies with right axillary lymph node biopsy, followed by immediate bilateral autologous deep inferior epigastric perforator (DIEP) flap-based breast reconstruction. Preoperatively, a computerized tomography angiogram was obtained for reconstructive preparation, which revealed a left adrenal mass. Ensuing work-up diagnosed a pheochromocytoma. Given the concern for breast cancer progression, the patient elected to proceed first with breast cancer surgery and reconstruction prior to addressing the adrenal tumor. Subsequently, 3 months later the patient was brought to the operating room for a laparoscopic left adrenalectomy for the pheochromocytoma. With complete pharmacologic abdominal relaxation, the abdomen proved too tight to accommodate sufficient pneumoperitoneum and the laparoscopy was aborted. The patient was evaluated in the outpatient setting for assessment of abdominal wall compliance at regular intervals. Five months later, the patient was taken back to the operating room where pneumoperitoneum was established without difficulty and the laparoscopic left adrenalectomy was performed without complications.

Conclusion: Pneumoperitoneum for laparoscopic surgery subsequent to autologous DIEP flap-based breast reconstruction may prove difficult as a result of loss of abdominal wall compliance. Prior to performing laparoscopy in such patients, surgeons should consider the details of the patient's previous reconstructive procedure and assess potential risk factors for difficulty with insufflation. Lastly, careful abdominal examination should be performed to indicate whether laparoscopy for elective procedures should be delayed until abdominal wall compliance normalizes.

Keywords: Abdominal insufflation, Breast reconstruction, Endocrine surgery, Microsurgery, Minimally invasive surgery

* Correspondence: mary.mcgrath@ucsf.edu
[1]Department of Surgery, Division of Plastic and Reconstructive Surgery,
University of California San Francisco, San Francisco, CA, USA
Full list of author information is available at the end of the article

Background

Laparoscopic abdominal surgery may prove difficult in patients who have undergone previous abdominal procedures. Routine anatomic landmarks may be distorted rendering safe trocar placement challenging. Intra- and retro-peritoneal scaring may increase technical difficulty. In addition, loss of abdominal wall compliance caused by abdominal wall fibrosis, removal of skin and soft tissue, fascial plication or the use of synthetic material may result in inadequate pneumoperitoneum [1–6].

Minimally invasive laparoscopic surgery is one of the most commonly performed procedures in general surgery with over 2 million cases performed annually in the United States [7]. The prevalence of breast reconstruction surgery following mastectomy for breast cancer has also increased [8–11]. In 2013, the American Society of Plastic Surgeons reported that 95,589 breast reconstructive procedures were performed [12]. Various breast reconstructive techniques exist, including several that involve autologous tissue transfer from the anterior abdominal wall.

The deep inferior epigastric perforator (DIEP) flap is a frequent autologous-based breast reconstructive option [12]. In this procedure, the deep inferior epigastric perforating artery and vein, along with the skin and soft tissues supplied by these vessels, is transferred to the chest wall with microvascular anastomoses to reconstruct the breast mound [13, 14].

We are presenting the first reported case of failed pneumoperitoneum for laparoscopy in a patient who had undergone previous DIEP flap-based breast reconstruction. Recommendations for recognizing and addressing loss of abdominal wall distensibility in patients who have had breast reconstruction with abdominal wall tissue are discussed.

Case presentation

A 55-year-old woman presented with recurrent invasive lobular carcinoma of the right breast following previous lumpectomy and partial irradiation for invasive lobular carcinoma. Ductal carcinoma in situ of the opposite left breast also had been treated in the past with lumpectomy. Given the patient history and the recurrence of disease in the right breast, bilateral skin- and nipple-sparing mastectomies with right axillary sentinel lymph node biopsy were planned. These would be followed by immediate bilateral autologous DIEP flap-based breast reconstructions.

Preoperatively, a computerized tomography angiogram was obtained to evaluate the perforator vascular anatomy of the anterior abdominal wall. This study showed a 2.5–3.0-cm left adrenal mass. Subsequent work-up diagnosed a pheochromocytoma. The patient was offered a laparoscopic adrenalectomy after alpha-blockade in addition to a genetic evaluation for hereditary causes of

pheochromocytoma. She was advised to undergo an adrenalectomy first before moving forward with oncologic and reconstructive breast surgery. However, given her concern for breast cancer progression, the patient preferred to proceed first with the breast cancer surgery and reconstruction to be followed with later surgery to address the adrenal tumor.

Under consultation with the patient's Endocrinologist, alpha-blockade (phenoxybenzamine) was initiated 2 weeks before surgery to prevent pheochromocytoma crisis and beta blockage (propanolol) was started 1 week later for heart rate control. Subsequently, bilateral skin- and nipple-sparing mastectomies were initiated with simultaneous abdominal tissue harvest for the reconstruction. Figure 1 a Doppler probe was used to identify the dominant perforators of the abdominal wall on each side of the midline. As the skin and soft tissue flap was developed, dissection on the right side in the suprafascial plane showed the perforating vessels to be small, measuring less than 1.0-mm in diameter. To avoid injury to these vessels, the

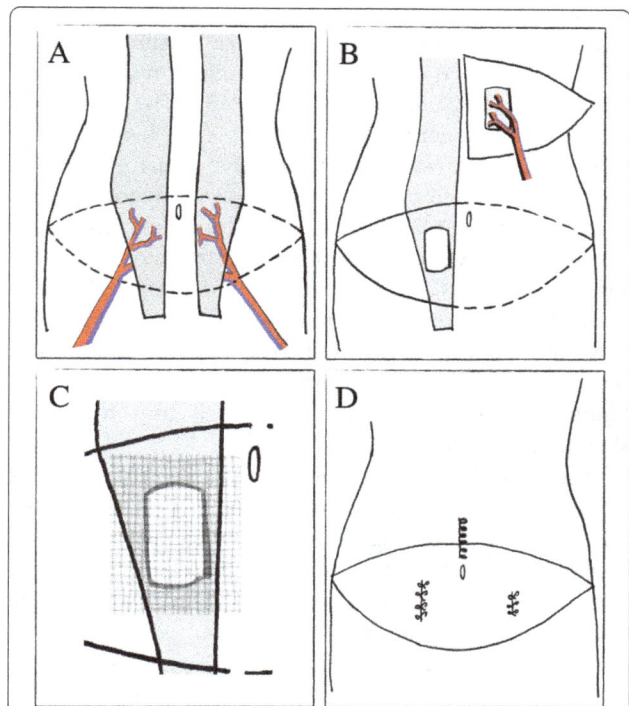

Fig. 1 Illustrations of Various Operative Stages of Patient's Breast Reconstruction. **a** Abdominal wall depicting bilateral rectus abdominis muscles (*grey*) with associated deep inferior epigastric arteries (*red*) and veins (*blue*). Dashed line indicates skin and soft tissue flaps harvested for breast reconstruction; **b** Right-sided DIEP flap used to recreate the left breast mound superimposed over left chest wall. Flap includes a portion of the right rectus abdominis muscle (*grey*) and rectus fascia to surround and protect the perforating vessels; **c** Small defect in right rectus abdominis muscle and fascia with a mesh underlay repair (hatched area reflects SeriScaffold® mesh); **d** Areas of rectus abdominis fascial plication

customary transmuscular dissection of the vessels was changed to include in the flap a 4 × 3-cm portion of the right rectus abdominis muscle and 4 × 2-cm portion of rectus fascia to surround and protect the vessels. On the left side, the perforating vessels to the flap also were small, but only a small cuff of rectus abdominis muscle and fascia was included in the flap. On both sides, only the deep inferior epigastric vessels were used for blood supply.

Following completion of the bilateral mastectomies, the internal mammary arteries and veins were isolated by removing a short segment of the third costal cartilage. The deep inferior epigastric vessels of the abdominal flaps were divided and microvascular anastomoses were performed between the deep inferior epigastric artery and vein and the internal mammary artery and vein on each side. With strong flow through the anastomoses, the flaps were deepithelialized (with the exception of a small skin paddle along the inframammary fold for postoperative monitoring), and inset in the mastectomy defects. The abdominal wall donor sites were then closed. Because the 4 × 3 cm segment of rectus abdominis muscle and fascia had been included on the right side to protect the vessels, the fascial closure was reinforced with a 4 × 6-cm piece of SeriScaffold® mesh (knitted, multi-filament, bioengineered silk) [15]. The mesh was placed as an underlay deep to the rectus fascia secured with 1 PDS mattress sutures, and the fascial edges were then approximated over the mesh with 0 Ethibond figure-of-eight sutures. On the left side, the rectus abdominis fascial closure was completed with 0 Ethibond and 1 PDS sutures. In order to prevent bulging in the upper abdomen where tissue had not been removed, the fascia was tightened by placating with an 0 PDS running suture. The remaining abdominal skin was advanced and closed in layers with exteriorization of the umbilicus through the skin in the midline (Fig. 2).

Three months later, the patient was brought to the Operating Room for a laparoscopic left adrenalectomy for the pheochromocytoma. Figure 3 with the patient in position and with complete pharmacologic abdominal relaxation, a Veress needle was placed for insufflation. However, the abdomen proved too tight to accommodate sufficient pneumoperitoneum. Given that inadequate abdominal wall distensibility was responsible for inadequate insufflation, rather than difficulty with Veress needle placement, open trocar placement was not undertaken. A laparoscopic retroperitoneal approach was not attempted because it also relies on creating working space through insufflation-mediated abdominal wall expansion [16–18]. Thus, the laparoscopy was aborted without incision. The adrenalectomy was not converted to an open procedure for several considerations: the patient's reluctance to proceed with an open intervention; because pharmacological management of pheochromocytoma via alpha

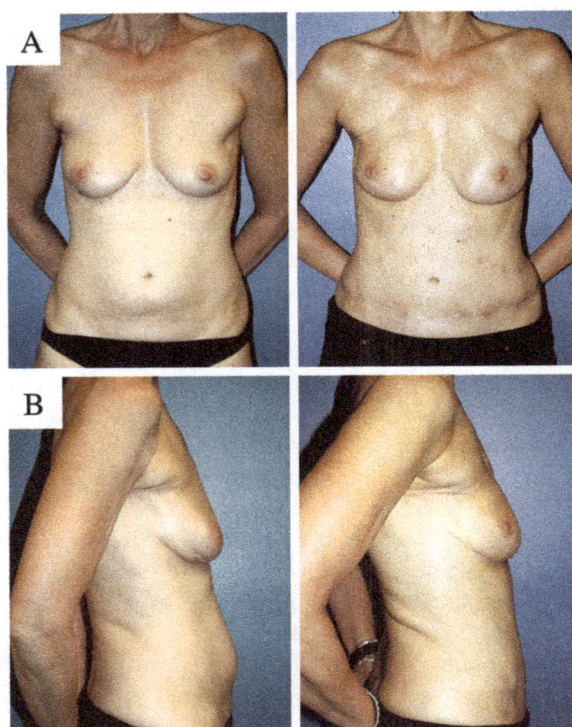

Fig. 2 Patient Photographs Pre and Post Breast Cancer Surgery and Reconstruction. **a** Frontal and **b** lateral views (*left*, pre-operative; *right*, post-operative). Note degree of abdominal wall tightening post-operatively

blockade rendered the procedure non-emergent [19, 20]; and the belief that primary closure would be troublesome.

While kept on pharmacological management of the pheochromocytoma, the patient was evaluated in the outpatient setting for assessment of abdominal wall compliance at regular intervals. Five months later, the patient's abdomen was felt to be compliant and she was taken back to the Operating Room for a laparoscopic left adrenalectomy. Pneumoperitoneum was established by Veress needle placement at Palmer's point and the abdomen accommodated 3 l of pneumoperitoneum. The left adrenalectomy proceeded routinely and the patient was discharged home the following day.

Discussion

This is the first report in the literature of an aborted laparoscopic procedure for failed pneumoperitoneum following autologous flap-based breast reconstruction. Given the frequency of laparoscopy and abdominal-based breast cancer reconstruction in current surgical practice, this case provides some insight into an important aspect of surgical disease management that has not been recognized or discussed in the literature.

Exposure of the surgical field during laparoscopic surgery is achieved by obtaining peritoneal access in order

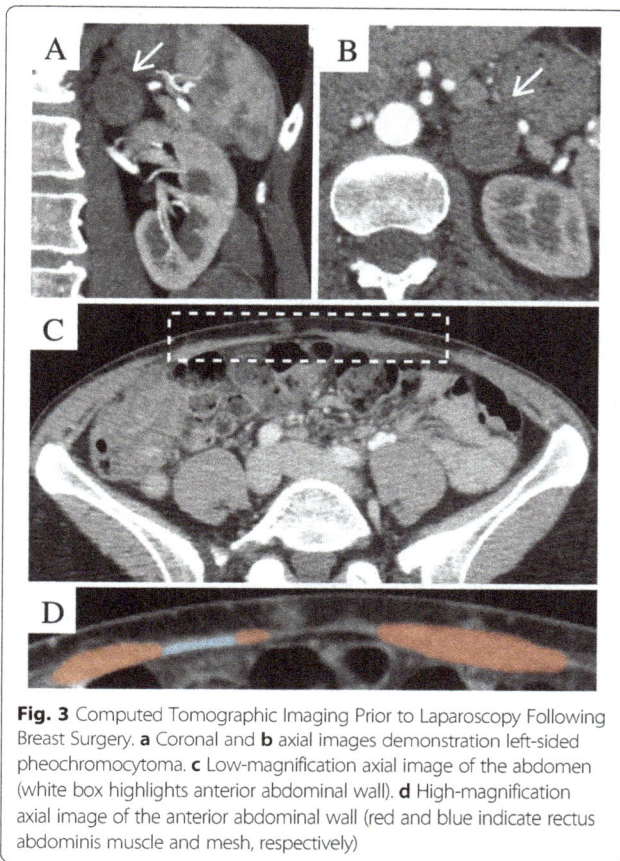

Fig. 3 Computed Tomographic Imaging Prior to Laparoscopy Following Breast Surgery. **a** Coronal and **b** axial images demonstration left-sided pheochromocytoma. **c** Low-magnification axial image of the abdomen (white box highlights anterior abdominal wall). **d** High-magnification axial image of the anterior abdominal wall (red and blue indicate rectus abdominis muscle and mesh, respectively)

to create a carbon dioxide pneumoperitoneum. This changes the abdominal wall shape from a cylinder to a dome and expands the abdominal wall surface by 15–20 % [21–23]. The factors that govern the degree of expansion of the surgical working space with pneumoperitoneum continue to be studied, but known factors include age and body size of individuals, as well as the effect of employing neuromuscular blockade, elevated intraabdominal pressures and pre-stretching of the abdominal wall [24].

Difficulties associated with performing laparoscopy in patients who have undergone prior abdominal wall surgery, such as abdominoplasty [1, 2, 4, 25], umbilical hernia repair [26] and transverse rectus abdominis myocutaneous flap-based breast reconstruction [27], along with techniques to overcome such challenges, have been described previously. First, the altered abdominal wall anatomy resulting from previous surgery makes safe and proper trocar placement challenging. The reconstructed umbilicus, which is often the anatomic landmark used to define the midline and inform placement of a Veress needle, may lie left or right of its native location [4]. In such cases, alternate stable landmarks can be used for reference, such as the xiphoid bone or the left subcostal pararectus region, Palmer's point [28]. In addition, others employ alternate

techniques for trocar placement, such as the modified open Hasson technique or the use of direct visual entry systems [25, 27, 29, 30].

Second, trocar perforation can be difficult in patients with previous abdominal surgery if the abdominal wall is fibrotic or scarred [2]. Operative modifications for safe and effective port placement in this setting include providing counter traction with towel clamps and using sharp dissection to perforate fibrosis [4].

Third, prior surgical procedures to tighten the abdominal wall, such as abdominoplasty, can prevent adequate pneumoperitoneum due to diminished abdominal wall compliance. This can result in working space deficiency. Loss of abdominal wall compliance was a major technical limitation described in a study detailing a technical approach to laparoscopic colectomy in patients who had previously undergone abdominoplasty [1]. The loss of abdominal wall compliance was thought secondary to fascial plication and skin removal [1, 4]. To recruit additional abdominal space, some advocate placing patients into the reverse Trendelenburg position with flexion of the legs at the hips [31].

In the present study, unsuccessful laparoscopic transperitoneal adrenalectomy was attempted 3 months following breast reconstruction. The patient's peritoneal cavity was accessed with a Veress needle but the abdominal wall was not sufficiently compliant to accommodate pneumoperitoneum. It is likely that several factors associated with the patient's body habitus and the DIEP flap-based breast reconstruction contributed to difficulty establishing pneumoperitoneum. The patient was nulliparous and slender with a 65.9-kg preoperative weight and 21.2 body mass index, and there was minimal fascial relaxation and little excess abdominal soft tissue. Removal of sufficient soft tissue for bilateral breast reconstruction meant that primary closure of the abdominal skin and soft tissue would necessarily be tight. This was exacerbated in this patient with the removal of a segment of rectus fascia and muscle to protect the small caliber perforating vessels to the abdominal wall. On the right side where rectus abdominis muscle and fascia were removed, the defect was repaired with placement of SeriScaffold® mesh beneath the fascia. Studies of synthetic mesh of various composition, including polypropylene, polyester and proline, show that abdominal mesh implantation diminishes abdominal wall compliance [32, 33]. Moreover, the abdominal wall fascia was plicated and therefore tightened at several points: superficial to the mesh underlay to reinforce the repair on the right, in the upper quadrants of the abdomen to reduce postoperatively bulging, and on the left where the small cuff of muscle was excised to protect the microvessels. Fascial plication tightens the abdominal wall, elevates intraabdominal pressures and in extreme cases has been shown to cause abdominal compartment syndrome

[34, 35]. Collectively, it is likely that removal of significant abdominal wall tissue in a slender patient, placement of abdominal wall mesh, and fascial plication all contributed to significantly decrease the abdominal wall compliance and preclude sufficient pneumoperitoneum.

Pharmacologic management of pheochromocytoma usually precedes other treatments because it can be immediately life threatening. Alpha-blockade is essential to normalize blood pressure, to expand contracted blood volume and to prevent severe intraoperative hypertension. Beta-blockade may also need to be employed to control heart rate, but only after establishing adequate alpha blockade to avoid unopposed alpha stimulation that can precipitate hypertensive crisis. Once the patient is stabilized medically, operative resection can proceed electively [19, 20, 36]. In this case it was the patient's preference to undergo breast cancer surgery and reconstruction prior to laparoscopic adrenalectomy, which was safe medically once the patient was fully alpha-blocked. In retrospect, however, delaying the breast surgery until after laparoscopy would have obviated the difficulties associated with abdominal wall compliance.

To date, the appropriate timing of laparoscopic surgery following abdominal wall-based breast reconstruction has not been discussed. In the present case, following the first aborted procedure, the patient was evaluated in the outpatient setting with serial abdominal exams. Over the course of 5 months, the patient's abdominal wall became notably softer and increasingly pliable. Subsequently, 8 months following breast reconstruction, the patient was taken to the Operating Room for a laparoscopic adrenalectomy where pneumoperitoneum was achieved without difficulty. This case shows that abdominal wall compliance after surgery changes impressively over time and that a return of abdominal wall pliability suitable for pneumoperitoneum is regained.

This report highlights an important area of investigative inquiry. It would be of interest to determine the time course of changes in abdominal wall compliance following abdominal wall surgery. Moreover, it would be important to determine whether objective measures and/or tools exist to assess abdominal wall compliance, similar to what has been described for burn scar assessment and softening [37–39].

For the surgeon scheduling a laparoscopic procedure for a patient who has had prior abdominal wall surgery, including development of flaps for breast reconstruction, preoperative evaluation may indicate that pneumoperitoneum will be problematic. If the laparoscopic procedure is elective, the surgery should be delayed. If not, the informed consent discussion should also include the possibility of aborted procedure for insufficient pneumoperitoneum, or the need for conversion to an open approach.

Conclusions

Pneumoperitoneum for laparoscopic surgery following autologous deep inferior epigastric (DIEP) perforator flap breast reconstruction may prove difficult as a result of loss of abdominal wall compliance. Surgeons should consider the details of the patient's breast reconstructive procedure in order to identify patients at risk for difficult pneumoperitoneum. Potential risk factors for difficulty with insufflation after breast reconstruction performed with abdominal tissue include: slender body habitus, nulliparous patient with minimal fascial relaxation, autologous flap-based reconstruction necessitating tight abdominal wall closure, placement of abdominal wall synthetic mesh, and fascial plication to tighten the remaining portions of the abdomen wall.

In the preoperative assessment of patients for laparoscopic surgery following abdominal wall-based breast reconstruction, history and careful abdominal exam to assess abdominal wall stiffness may indicate that laparoscopy for elective procedures should be delayed until abdominal wall compliance normalizes.

Abbreviations
DIEP: deep inferior epigastric perforator.

Competing interests
GMK has received research support from Allergan and is also a speaker for Allergan, LifeCell and Novadaq. DSC is a consultant for Mentor and LifeCell. None of the other authors has a financial interest in any of the products, devices or drugs mentioned in this manuscript.

Authors' contributions
MHM, QD and DMB conceived the study, acquired the data and drafted the manuscript; MHM, QD, DMB, GMK and DSC performed analysis and interpretation of data and provided critical revision; QD, GMK and DSC treated the patient. All authors read and approved the final manuscript.

Authors' information
Not applicable.

Acknowledgements
Thank you to Dr. Emily Morell Balkin for her artistic illustrations as well as to Dr. Robert Bell for his thoughtful discussion related to attempted abdominal insufflation in the setting of poor abdominal wall compliance.

Funding
This work was supported by the UCSF Open Access Publishing Fund.

Author details
[1]Department of Surgery, Division of Plastic and Reconstructive Surgery, University of California San Francisco, San Francisco, CA, USA. [2]Department of Surgery, Section of Endocrine Surgery, University of California San Francisco, San Francisco, CA, USA. [3]Department of Plastic Surgery, California-Pacific Medical Center, San Francisco, CA, USA.

References

1. Atallah S, Albert M, Felix O, Izfar S, Debeche-Adams T, Larach S. The technical approach to laparoscopic colectomy in patients who have undergone prior abdominoplasty. Tech Coloproctol. 2013;17(1):111–6.
2. Bisson MA, Breeson AJ, Henderson HP. Failed pneumoperitoneum post abdominoplasty. Eur J Plast Surg. 2007;30(3):147–8.
3. Dodson MG. The treatment of failed laparoscopy using open laparoscopy. Int J Gynaecol Obstet. 1984;22(4):331–4.
4. Karip B, Altun H, Iscan Y, Bazan M, Celik K, Ozcabi Y, Agca B, Memisoglu K. Difficulties of bariatric surgery after abdominoplasty. Case Rep Surg. 2014; 2014:620175.
5. Morris L, Ituarte P, Zarnegar R, Duh QY, Ahmed L, Lee J, Inabnet W 3rd, Meyer-Rochow G, Sidhu S, Sywak M, et al. Laparoscopic adrenalectomy after prior abdominal surgery. World J Surg. 2008;32(5):897–903.
6. Peterson EP, Behrman SJ. Laparoscopic tubal sterilization. Am J Obstet Gynecol. 1971;110(1):24–31.
7. Fuller J, Ashar BS, Carey-Corrado J. Trocar-associated injuries and fatalities: an analysis of 1399 reports to the FDA. J Minim Invasive Gynecol. 2005;12(4): 302–7.
8. Gomez SL, Lichtensztajn D, Kurian AW, Telli ML, Chang ET, Keegan TH, Glaser SL, Clarke CA. Increasing mastectomy rates for early-stage breast cancer? Population-based trends from California. J Clin Oncol. 2010;28(10):e155–7. author reply e158.
9. Howard-McNatt MM. Patients opting for breast reconstruction following mastectomy: an analysis of uptake rates and benefit. Breast Cancer (Dove Med Press). 2013;5:9–15.
10. Kummerow KL, Du L, Penson DF, Shyr Y, Hooks MA. Nationwide trends in mastectomy for early-stage breast cancer. JAMA Surg. 2015;150(1):9–16.
11. McGuire KP, Santillan AA, Kaur P, Meade T, Parbhoo J, Mathias M, Shamehdi C, Davis M, Ramos D, Cox CE. Are mastectomies on the rise? A 13-year trend analysis of the selection of mastectomy versus breast conservation therapy in 5865 patients. Ann Surg Oncol. 2009;16(10):2682–90.
12. Surgeons ASoP. 2013 Plastic Surgery Statistics Report. 2013.
13. Allen RJ, Treece P. Deep inferior epigastric perforator flap for breast reconstruction. Ann Plast Surg. 1994;32(1):32–8.
14. Guerra AB, Metzinger SE, Bidros RS, Rizzuto RP, Gill PS, Nguyen AH, Dupin CL, Allen RJ. Bilateral breast reconstruction with the deep inferior epigastric perforator (DIEP) flap: an experience with 280 flaps. Ann Plast Surg. 2004; 52(3):246–52.
15. Serica Technologies, Inc. Section 510(k) Summary (SeriScaffold Surgical Mesh). U.S. Department of Health and Human Services, Food and Drug Administration. http://www.accessdata.fda.gov/cdrh_docs/pdf8/K080442.pdf.
16. Walz MK, Alesina PF, Wenger FA, Deligiannis A, Szuczik E, Petersenn S, Ommer A, Groeben H, Peitgen K, Janssen OE, et al. Posterior retroperitoneoscopic adrenalectomy–results of 560 procedures in 520 patients. Surgery. 2006;140(6):943–8. discussion 948–950.
17. Hisano M, Vicentini FC, Srougi M. Retroperitoneoscopic adrenalectomy in pheochromocytoma. Clinics (Sao Paulo). 2012;67 Suppl 1:161–7.
18. Walz MK, Alesina PF, Wenger FA, Koch JA, Neumann HP, Petersenn S, Schmid KW, Mann K. Laparoscopic and retroperitoneoscopic treatment of pheochromocytomas and retroperitoneal paragangliomas: results of 161 tumors in 126 patients. World J Surg. 2006;30(5):899–908.
19. Lenders JW, Duh QY, Eisenhofer G, Gimenez-Roqueplo AP, Grebe SK, Murad MH, Naruse M, Pacak K, Young WF Jr. Pheochromocytoma and paraganglioma: an endocrine society clinical practice guideline. J Clin Endocrinol Metab. 2014;99(6):1915–42.
20. Scholten A, Cisco RM, Vriens MR, Cohen JK, Mitmaker EJ, Liu C, Tyrrell JB, Shen WT, Duh QY. Pheochromocytoma crisis is not a surgical emergency. J Clin Endocrinol Metab. 2013;98(2):581–91.
21. Song C, Alijani A, Frank T, Hanna G, Cuschieri A. Elasticity of the living abdominal wall in laparoscopic surgery. J Biomech. 2006;39(3):587–91.
22. Song C, Alijani A, Frank T, Hanna GB, Cuschieri A. Mechanical properties of the human abdominal wall measured in vivo during insufflation for laparoscopic surgery. Surg Endosc. 2006;20(6):987–90.
23. Srivastava A, Niranjan A. Secrets of safe laparoscopic surgery: Anaesthetic and surgical considerations. J Minim Access Surg. 2010;6(4):91–4.
24. Vlot J, Staals LM, Wijnen RM, Stolker RJ, Bax KN. Optimizing working space in laparoscopy: CT measurement of the influence of small body size in a porcine model. J Pediatr Surg. 2015;50(3):465–71.
25. Cassaro S, Leitman IM. A technique for laparoscopic peritoneal entry after abdominoplasty. J Laparoendosc Adv Surg Tech A. 2013;23(12):990–1.
26. Vellinga TT, De Alwis S, Suzuki Y, Einarsson JI. Laparoscopic entry: the modified alwis method and more. Rev Obstet Gynecol. 2009;2(3):193–8.
27. Tsahalina E, Crawford R. Laparoscopic surgery following abdominal wall reconstruction: description of a novel method for safe entry. BJOG. 2004; 111(12):1452–3.
28. Tufek I, Akpinar H, Sevinc C, Kural AR. Primary left upper quadrant (Palmer's point) access for laparoscopic radical prostatectomy. Urol J. 2010;7(3):152–6.
29. Ahmad G, O'Flynn H, Duffy JM, Phillips K, Watson A. Laparoscopic entry techniques. Cochrane Database Syst Rev. 2012;2:CD006583.
30. Altun H, Banli O, Karakoyun R, Boyuk A, Okuducu M, Onur E, Memisoglu K. Direct trocar insertion technique for initial access in morbid obesity surgery: technique and results. Surg Laparosc Endosc Percutan Tech. 2010;20(4):228–30.
31. Mulier JP, Dillemans B, Van Cauwenberge S. Impact of the patient's body position on the intraabdominal workspace during laparoscopic surgery. Surg Endosc. 2010;24(6):1398–402.
32. Junge K, Klinge U, Prescher A, Giboni P, Niewiera M, Schumpelick V. Elasticity of the anterior abdominal wall and impact for reparation of incisional hernias using mesh implants. Hernia. 2001;5(3):113–8.
33. Muller M, Klinge U, Conze J, Schumpelick V. Abdominal wall compliance after Marlex mesh implantation for incisional hernia repair. Hernia. 1998;2:113–7.
34. Graca Neto L, Araujo LR, Rudy MR, Auersvald LA, Graf R. Intraabdominal pressure in abdominoplasty patients. Aesthetic Plast Surg. 2006;30(6):655–8.
35. Izadpanah A, Karunanayake M, Petropolis C, Deckelbaum DL, Luc M. Abdominal compartment syndrome following abdominoplasty: A case report and review. Indian J Plast Surg. 2014;47(2):263–6.
36. Garg MK, Kharb S, Brar KS, Gundgurthi A, Mittal R. Medical management of pheochromocytoma: Role of the endocrinologist. Indian J Endocrinol Metab. 2011;15 Suppl 4:S329–36.
37. Cleary C, Sanders AK, Nick TG. Reliability of the skin compliance device in the assessment of scar pliability. J Hand Ther. 2007;20(3):232–7. quiz 238.
38. Fearmonti R, Bond J, Erdmann D, Levinson H. A review of scar scales and scar measuring devices. Eplasty. 2010;10:e43.
39. Lye I, Edgar DW, Wood FM, Carroll S. Tissue tonometry is a simple, objective measure for pliability of burn scar: is it reliable? J Burn Care Res. 2006;27(1):82–5.

15

Clinical value of a prophylactic minitracheostomy after esophagectomy: analysis in patients at high risk for postoperative pulmonary complications

Yayoi Sakatoku, Masahide Fukaya*, Kazushi Miyata, Keita Itatsu and Masato Nagino

Abstract

Background: The aim of this study is to evaluate the clinical value of a prophylactic minitracheostomy (PMT) in patients undergoing an esophagectomy for esophageal cancer and to clarify the indications for a PMT.

Methods: Ninety-four patients who underwent right transthoracic esophagectomy for esophageal cancer between January 2009 and December 2013 were studied. Short surgical outcomes were retrospectively compared between 30 patients at high risk for postoperative pulmonary complications who underwent a PMT (PMT group) and 64 patients at standard risk without a PMT (non-PMT group). Furthermore, 12 patients who required a delayed minitracheostomy (DMT) due to postoperative sputum retention were reviewed in detail, and risk factors related to a DMT were also analyzed to assess the indications for a PMT.

Results: Preoperative pulmonary function was lower in the PMT group than in the non-PMT group: FEV1.0 (2.41 vs. 2.68 L, $p = 0.035$), and the proportion of patients with FEV1.0% <60 (13.3% vs. 0%, $p = 0.009$). No between-group differences were observed in the proportion of patients who suffered from postoperative pneumonia, atelectasis, or re-intubation due to respiratory failure. Of the 12 patients with a DMT, 11 developed postoperative pneumonia, and three required re-intubation due to severe pneumonia. Multivariate analysis revealed FEV1.0% <70% and vocal cord palsy were independent risk factors related to a DMT.

Conclusion: A PMT for high-risk patients may prevent an increase in the incidence of postoperative pneumonia and re-intubation. The PMT indications should be expanded for patients with vocal cord palsy or mild obstructive respiratory disturbances.

Keywords: Minitracheostomy, Postoperative pneumonia, Esophagectomy

Background

In Japan, the standard surgical procedure for esophageal cancer is subtotal esophagectomy with extended lymph node dissection, which requires the skeletonization of the upper mediastinal structures. This procedure is highly invasive, with high morbidity and mortality rates [1, 2]. Postoperative pneumonia is the most serious complication after esophagectomy and is a major risk factor for in-hospital mortality [3]. Impairment of the swallowing function due to cervical lymph node dissection and vocal cord palsy resulting from para-laryngeal nerve lymph node dissection both cause pulmonary aspiration. The impairment of postoperative pulmonary function and postoperative chest pain induce difficulty in expectoration, which can lead to sputum retention and postoperative pneumonia.

Although bronchoscopic aspiration is typically performed for sputum retention, this procedure requires trained bronchoscopists; a significant delay often occurs from onset to treatment. Bronchoscopic aspiration places a large burden on patients. Local anesthetic administered to the mucous membranes of the pharynx, larynx, and trachea often

* Correspondence: mafukaya@med.nagoya-u.ac.jp
Division of Surgical Oncology, Department of Surgery, Nagoya University
Graduate School of Medicine, 65 Tsurumai-cho, Showa-ku, Nagoya 466-8550,
Japan

induces the pulmonary aspiration of intraoral bacteria. However, a minitracheostomy allows nursing staff without specialized training to have immediate access to the bronchial tree. The introduction of a catheter into the trachea through the minitracheostomy typically evokes an effective cough that helps clear secretions.

Previous authors have reported that a prophylactic minitracheostomy (PMT) helps prevent postoperative pulmonary complications in patients who undergo pulmonary resection for lung cancer [4–8]. However, given the limited number of available reports, the clinical value of a PMT is unclear in patients undergoing an esophagectomy. Since January 2009, we have used a PMT in patients at a high risk for postoperative pulmonary complications to decrease these complications. The aim of this study was to evaluate the clinical value of a PMT in patients undergoing an esophagectomy for esophageal cancer and to clarify the indications for a PMT.

Methods
Patients
From January 2009 to December 2013, 99 patients underwent a right transthoracic esophagectomy via muscle sparing thoracotomy (MST) as reported previously [9]. Of these, two patients with a previous laryngectomy and one patient with a synchronous laryngectomy were excluded. Two other patients who underwent a tracheostomy for delayed extubation were also excluded. Thus, the remaining 94 patients were subjected to analysis. The ethical committee of Nagoya University Hospital approved our study (No. 2016–0361); written informed consent was obtained from all patients.

Surgical procedures
All patients underwent a right transthoracic esophagectomy via MST with mediastinal lymphadenectomy, including bilateral recurrent laryngeal nerve lymph node dissection and laparotomy for dissecting abdominal lymph nodes, to establish a reconstructive conduit. Thoracotomy was followed by laparotomy in patients with borderline resectable tumors, while laparotomy was followed by thoracotomy in all other patients. The gastric tube was selected as the primary reconstructive conduit. The percutaneous route was chosen in patients who were older or who had liver cirrhosis, and the retrosternal route was used in patients with possible residual tumors (R1/2 resection). In the other patients, the choice of the reconstruction route that was used depended on the surgeon's preference. Reconstruction with a pedicled jejunum was performed via the percutaneous route in all patients who had previously undergone or synchronously underwent gastrectomy.

Prophylactic minitracheostomy
The tracheal tube was routinely extubated on the first postoperative day if the general condition of the patients was stable. The degree of vocal cord palsy was evaluated by bronchoscopy in all patients just after extubation, and a PMT was subsequently performed using a Minitrach II® (SIMS Portex, Hythe, Kent, UK) with the percutaneous Seldinger technique for patients at high risk of postoperative pulmonary complications. These patients included elderly patients over 80 years of age, patients with vocal cord palsy and the presence of a slit between the vocal cords, patients with low pulmonary function [(a forced expiratory volume in 1 s (FEV1.0) <1.5 L or a percent predicted forced expiratory volume in 1 s (FEV1.0%) <60%)], patients with preoperative pneumonia, including interstitial pneumonia, and patients with aspiration noted in an upper gastrointestinal image (Table 1). Routine prophylactic aspiration by bronchoscopy was never performed. A mini-tracheal tube was extubated unless the patients developed pulmonary aspiration after the start of oral intake. A total of 30 patients underwent a PMT; 16 patients were selected to undergo a PMT before surgery, and the remaining 14 patients underwent a PMT after surgery. We performed a delayed minitracheostomy (DMT) following bronchoscopic aspiration for patients with postoperative sputum retention despite the presence of vocal cord palsy.

Perioperative care
All patients received intravenous injections of methylprednisolone to attenuate the inflammatory responses as follows: 250 mg intravenously 1 h before the start of surgery, 125 mg on day 1, and 80 mg on day 2. One epidural catheter was intubated between the fifth and sixth thoracic vertebra, and another epidural catheter was intubated between the ninth and tenth thoracic vertebra. Continuous epidural anesthesia with fentanyl and ropivacaine or levobupivacaine was used until day 6. An intravenous drip injection of pentazocine (15 mg) or buprenorphine (3 mg) was administered as needed until day 10. An injection of loxoprofen or pregabalin was administered via feeding

Table 1 Indication of prophylactic minitracheostomy

Indication	Number of patients
Preoperative	
Old age	2
Low pulmonary function	5
Preoperative pneumonia	5
Aspiration	3
Low pulmonary function + Aspiration	1
Postoperative	
Vocal cord palsy	14

tube from day 11 until the start of oral intake. Computed tomography (CT) was performed on day 7 in all patients. Atelectasis was assessed by radiological evidence of plate atelectasis, labor collapse, or total lung collapse as shown on the CT image.

Postoperative complications were defined as any event requiring specific medical or surgical treatment and were assessed according to the Clavien-Dindo classification [10]. A PMT was not considered to be a grade 3 pulmonary complication.

Statistical analyses

The results are expressed as the median (range). Fisher's exact probability test and the Mann-Whitney U test were used for analysis as appropriate. Univariate and multivariate analyses were performed using a logistic regression model to identify the independent factors that were associated with postoperative pneumonia. In the multivariate analysis, the factors that showed a p value of <0.200 in the univariate analysis were selected and subjected to a stepwise logistic regression analysis. All statistical analyses were performed with SPSS software version 20.0 J. The two-sided p values were calculated and are presented. A p value of <0.05 was considered statistically significant.

Results

Patient characteristics

No significant differences were observed between the PMT and non-PMT groups in terms of the age, gender, tumor location, clinical stage, or proportion of patients who underwent preoperative chemotherapy, preoperative chemoradiotherapy, or a salvage operation (Table 2). Regarding the preoperative pulmonary function, the FEV1.0 was significantly lower in the PMT group than that in the non-PMT group. The proportion of patients with FEV1.0% less than 60% was significantly higher in the PMT group than that in the non-PMT group.

Surgical procedures

The surgical procedures are summarized in Table 3. No between-group differences were observed in the proportion of patients requiring cervical lymph node dissection, a reconstructive organ, a reconstructive route, and an anastomotic portion. The operative time and blood loss were similar between the two groups.

Postoperative outcomes

The duration of intubation was significantly longer in the PMT group than in the non-PMT group (Table 4). No significant differences were observed between the two groups in terms of the incidence of grade 2 postoperative pneumonia and atelectasis. Of the 64 non-PMT patients, 12 patients required a DMT due to postoperative

Table 2 Patients' characteristics

Variables	PMT group (n = 30)	Non-PMT group (n = 64)	P
Age [year]	68.5 (51–86)	65.0 (43–78)	0.071
Gender (male/female)	23/7	57/7	0.131
Location of tumor, n (%)			0.413
Ut	6 (20.0)	6 (9.4)	
Mt	13 (43.3)	36 (56.2)	
Lt	9 (30.3)	16 (25.0)	
Ae	2 (6.7)	6 (9.4)	
cStage (UICC 7th), n (%)			0.153
I	5 (16.7)	25 (39.1)	
II	10 (33.3)	14 (21.9)	
III	12 (40.0)	20 (31.2)	
IV	3 (10.0)	5 (7.8)	
Neoadjuvant chemotherapy, n (%)	14 (46.7)	26 (40.6)	0.652
Neoadjuvant chemoradiotherapy, n (%)	6 (20.0)	5 (7.8)	0.099
Salvage operation, n (%)	1 (3.3)	4 (6.3)	1.000
Preoperative pulmonary function			
VC [L]	3.51 (2.03–5.43)	3.66 (2.05–5.57)	0.113
%VC	114 (67–134)	110 (76–166)	0.703
FEV1.0 [L]	2.41 (1.11–3.36)	2.68 (1.59–4.13)	0.035
FEV1.0%	71.5 (53.2–91.3)	76.4 (60.2–93.8)	0.160
FEV1.0% < 60%, n (%)	4 (13.3)	0	0.009

PMT prophylactic minitracheostomy

sputum retention, and seven required re-intubation. The incidence of vocal cord palsy was significantly higher in the PMT group than that in the non-PMT group because a PMT was performed for patients with vocal cord palsy and the presence of a slit between the vocal cords. No between-group differences were observed in terms of paroxysmal tachycardia or anastomotic leakage. The lengths of postoperative hospital stays were not different. One patient died of severe pneumonia on day 34 in the non-PMT group.

Regarding patients with vocal cord palsy, in two patients who underwent the resection of unilateral recurrent nerve involved in metastatic lymph node, ansa cervicalis-recurrent nerve anastomosis was performed simultaneously. Though the vocal palsy was permanent, they kept relatively good phonating function and swallowing function without aspiration. All the other patients with vocal code palsy recovered conservatively within 6 months after the operation. All patients with postoperative aspiration became orally ingestible by swallowing rehabilitation.

Next, we reviewed in detail the 12 patients who underwent a DMT (Table 5). Of these patients, seven had mild obstructive respiratory disturbances, and five had vocal cord palsy. Co-morbidities with liver cirrhosis, heart failure, failed smoking cessation, and walking difficulty were also found.

Table 3 Surgical procedures

Variables	PMT group (n = 30)	Non-PMT group (n = 64)	P
Cervical lymph node dissection, n (%)	24 (80.0)	52 (81.3)	1.000
Reconstructed organ, n (%)			0.064
Stomach	27 (90.0)	46 (71.9)	
Jejunum	3 (10.0)	18 (28.1)	
Reconstructive route, n (%)			0.229
Percutaneous	7 (23.4)	20 (31.2)	
Retrosternal	10 (33.3)	11 (17.2)	
Postmediastinal	13 (43.3)	33 (51.6)	
Anastomotic portion			
Cervical / Intrathoracic	23 / 7	40 / 24	0.240
Operative time [min]	540 (406–732)	584 (306–975)	0.084
Blood loss [ml]	1057 (262–2567)	964 (269–6698)	0.320
Blood transfusion, n (%)	19 (63.3)	33 (51.6)	0.374

PMT prophylactic minitracheostomy

When the 12 patients with a DMT were compared with the 52 patients without a DMT, significant between-group differences were observed in terms of the following parameters: the incidence of postoperative pneumonia (11/12 vs. 14/42, $p < 0.001$, atelectasis (9/12 vs. 11/52, $p < 0.001$), and postoperative hospital stay [50 (18–137) vs. 24 (14–224) days, $p = 0.008$].

Of the 12 patients who received a DMT, three required re-intubation due to severe pneumonia. However, of the 52 patients without a DMT, four underwent re-intubation. These four patients did not undergo a minitracheostomy before re-intubation due to sudden respiratory failure or acute progressive severe pneumonia.

Table 4 Postoperative outcomes

Variables	PMT group (n = 30)	Non-PMT group (n = 64)	P
Extubation of tracheal tube [POD]	2 (1–6)	1 (1–11)	0.002
Pulmonary complications, n (%)			
Postoperative pneumonia (≧CD2)	8 (26.7)	25 (39.1)	0.258
Atelectasis[a]	10 (33.3)	26 (40.6)	0.495
Re-intubation	0	7 (10.9)	0.093
Other complications, n (%)			
Vocal cord palsy	16 (53.3)	12 (18.8)	0.001
Paroxysmal tachycardia	7 (23.3)	13 (20.3)	0.790
Anastomotic leakage	0	8 (12.5)	0.052
Any complication (≧CD3a), n (%)	5 (16.7)	21 (32.8)	0.137
90-day mortality, n (%)	0	1 (1.6)	1.000
Postoperative hospital day [days]	28 (16–97)	30 (14–226)	0.460

PMT prophylactic minitracheostomy, *CD* Clavien-Dindo classification
[a]diagnosed by computed tomography

Table 5 The characteristics of the patients with delayed minitracheostomy

	Age	FEV1.0% < 70	Vocal cord palsy	Others factors
1	60–69			Failure to cease tobacco
2	60–69	O	O	
3	60–69	O		Liver cirrhosis (ICGR15 = 19%)
4	60–69		O	
5	70–79	O		Walking difficulty
6	70–79			Heart failure (EF48%)
7	40–49			Failure to control pain
8	70–79	O	O	
9	70–79	O		
10	60–69		O	Liver cirrhosis (ICGR15 = 25%)
11	60–69	O		
12	70–79	O	O	

ICGR15 indocyanine green retention time 15 min, *EF* ejection fraction

Logistic regression analysis of the risk factors related to DMT

The risk factors related to a DMT were analyzed using univariate and multivariate logistic regression analyses in the 64 non-PMT patients (Table 6). Nine possible risk factors were included in the analysis. The dysfunction of other organs was defined as a history of ischemic heart disease or heart failure, cerebrovascular disease, liver cirrhosis (indocyanine green retention time at 15 min >15%), or renal failure (serum creatinine level > 1.5 mg/dl). Among these potential risk factors, multivariate analysis identified FEV1.0% < 70% and vocal cord palsy as independent risk factors.

Discussion

Our results demonstrated that the incidence of postoperative pulmonary complications in high-risk patients (the PMT group) was at least equivalent to that in the standard-risk patients (the non-PMT group). A noteworthy observation was that no patient required re-intubation in the PMT group. A PMT may prevent an increase in the incidence of postoperative pneumonia and re-intubation in patients at high risk for pulmonary complications. Although no complications related to a PMT were reported in this study, severe complications associated with a minitracheostomy have been reported, such as membranous tracheal injury, bleeding from the anterior cervical vein, hoarseness, and obstructive sub-glottic granuloma after removal of a minitracheostomy tube [11–13]. A minitracheostomy may prevent elevation of the larynx during swallowing and impair the swallowing function. Therefore, a PMT should be restricted to high-risk patients, and it is important to appropriately select patients requiring a PMT.

Table 6 Uni-and multivariate analyses for risk factors related to delayed mini-tracheostomy

Variables	n	DMT n (%)	Univariate P	Multivariate HR (95%-CI)	P
Age			0.238		
75>	55	9 (16.4)			
≧75	9	3 (33.3)			
Brinkman Index			0.968		
800>	37	7 (18.9)			
≧800	27	5 (18.5)			
FEV1.0%			0.061		0.032
≧70	42	5 (11.9)		1	
<70	22	7 (31.8)		5.06 (1.15–22.21)	
Clinical stage (UICC 7th)			0.838		
I	25	5 (20.0)			
II III IV	39	7 (17.9)			
Preoperative chemoradiotherapy			0.533		
Absent	55	11 (20.0)			
Present	9	1 (11.1)			
Cervical lymph node dissection			0.162		
Absent	12	4 (33.3)			
Present	52	8 (15.4)			
Reconstructive organs			0.790		
Stomach	46	9 (19.6)			
Jejunum	18	3 (16.7)			
Vocal cord palsy			0.032		0.017
Absent	52	7 (13.5)		1	
Present	12	5 (41.7)		6.90 (1.41–33.85)	
Dysfunction of other organs			0.073		
Absent	54	8 (14.8)			
Present	10	4 (40.0)			

DMT delayed mini-tracheostomy, *HR* hazard ratio, *CI* confidence interval

Regarding our PMT indications in this study, age, low pulmonary function, and vocal cord palsy were reported to be associated with postoperative pneumonia after esophagectomy [14, 15]. Aspiration of oral bacteria is commonly known to cause postoperative pneumonia [16]. Vocal cord palsy with a slit and reduced swallowing function with aspiration on the upper gastrointestinal image were therefore included as indications for a PMT. In patients with preoperative pneumonia including interstitial pneumonia, worsening of this condition due to an esophagectomy can be lethal; thus, preoperative pneumonia was also included as an indication for PMT.

A routine tracheostomy may be safer than a minitracheostomy when emergency airway management is needed. However, a tracheostomy leads to temporary voicelessness, which is stressful for patients and causes impairment of the swallowing function due to the restriction of the elevation movement of the larynx during swallowing. Moreover, a tracheostomy can occasionally cause severe complications such as recurrent

laryngeal nerve injury, tracheoesophageal fistula, or tracheo-brachiocephalic artery fistula. We propose that a prophylactic tracheostomy is too invasive.

In this study, none of the 30 patients who received a PMT according to our indications required re-intubation, whereas 12 of the non-PMT patients required a DMT due to postoperative sputum retention, and three developed severe pneumonia and required re-intubation. A multivariate analysis revealed that FEV1.0% <70% and vocal cord palsy were independent risk factors related to a DMT. Therefore, the indications for a PMT should be expanded for such patients despite the presence of a slit between the vocal cords. After this analysis, we expanded the indications for a PMT.

Although we focused on pulmonary function and aspiration to define the indications for a PMT, the DMT group included patients with health problems other than pulmonary function, such as liver cirrhosis, heart failure, and walking difficulty. In the prospective randomized trial reported by Pramod et al. [6, 17], the indications for a PMT included ischemic heart disease and cerebrovascular disease, which are likely to be exacerbated by postoperative hypoxia. In their study, some patients developed acute myocardial infarction or cerebellar infarction secondary to sputum retention. In addition to pulmonary function and aspiration, other organ disorders, such as heart failure, ischemic heart disease, liver cirrhosis, cerebrovascular disease, and performance status should be considered for a PMT.

In the present study, 11 of the 12 patients with a DMT due to postoperative sputum retention developed postoperative pneumonia, and three patients progressed to severe pneumonia. These observations demonstrate that a DMT after postoperative sputum retention cannot prevent postoperative pneumonia. In patients with sputum retention, oral bacteria may have dripped into the bronchial tree gradually due to postoperative vocal cord palsy and an impairment of swallowing function immediately after extubation. Thus, when sputum retention occurs, a pulmonary infection may have already developed. It is therefore important to prophylactically perform a minitracheostomy.

Some limitations were associated with this study. First, this is a retrospective study with only a small number of patients. Second, most of our patients underwent cervical lymph node dissection which is not generally performed in western country. Cervical lymph node dissection was reported to increase the incidence of vocal cord palsy [1] and impair swallowing function [18], and may lead to the increase of the incidence of postoperative pneumonia. Therefore, our results do not apply to patients without cervical lymph node dissection, and it may be necessary to reconsider the indications for a PMT for patients without cervical lymph node dissection. Third, all study patients underwent an open thoracotomy.

The incidence of pulmonary complication in open thoracotomy has been reported to be 12.5 to 39.66% [19]. The incidence of postoperative pneumonia in our study was 35.1%, and not particularly high, compared with open thoracotomy groups in the other studies. However, thoracoscopic esophagectomy has recently become popular and has been reported to reduce pulmonary complications compared to open thoracotomy [19–21]. It may be necessary to reconsider the PMT indications also for patients receiving thoracoscopic esophagectomy. Fourth, because this study did not compare two groups with the same condition, no conclusive results can be drawn from this comparison. A prospective randomized study comparing a PMT group and a non-PMT group of patients at high risk for pulmonary complications is needed.

Conclusion

A PMT for patients at high risk for postoperative pulmonary complications may be effective for preventing an increase in the incidence of postoperative pneumonia and re-intubation. The indications for a PMT should be expanded for patients with mild obstructive respiratory disturbances or vocal cord palsy despite the presence of a slit between the vocal cords.

Abbreviations
CT: Computed tomography; DMT: Delayed minitracheostomy; MST: Muscle sparing thoracotomy; PMT: prophylactic minitracheostomy

Acknowledgements
The authors acknowledge all the medical and surgical staffs that took care of the patients.

Funding
All authors report no source of funding for conducting this manuscript.

Availability of data and materials
The database of this study may provide insight in clinical and personal information about our patients. Therefore, these data cannot be made publically available unless the approval of the ethical committee of our hospital is obtained.

Authors' contributions
MF, KM, KI, and YS performed the surgery, and took charge of postoperative care. MF and MN analyzed these clinical data. YS prepared the manuscript. MF and MN assisted in drafting the manuscript and reviewed the article. All authors read and approved the final manuscript.

Competing interests
All authors declare that they have no competing interests.

References
1. Fujita H, Kakegawa T, Yamana H, Shima I, Toh Y, Tomita Y, Fujii T, Yamasaki K, Higaki K, Noake T, et al. Mortality and morbidity rates, postoperative course, quality of life, and prognosis after extended radical lymphadenectomy for esophageal cancer. Comparison of three-field lymphadenectomy with two-field lymphadenectomy. Ann Surg. 1995;222(5):654–62.
2. Nishimaki T, Suzuki T, Suzuki S, Kuwabara S, Hatakeyama K. Outcomes of extended radical esophagectomy for thoracic esophageal cancer. J Am Coll Surg. 1998;186(3):306–12.
3. Fang W, Kato H, Tachimori Y, Igaki H, Sato H, Daiko H. Analysis of pulmonary complications after three-field lymph node dissection for esophageal cancer. Ann Thorac Surg. 2003;76(3):903–8.
4. Issa MM, Healy DM, Maghur HA, Luke DA. Prophylactic minitracheotomy in lung resections. A randomized controlled study. J Thorac Cardiovasc Surg. 1991;101(5):895–900.
5. Randell TT, Tierala EK, Lepantalo MJ, Lindgren L. Prophylactic minitracheostomy after thoracotomy: a prospective, random control, clinical trial. The European journal of surgery =. Acta Chir. 1991;157(9):501–4.
6. Bonde P, Papachristos I, McCraith A, Kelly B, Wilson C, McGuigan JA, McManus K. Sputum retention after lung operation: prospective, randomized trial shows superiority of prophylactic minitracheostomy in high-risk patients. Ann Thorac Surg. 2002;74(1):196–202. discussion 202-193
7. Abdelaziz M, Naidu B, Agostini P. Is prophylactic minitracheostomy beneficial in high-risk patients undergoing thoracotomy and lung resection? Interact Cardiovasc Thorac Surg. 2011;12(4):615–8.
8. Beach L, Denehy L, Lee A. The efficacy of minitracheostomy for the management of sputum retention: a systematic review. Physiotherapy. 2013;99(4):271–7.
9. Miyata K, Fukaya M, Itatsu K, Abe T, Nagino M. Muscle sparing thoracotomy for esophageal cancer: a comparison with posterolateral thoracotomy. Surg Today. 2015;
10. Dindo D, Demartines N, Clavien PA. Classification of surgical complications: a new proposal with evaluation in a cohort of 6336 patients and results of a survey. Ann Surg. 2004;240(2):205–13.
11. Wain JC, Wilson DJ, Mathisen DJ. Clinical experience with minitracheostomy. Ann Thorac Surg. 1990;49(6):881–5. discussion 885-886
12. Browne J, McShane D, Donnelly M. An unusual complication of minitracheostomy. Eur J Anaesthesiol. 1999;16(8):571–3.
13. Ohtsuka T, Nomori H, Watanabe K, Kaji M, Naruke T, Suemasu K. Obstructive subglottic granuloma after removal of a minitracheostomy tube. Ann Thorac Cardiovasc Surg. 2006;12(4):265–6.
14. Ferguson MK, Durkin AE. Preoperative prediction of the risk of pulmonary complications after esophagectomy for cancer. J Thorac Cardiovasc Surg. 2002;123(4):661–9.
15. Gockel I, Kneist W, Keilmann A, Junginger T. Recurrent laryngeal nerve paralysis (RLNP) following esophagectomy for carcinoma. Eur J Surg Oncol. 2005;31(3):277–81.
16. Akutsu Y, Matsubara H, Okazumi S, Shimada H, Shuto K, Shiratori T, Ochiai T. Impact of preoperative dental plaque culture for predicting postoperative pneumonia in esophageal cancer patients. Dig Surg. 2008;25(2):93–7.
17. Bonde P, McManus K, McAnespie M, McGuigan J. Lung surgery: identifying the subgroup at risk for sputum retention. Eur J Cardio Thorac Surg. 2002;22(1):18–22.
18. Yasuda T, Yano M, Miyata H, Yamasaki M, Takiguchi S, Fujiwara Y, Doki Y. Evaluation of dysphagia and diminished airway protection after three-field esophagectomy and a remedy. World J Surg. 2013;37(2):416–23.
19. Guo W, Ma X, Yang S, Zhu X, Qin W, Xiang J, Lerut T, Li H. Combined thoracoscopic-laparoscopic esophagectomy versus open esophagectomy: a meta-analysis of outcomes. Surg Endosc. 2016;30(9):3873–81.
20. Tsujimoto H, Takahata R, Nomura S, Yaguchi Y, Kumano I, Matsumoto Y, Yoshida K, Horiguchi H, Hiraki S, Ono S, et al. Video-assisted thoracoscopic surgery for esophageal cancer attenuates postoperative systemic responses and pulmonary complications. Surgery. 2012;151(5):667–73.
21. Kubo N, Ohira M, Yamashita Y, Sakurai K, Toyokawa T, Tanaka H, Muguruma K, Shibutani M, Yamazoe S, Kimura K, et al. The impact of combined thoracoscopic and laparoscopic surgery on pulmonary complications after radical esophagectomy in patients with resectable esophageal cancer. Anticancer Res. 2014;34(5):2399–404.

16

Successful joint preservation of distal radius osteosarcoma by *en bloc* tumor excision and reconstruction using a tumor bearing frozen autograft

Takashi Higuchi, Norio Yamamoto, Katsuhiro Hayashi, Akihiko Takeuchi*⬥, Kensaku Abe, Yuta Taniguchi, Yoshihiro Araki, Kaoru Tada and Hiroyuki Tsuchiya

Abstract

Background: The wrist joint is an extremely rare site for osteosarcoma. Joint structure preservation to maintain good limb function is well described in case of knee osteosarcoma, whereas it is not described in case of wrist joint osteosarcoma. In this report, we present the first case of joint preservation surgery to treat distal radius osteosarcoma using a tumor bearing autograft treated with liquid nitrogen.

Case presentation: A 46-year-old male presented with swelling and pain in the right wrist and was diagnosed with conventional osteosarcoma of the distal radius. The patient responded well to neoadjuvant chemotherapy and the tumor shrank remarkably. Wide tumor excision to preserve the radiocarpal joint and reconstruction with a tumor bearing frozen autograft were performed. Partial bone union was detected 3 months postoperatively and complete bone union was detected 9 months postoperatively. Following the surgery, there was immediate commencement of the range of motion (ROM) training in both the wrist and fingers. At the final postoperative follow-up of 41 months, the patient had normal ROM in the wrist, fingers, and forearms, with a score of 100% in the Musculoskeletal Tumor Society (MSTS) score and was disease free.

Conclusion: We present the first case in which *en bloc* tumor excision with joint preservation of the wrist and reconstruction using a tumor bearing frozen autograft were performed. The surgery yielded excellent hand, wrist, and forearm function at the final follow-up.

Keywords: Osteosarcoma, Distal radius, Joint preservation, Liquid nitrogen, Recycled autograft

Background

Osteosarcomas are the most common of primary malignant bone tumors. The most common site of the disease is the metaphyseal bone around the knee [1]. On the other hand, osteosarcoma of the wrist is extremely rare; it has been reported that only < 1% of osteosarcomas arise in the distal radius [1]. Recent advances in multimodality therapy have resulted in limb-sparing surgery being the standard for high-grade osteosarcomas. Furthermore, for select patients, joint-sparing surgery is possible, allowing preservation of the joint structure in an effort to maintain normal limb function [2]. Several case series have reported the usefulness of sparing the knee joint in osteosarcoma in maintaining the function of the knee [3–5], whereas reports regarding wrist joint sparing surgery in osteosarcoma are few. This report presents a successful case of a distal radius osteosarcoma treated by *en bloc* resection and reconstructed with a tumor bearing autograft treated by liquid nitrogen. This surgery resulted in the preservation of the radiocarpal joint, and yielded normal function after the surgery. So, far, this report is the first to describe a wrist joint sparing surgery in distal radius osteosarcoma using a recycled bone graft technique.

* Correspondence: a_take@med.kanazawa-u.ac.jp
Department of Orthopaedic Surgery, Graduate School of Medical Science, Kanazawa University, 13-1 Takara-machi, Kanazawa 920-8641, Japan

Case presentation

A 46-year-old Japanese male patient was referred to our hospital with pain and swelling of the right wrist that had persisted for approximately 3 months. A plain radiograph (Fig. 1a), though hard to discern, and a computed tomography (CT) scan (Fig. 1b, c) of the forearm revealed a periosteal reaction at the dorsal site of the right distal radius. Gadolinium contrast magnetic resonance imaging (MRI) revealed a large soft tissue extension between the radius and the ulna, which was strongly enhanced and continued to an intramedullary enhanced lesion, suggesting that the high-grade malignant tumor arising from intramedullary bone extended widely to the soft tissue. There was no clear bone infiltration into the ulna (Fig. 1d, e). No distant metastasis was detected. The pathological diagnosis from the open biopsy was conventional osteosarcoma (Fig. 1f), and six courses of neoadjuvant chemotherapy with intravenous cisplatin (120 mg/m2) and doxorubicin (30 mg/m2/day × 2 days) were administered according to our chemotherapy

regimen [6]. As chemotherapy progressed, the swelling and restricted range of motion (ROM) of the forearm was reduced, with the difference between the left and right wrists disappearing completely after six courses. Preoperatively, the extraosseous lesion appeared greatly shrunken, represented by only a slight signal contrast within the intraosseous membrane. This was confirmed by CT (Fig. 2a) and MRI (Fig. 2b, c), and the response to chemotherapy was considered complete. Wide tumor excision and reconstruction with a tumor bearing frozen autograft was performed. Briefly, a longitudinal dorsal incision was performed and an osteotomy of the distal part of the radius was made 1 cm proximal from the epiphysis to preserve the joint with securing the bony margin according to the preoperative planning using MRI gadolinium enhancement analyses (Fig. 3a). The osteotomy of the proximal part of the radius was made 2 cm proximal from the tumor on the basis of the preoperative MRI and an intercalary resection of the tumor-bearing bone was performed (Fig. 3b). The soft

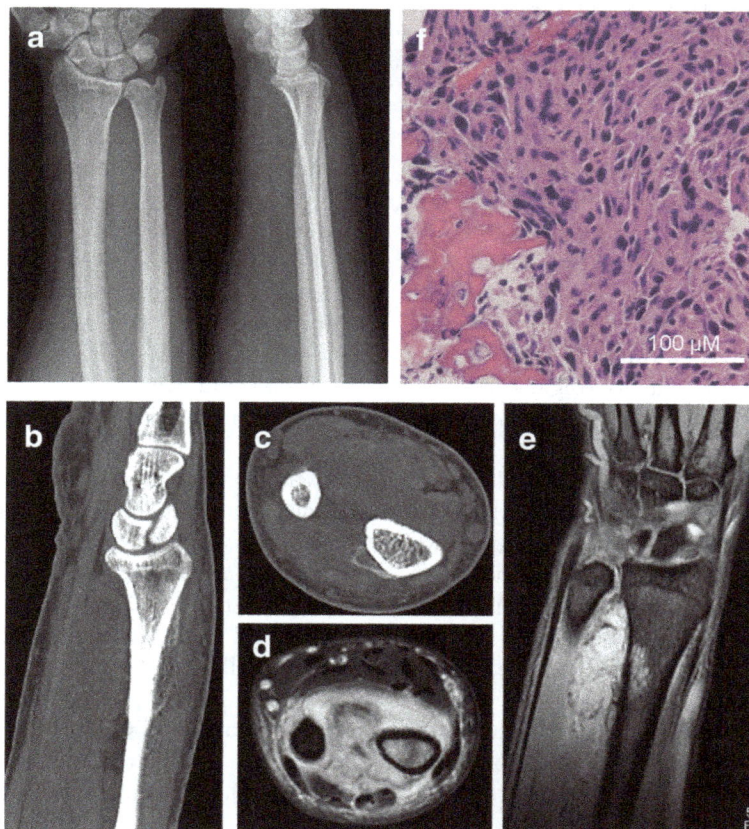

Fig. 1 Before neoadjuvant chemotherapy. **a** Plain radiography. Mild cortical irregularity was detected at the ulnar side of the radius. **b, c** CT: (**b**) sagittal and (**c**) axial images (bone condition). A periosteal reaction was detected at the dorsal radius. **d, e** Gadolinium contrast MRI: (**d**) axial and (**e**) coronal images. A huge extraskeletal tumor surrounding the radius was strongly enhanced. **f** Hematoxylin-Eosin staining of the specimen from open biopsy. Highly dense tumor cells with strong nuclear atypia or atypical mitosis, and tumoral osteoid were detected. No cartilage formation was detected

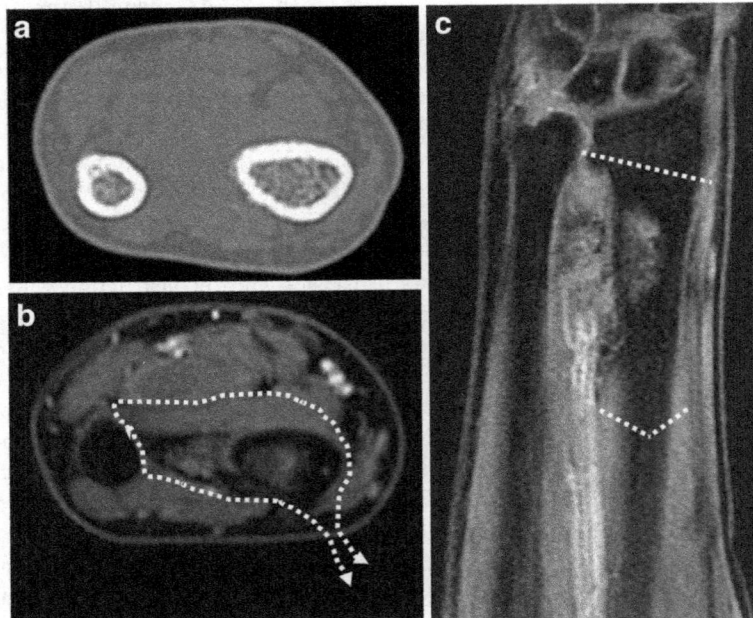

Fig. 2 After neoadjuvant chemotherapy. **a** CT axial image (bone condition). Periosteal reaction was detected prior to chemotherapy. **b**, **c** Gadolinium contrast MRI; (**b**) axial and (**c**) coronal images. The soft tissue extension of the tumor shrunk remarkably and a small enhanced lesion was detected in the radius and intraosseous membrane. The dotted arrow indicates the resection range including the radius, intraosseous membrane, and pronator quadratus muscle. The dotted line indicates the osteotomy line of the radius

tissue, including the complete pronator quadratus muscle, intraosseous membrane, and periosteum of the ulna where the soft-tissue extension of the tumor originally existed before chemotherapy, was peeled from the ulna and excised with the tumor bearing bone. After stripping the soft tissue, the tumor bearing bone was frozen in liquid nitrogen for 20 min (Fig. 3c, d), thawed at room temperature for 15 min, rinsed in distilled water for 15 min, and then returned to its original site. The frozen autograft was reconstructed with a long volar plate approached from a dorsal incision (Acu-Loc 2 extension plate, Acumed, LLC., OR., USA), and a small volar incision was made in order to insert the distal screws (Fig. 4a, b). Postoperative partial bone union was detected at 3 months and complete bone union was detected at 9 months, both of which were confirmed by plural direction radiography (Fig. 4c, d). Following the surgery, ROM training of both the wrist and fingers commenced immediately and the patient achieved normal ROM with active dorsiflexion of the affected wrist to 85° (Fig. 5a), palmar flexion to 80° (Fig. 5b), and both pronation and supination of the affected forearm to 90° within 9 months after the surgery (Fig. 5c, d). Postoperative functional results were as follows: 100% in the Musculoskeletal Tumor Society (MSTS) score, 12.5 in the Disabilities of the Arm, Shoulder and Hand (DASH) score and 93.5 in the Toronto Extremity Salvage Score (TESS). The Short Form-36 (SF-36) scores accounted for

39.5 of the Physical component summary, 66.6 of the Mental component summary, and 33.4 of the Role/Social component summary at the final postoperative follow-up of 41 months. The patient was discharged after 3 courses of adjuvant chemotherapy. These were administered as neoadjuvant chemotherapy, as the histological evaluation of surgical specimens diagnosed the patient as a good responder (classified as grade III/IV in the Rosen and Huvos evaluation system). At the final follow-up, the patient was found to be disease free.

Discussion and conclusions

Although the distal radius is an extremely uncommon skeletal site for osteosarcoma, it is not a rare site for benign bone tumors such as giant cell tumors of bone [1]. Even patients with distal radius giant-cell tumors have experienced local recurrence, with subsequent surgeries required following treatment failures. Wang et al. reported that among 27 patients receiving wrist arthrodesis for Campanacci Grade III giant cell tumors of distal radius, 11 patients required additional surgical procedures (41%) (8 for complications (30%) and 3 for local recurrences (11%)) [7]. This finding underscores the difficulty in treating osteosarcomas, very aggressive tumors that require wider margins to treat than giant cell tumors in this site. Many reconstructive procedures for massive defects following the *en bloc* excision of the tumor in the distal radius, including arthrodesis using

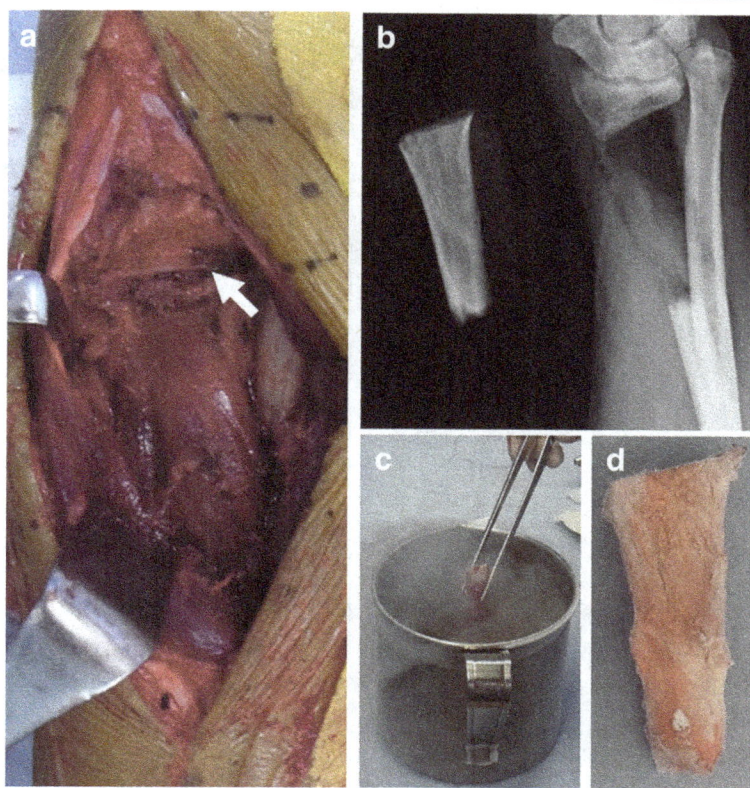

Fig. 3 Intraoperative photos (**a**) The dorsal approach at the flexible side of the radiocarpal joint. The tumor bearing bone was resected with a biopsy tract, pronator quadratus muscle, and intraosseous membrane. The main extensor and flexor tendons were preserved. **b** Intraoperative radiograph of the tumor bearing bone resected along the planned osteotomy line. **c** The tumor bearing bone was frozen in liquid nitrogen. **d** After freezing

corticocancellous graft (e.g., iliac crest graft [7], free fibular graft [8, 9]), or ulnar translocation [10]), radial carpal arthroplasty using free fibular head transfer [11, 12], osteoarticular allografts [13], and prosthesis [14, 15] have been reported.

Arthrodesis provides stability at the expense of wrist motion, which may cause impairment in daily life activities. However, if the carpal bones can be preserved, partial arthrodesis (radio-scapho-lunate arthrodesis) is preferred to reduce restrictions in wrist motion to a greater extent than in total arthrodesis [8]. For osteochondral defects, ulnar translocations are less invasive than corticocancellaous grafts in terms of the donor site. However, stress fracture is a potential problem in these grafts, and approximately half of the patients report stress fractures [9].

Several wrist arthroplasty techniques that preserve wrist motion have been reported [11–15]. Wrist prosthesis has been reported and found to result in satisfactory postoperative function [14, 15]. However, limited availability, infection, aseptic loosening, and dorsal subluxation of the ulnar head are the major problems in custom prostheses [15]. Fibular head transfer, along with the shaft, is an attractive method for the replacement of the radiocarpal joint, but the procedure is technically

demanding and complications include progressive degenerative changes, bony collapse due to poor vascularity of the fibular head, and volar subluxation resulting from incongruity between the fibular head and the proximal carpal row [12]. These complications, in addition to limited availability, are also problematic in arthroplasty with osteoarticular allografts [13]. Overall, wrist arthroplasty may provide better wrist ROM, at least in the short-term. However, this may come at the expense of wrist stability when compared to wrist arthrodesis. Zhu et al. compared the functional outcomes of 14 distal radius giant cell tumors treated by partial wrist arthrodesis using fibular grafts or arthroplasty using fibular head grafts and found that there were significant differences in flexion-extension; the average wrist ROM of the 7 patients that underwent partial arthrodesis were 55.9° of total flexion-extension and 127.6° of total pronation-supination, whereas the average wrist ROM of the 7 patients that underwent wrist arthroplasty were 71.6° of total flexion-extension and 140° of total pronation-supination [16].

To maintain wrist function and to avoid complications associated with wrist arthrodesis or arthroplasty, preserving the wrist joint by maintaining the epiphysis of the

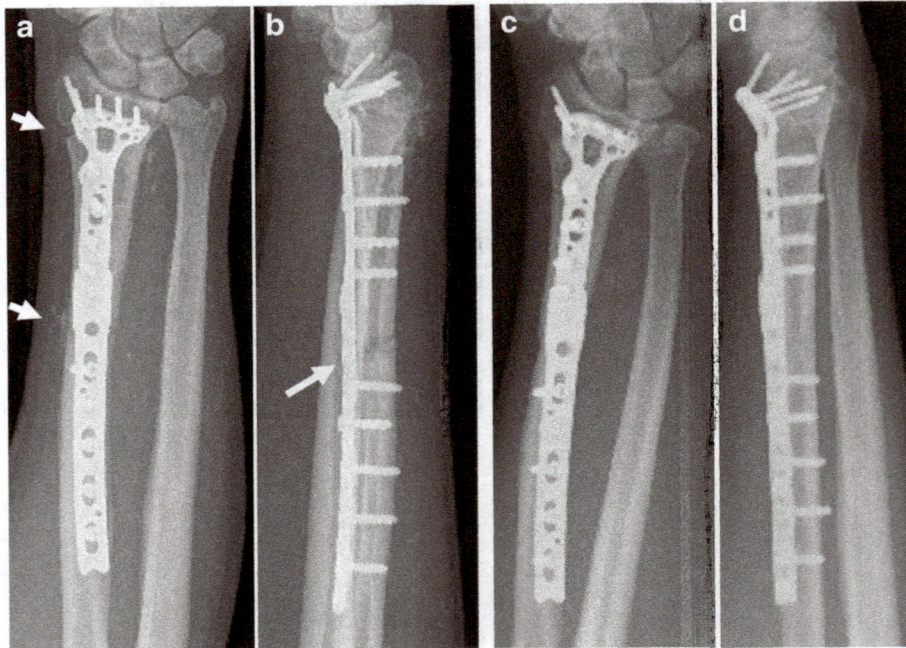

Fig. 4 a, **b** Postoperative radiographs. Arrows indicate the osteotomy line. **c**, **d** Radiographs of the final follow-up. The bone was completely united and the osteotomy line was obscured

radius is an ideal method in select patients. There is only one report from Yu et al. that mentions wrist joint preserving surgery in osteosarcoma [17]. In this study, the affected limb was reconstructed with a free fibular shaft after *en bloc* intercalary resection of the tumor bone. In a distal radius osteosarcoma case with a short follow-up period, good postoperative function (active dorsiflexion of the affected wrist was to 90° and palmar flexion was to 45°) was found. The author determined that preserving

the joint surface could maintain wrist stability and positively affect wrist function [17]. The present case is the second report that involves wrist joint preservation in distal radial osteosarcoma, and the first case to use a recycled bone technique for reconstruction.

The advantages of autograft recycling include perfect fitness to the original site, good availability, lack of the requirement for a bone bank, the capacity for biological reconstruction, lack of disease transmission, reduced

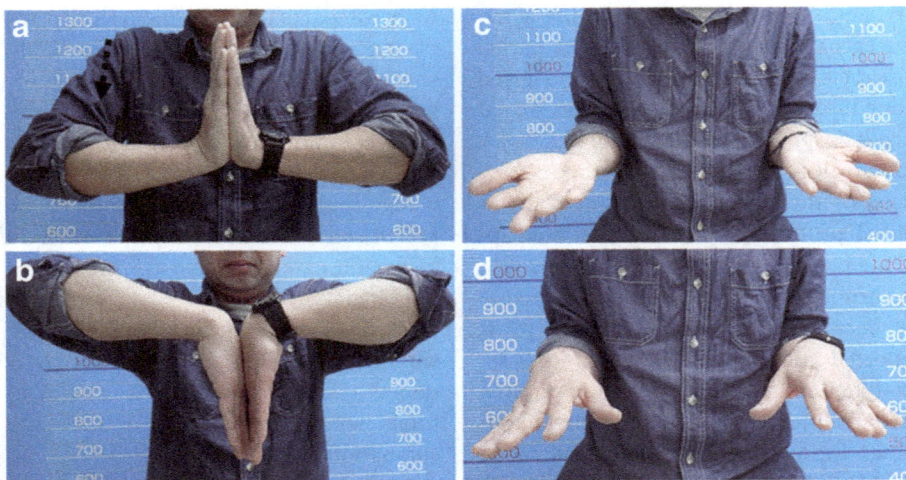

Fig. 5 Range of motion of the wrist and forearm at the final follow-up. **a** Dorsiflexion of the right wrist was 85°; (**b**) palmar flexion was 80°; (**c**) pronation of the right forearm was 90°; and (**d**) supination was 90°

immunological response, soft tissue and ligament attachment capabilities, and the availability of a massive bone stock [18]. In 1999, we initially developed our tumor-bearing frozen autograft technique, and have since reported its usefulness [18, 19]. The advantages of frozen autografts include simplicity and the possibility of preserving proteins, including bone morphogenetic proteins (BMPs), which lead to an increased rate of osteoinduction and osteoconduction [20]. In the present study, the frozen bone was united and well preserved at the final follow-up, and the patient was able to achieve normal wrist flexion and extension (dorsiflexion of the affected wrist was to 85° and palmar flexion was to 80°). Furthermore, the patient was able to achieve normal forearm rotation (both pronation and supination to 90°).

Pronation and supination of the forearm play a main role in turning the hand toward an object and are the movements frequently used in daily life [21]. These forearm rotation movements require the anatomical alignment of both the radius and ulna in addition to intact wrist and elbow joints [21, 22]. The misalignment of the radius may lead to radioulnar impingement, increased tension in the interosseous membrane, or contracture of the soft tissues, which have been reported as the main causes for loss of forearm rotation [22, 23]. Using fibular grafting for reconstruction following *en bloc* excision of tumor bone may cause axial malalignment in the forearm, which causes ulnar impingement and worsens forearm rotation [9]. In addition to axial malalignment, shortening of the radius can also induce a severe loss in forearm rotation. Bronstein et al. reported in their cadaveric study that a radial shortening of 10 mm reduced forearm pronation by 47% and supination by 29% [23]. Because the function of the forearm is strongly dependent on the osseous anatomical alignment of the radius, recycled bone, including frozen autografts, can be perfectly matched to the original site and can reproduce the proper anatomical alignment. Therefore, they are more favorable than other reconstructive materials such as fibular allografts or prostheses for reconstruction in forearm tumor surgery. In the present case, we were able to reconstruct the anatomical osseous alignment of the radius by frozen autograft with preservation of the intact ulna, thus enabling the patient to achieve normal forearm rotation.

From the present case, we demonstrated that joint preservation surgery with reconstruction using frozen autografts showed satisfactory results in terms of the function of the affected limb in a case of forearm tumor. However, this technique must be applied to select patients, i.e., those with metaphyseal osteosarcoma with an articular surface, a subchondral bone, a collateral metaphyseal cortex preserved after adequate excision of the tumor, and joints in which internal fixation with plates and screws is possible. In addition, it is important that the patient achieves a good response to neoadjuvant chemotherapy to secure the negative margin. Decke et al., in their series of 39 osteosarcomas of the hand and forearm, reported that the mean overall survival rate in patients with wide or radical tumor resection was higher (88.0%) than in patients in with narrow margins of resection (75.0%) [24]. However, achieving wide tumor resection at the distal forearm is challenging because of the small size of the muscle and expandable soft tissue. Therefore, the surgeon should not hesitate to choose other surgical options, including wrist joint sacrificing surgery or amputation, if the neoadjuvant chemotherapy is not effective or a wide margin is not possible [24]. In the present case, the neoadjuvant chemotherapy was very effective and the soft tissue tumor shrunk remarkably, enabling a secured margin for preservation of the wrist joint, and there were neither local nor distant recurrences found during follow-up.

In conclusion, a wrist joint preservation surgery with tumor bearing frozen autograft reconstruction was successful and resulted in satisfactory functioning of the hand, wrist, and forearm at the final follow-up.

Abbreviations
CT: Computed tomography; DASH score: Disabilities of the Arm, Shoulder and Hand score; MRI: Magnetic resonance imaging; MSTS score: Musculoskeletal Tumour Society score; ROM: Range of motion; SF-36: Short Form-36; TESS: Toronto Extremity Salvage Score

Acknowledgements
Not applicable.

Funding
There is no funding source.Authors' contributions.

Author's contributions
T.H. participated in the surgery, and was involved in data collection, case analysis and writing the manuscript. A.T. participated in the surgery, followed up the patient, and was involved in data collection, case analysis and writing the manuscript. N.Y., K.H., K.A., Y.T., and Y.A. assisted in drafting the manuscript and reviewed the article. K.T. participated in the surgery and followed up the patient. H.T. performed surgery and followed up the patient. All authors read and approved the final manuscript.

Competing interests
No benefits in any form have been received or will be received from a commercial party related directly or indirectly to the subject of this article.

References
1. Unni KK, Inwards CY. Dahlin's bone tumors: general aspects and data on 10,165 cases. 6th ed. Philadelphia: Lippincott Williams & Wilkins; 2010.
2. Tsuchiya H, Abdel-Wanis M, Kitano S, Sakurakichi K, Yamashiro T, Tomita K. The natural limb is best: joint preservation and reconstruction by distraction osteogenesis for high-grade juxta-articular osteosarcomas. Anticancer Res. 2002;22:2373–6.

3. Higuchi T, Yamamoto N, Nishida H, Hayashi K, Takeuchi A, Kimura H, Miwa S, Inatani H, Shimozaki S, Kato T, Aoki Y, Abe K, Taniguchi Y, Tsuchiya H. Knee joint preservation surgery in osteosarcoma using tumour-bearing bone treated with liquid nitrogen. Int Orthop. 2017;41(10):2189–97. https://doi.org/10.1007/s00264-017-3499-x.

4. Aponte-Tinao L, Ayerza MA, Muscolo DL, Farfalli GL. Survival, recurrence, and function after epiphyseal preservation and allograft reconstruction in osteosarcoma of the knee. Clin Orthop Relat Res. 2015;473:1789–96.

5. Betz M, Dumont CE, Fuchs B, Exner GU. Physeal distraction for joint preservation in malignant metaphyseal bone tumors in children. Clin Orthop Relat Res. 2012;470:1749–54.

6. Tsuchiya H, Tomita K, Mori Y, Asada N, Yamamoto N. Marginal excision for osteosarcoma with caffeine assisted chemotherapy. Clin Orthop Relat Res. 1999;358:27–35.

7. Wang T, Chan CM, Yu F, Li Y, Niu X. Does wrist arthrodesis with structural iliac crest bone graft after wide resection of distal radius giant cell tumor result in satisfactory function and local control? Clin Orthop Relat Res. 2017;475(3):767–75.

8. Bickert B, Ch H, Germann G. Fibulo-scapho-lunate arthrodesis as a motion-preserving procedure after tumour resection of the distal radius. J Hand Surg Br. 2002;27(6):573–6.

9. Lackman RD, McDonald DJ, Beckenbaugh RD, Sim FH. Fibular reconstruction for giant cell tumor of the distal radius. Clin Orthop Relat Res. 1987;(218):232-238.

10. Puri A, Gulia A, Agarwal MG, Reddy K. Ulnar translocation after excision of a Campanacci grade-3 giant-cell tumour of the distal radius: an effective method of reconstruction. J Bone Joint Surg Br. 2010;92(6):875–9.

11. Peng-Fei S, Yu-Hua J. Reconstruction of distal radius by fibula following excision of grade III giant cell tumour: follow-up of 18 cases. Int Orthop. 2011;35(4):577–80.

12. Usui M, Murakami T, Naito T, Wada T, Takahashi T, Ishii S. Some problems in wrist reconstruction after tumor resection with vascularized fibular-head graft. J Reconstr Microsurg. 1996;12:81–8.

13. Bianchi G, Donati D, Staals EL, Mercuri M. Osteoarticular allograft reconstruction of the distal radius after bone tumour resection. J Hand Surg Br. 2005;30(4):369–73.

14. Natarajan MV, Chandra Bose J, Viswanath J, Balasubramanian N, Sameer M. Custom prosthetic replacement for distal radial tumours. Int Orthop. 2009;33(4):1081–4.

15. Wang B, Wu Q, Liu J, Chen S, Zhang Z, Shao Z. What are the functional results, complications, and outcomes of using a custom unipolar wrist hemiarthroplasty for treatment of grade III giant cell tumors of the distal radius? Clin Orthop Relat Res. 2016;474(12):2583–90.

16. Zhu Z, Zhang C, Zhao S, Dong Y, Zeng B. Partial wrist arthrodesis versus arthroplasty for distal radius giant cell tumours. Int Orthop. 2013;37(11):2217–23.

17. Yu X, Xu S, Xu M, Yuan Y. Osteosarcoma of the distal radius treated by en bloc resection and reconstruction with a fibular shaft preserving the radiocarpal joint: a case report. Oncol Lett. 2014;7(5):1503–6.

18. Tsuchiya H, Wan SL, Sakayama K, Yamamoto N, Nishida H, Tomita K. Reconstruction using an autograft containing tumour treated by liquid nitrogen. J Bone Joint Surg Br. 2005;87(2):218–25.

19. Igarashi K, Yamamoto N, Shirai T, Hayashi K, Nishida H, Kimura H, et al. The long-term outcome following the use of frozen autograft treated with liquid nitrogen in the management of bone and soft-tissue sarcomas. J Bone Joint Surg Br. 2014;96:555–61.

20. Takata M, Sugimoto N, Yamamoto N, Shirai T, Hayashi K, Nishida H, et al. Activity of bone morphogenetic protein-7 after treatment at various temperatures: freezing vs. pasteurization vs. allograft. Cryobiology. 2011;63:235–9.

21. Norkin CC, Levangie PK. Joint structure and function: a comprehensive analysis. 5th ed. Philadelphia: FA Davis; 2011.

22. Dumont CE, Thalmann R, Macy JC. The effect of rotational malunion of the radius and the ulna on supination and pronation. J Bone Joint Surg Br. 2002;84(7):1070–4.

23. Bronstein A, Heaton D, Tencer AF, Trumble TE. Distal radius malunion and forearm rotation: a cadaveric study. J Wrist Surg. 2014;3(1):7–11.

24. Daecke W, Bielack S, Martini AK, Ewerbeck V, Jürgens H, Kotz R, et al. Osteosarcoma of the hand and forearm: experience of the cooperative osteosarcoma study group. Ann Surg Oncol. 2005;12(4):322–31.

17

Evaluation of resection of the gastroesophageal junction and jejunal interposition (Merendino procedure) as a rescue procedure in patients with a failed redo antireflux procedure. A single-center experience

Apostolos Analatos[1,2,3]* (iD), Mats Lindblad[1], Ioannis Rouvelas[1], Peter Elbe[1], Lars Lundell[1], Magnus Nilsson[1], Andrianos Tsekrekos[1] and Jon A. Tsai[1]

Abstract

Background: Primary antireflux surgery has high success rates but 5 to 20% of patients undergoing antireflux operations can experience recurrent reflux and dysphagia, requiring reoperation. Different surgical approaches after failed fundoplication have been described in the literature. The aim of this study was to evaluate resection of the gastroesophageal junction with jejunal interposition (Merendino procedure) as a rescue procedure after failed fundoplication.

Methods: All patients who underwent a Merendino procedure at the Karolinska University Hospital between 2004 and 2012 after a failed antireflux fundoplication were identified. Data regarding previous surgical history, preoperative workup, postoperative complications, subsequent investigations and re-interventions were collected retrospectively. The follow-up also included questionnaires regarding quality of life, gastrointestinal function and the dumping syndrome.

Results: Twelve patients had a Merendino reconstruction. Ten patients had undergone at least two previous fundoplications, of which one patient had four such procedures. The main indication for surgery was epigastric and radiating back pain, with or without dysphagia. Postoperative complications occurred in 8/12 patients (67%). During a median follow-up of 35 months (range 20–61), four (25%) patients had an additional redo procedure with conversion to a Roux-en-Y esophagojejunostomy within 12 months, mainly due to obstructive symptoms that could not be managed conservatively or with endoscopic techniques. Questionnaires scores were generally poor in all dimensions.

Conclusions: In our experience, the Merendino procedure seems to be an unsuitable surgical option for patients who require an alternative surgical reconstruction due to a failed fundoplication. However, the small number of patients included in this study as well as the small number of participants who completed the postoperative workout limits this study.

Keywords: Gastroesophageal reflux, Reoperation, Quality of life, Jejunal interposition, Merendino procedure

* Correspondence: apanalat@gmail.com
[1]Centre for Digestive Diseases, Karolinska University Hospital and Division of Surgery, Department of Clinical Intervention and Technology (CLINTEC), Karolinska Institutet, Stockhom, Sweden
[2]Department of Surgery, Nyköping Hospital, Nyköping, Sweden
Full list of author information is available at the end of the article

Background

Fundoplication in patients with chronic gastroesophageal reflux disease (GERD) is generally followed by excellent short- and long-term results [1–5]. Failures are, however, unavoidable and present with recurrent reflux symptoms, postprandial pain, dysphagia and delayed gastric emptying [6]. A variety of different mechanisms may cause these symptoms such as recurrent hiatal hernia, dislocation of the fundoplication, vagus nerve damage and/or other morphological abnormalities in the hiatus [7, 8]. The problem with many of these symptoms (with the exception of acid reflux), appearing after a defective surgical repair, is that the result of conservative treatment is usually poor which consequently leads to the need for another fundoplication, with the aim to achieve a durable repair [9, 10]. With very few exceptions, the reported postoperative morbidity is significantly higher after redo surgery, which is due to the complexity of the anatomical region, postoperative scarring and deformation [11–15]. If severe symptoms recur after a second or third fundoplication remedial surgical interventions have been advocated including total gastrectomy or gastric bypass [16, 17]. The outcome of these procedures has often been reported as good to excellent but a substantial publication bias in favour of respective surgical intervention may be present. In addition, a number of potentially relevant factors have to be taken into consideration. Maintenance of the gastrointestinal continuity with preservation of the duodenal and proximal jejunum contact with ingested food particles and prevention of reflux into the esophagus are critically important factors as well as the role of the gastric reservoir, which may be relevant for preventing post-gastrectomy symptoms. An additional symptom component, which may be prevalent, is chronic epigastric pain radiating to the back with or without exacerbation after ingestion of food. The mechanisms behind these complaints are poorly understood, but the need for surgical clearance and resection has been advocated [18].

Resection of the gastroesophageal junction with interposition of a jejunal segment between the distal esophagus and the remnant stomach (Merendino procedure) has been used in various clinical situations, mainly in patients with peptic strictures during the pre-proton pump inhibitor era and more recently for early Barrett cancer, where encouraging results have been reported [19–22]. Proximal gastrectomy with jejunal interposition for non-advanced proximal gastric cancer, which is similar to the Merendino procedure, is performed mainly in the Far East and has been shown to induce fewer post gastrectomy symptoms as compared to total gastrectomy with Roux-en-Y reconstruction, without adding more postoperative complications [23, 24]. Therefore, the Merendino procedure may have the potential to offer significant advantages in challenging post-fundoplication situations. Hereby, we report a single institution's experience of this reconstruction method in patients with a history of failed redo antireflux surgery.

Methods

Identification and inclusion of patients

All patients who underwent a Merendino procedure between 2004 and 2012 at the Karolinska University Hospital, for other causes than cancer, were identified via the computerised patient records and registries for surgical procedures (Take Care, Orbit, HOPA). Patient records were reviewed and data regarding previous surgical history, preoperative workup, postoperative complications, subsequent investigations and re-interventions were collected. In 2013 all study patients, who still had an intact Merendino reconstruction were contacted and asked to participate in a follow-up with questionnaire regarding quality of life, gastrointestinal symptoms and the dumping syndrome. During the course of the management of all GERD patients, barium swallow, esophageal manometry and ambulatory 24-h pH measurement had previously been performed. The Stockholm Local Ethics Committee had approved this study and all patients who participated in the study gave their written informed consent.

Surgical procedure

Resection of the distal esophagus, cardia and proximal stomach with jejunal interposition was done via an upper midline laparotomy. A wide phrenotomy was usually performed to expose the lower posterior mediastinum and allow a safe dissection of the distal esophagus proximal to the area of previous fundoplication, which typically contained abundant scar tissue and in one case a large epiphrenic diverticulum. The dissection of the proximal stomach was also performed beyond the area of the fundoplication. After division of the distal esophagus and the fundus of the stomach, a 30 cm pedunculated, isoperistaltic jejunal segment was prepared and hand-sutured end to side to the distal esophagus and end to side to the minor curvature side of the body of the stomach with absorbable interrupted sutures (Fig. 1). In 4 patients a pyloroplasty was also added. In order to protect the jejunum from refluxed gastric content, either a posterior or anterior fundoplication was created by use of the most oral portion of the major curvature side of the remaining stomach. All patients also had a feeding jejunostomy tube placed for temporary enteral nutrition.

QoL and symptom questionnaires

Patients eligible for the postoperative questionnaires received information about the study by telephone and then received three questionnaires by mail – the Quality Of Life in Reflux And Dyspepsia (QOLRAD), the Gastrointestinal Symptom Rating Scale (GSRS) and the Dumping Symptom Rating Scale (DSRS)

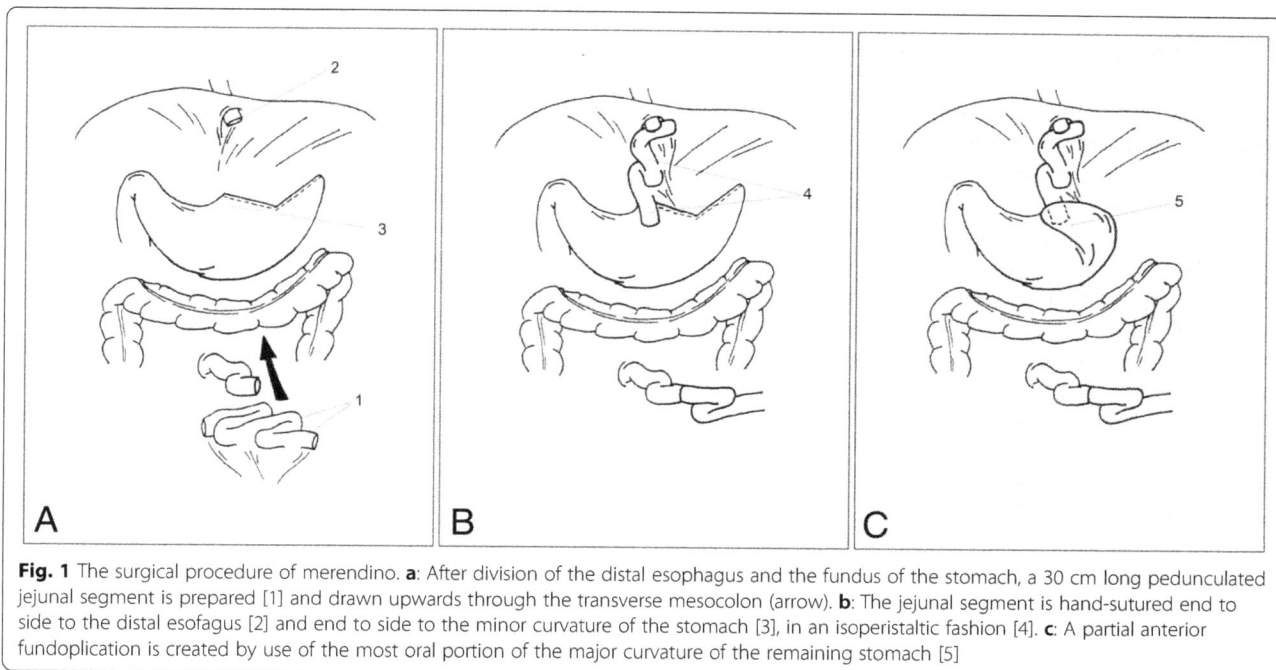

Fig. 1 The surgical procedure of merendino. **a**: After division of the distal esophagus and the fundus of the stomach, a 30 cm long pedunculated jejunal segment is prepared [1] and drawn upwards through the transverse mesocolon (arrow). **b**: The jejunal segment is hand-sutured end to side to the distal esofagus [2] and end to side to the minor curvature of the stomach [3], in an isoperistaltic fashion [4]. **c**: A partial anterior fundoplication is created by use of the most oral portion of the major curvature of the remaining stomach [5]

instruments [25–27]. The QOLRAD questionnaire includes 25 questions divided into 5 dimensions: emotional distress, sleep disturbance, vitality, food/drink problems and physical/social function and is rated on a seven-point graded Likert scale, with low values indicating a more severe impact on daily functioning. Symptoms related to general gastrointestinal symptoms were assessed by GSRS, which is a disease specific instrument of 15 items combined in 5 different symptom-categories such as reflux, abdominal pain, indigestion, diarrhoea and constipation. The GSRS also has a seven-point graded Likert-type scale in which each symptom-cluster can take a score from 1 to 7, where 1 represents absence of symptoms and 7 very intense symptoms. The dumping syndrome (DS) was scored by the newly developed DSRS questionnaire. This includes questions regarding 11 typical symptoms (fatigue, palpitations, sweating/flushing, cold sweats/paleness, need to lie down, diarrhoea, nausea/vomiting, stomach cramp, fainting esteem, pain and vomiting) associated with the DS of which 9 items represents symptoms that occur after meals. The severity of each symptom during the past week is graded on a seven-point Likert-scale where 1 represents "no trouble at all" and 7 "very severe problems". The frequency of 9 of the DS symptoms in the last 2 weeks is measured on a six-point Likert-scale where 1 represents "no trouble at all" and 6 "several times a day". The mean of the severity items is the severity score and the mean of the frequency items is the frequency score and the total DSRS score is calculated by multiplying the severity score with the frequency score.

Manometry of the esophagus and the interposed jejunal segment

Esophageal manometry investigations of the esophagus and the interposed jejunal segment were performed at the Karolinska University Hospital. A solid state High Resolution Manometry (HRM) assembly with 36 solid-state sensors spaced at 1-cm intervals was used (Sierra Scientific Instruments Inc., Los Angeles, CA) [28]. Each sensor is circumferentially sensitive and zeroed to atmospheric pressure. The HRM assembly was passed transnasally and positioned to record from the native esophagus, through the interposed jejunal segment into the gastric reservoir. The manometric protocol included a 5-min period to assess basal pressures and ten 10-mL water swallows. Manometric data were analyzed using both ManoView analysis software (Sierra Scientific Instruments Inc., Los Angeles, CA) and custom programs written in Matlab (The MathWorks Inc., Natick, MA).

Statistics

All the collected data were stored in a database and analyzed using SPSS statistical software. Data are presented as median and range. Body weight before surgery and at follow-up was compared using the Mann-Whitney test. A p-value less than 0.05 was considered statistically significant.

Results
Previous surgical history, indications for Merendino procedure and preoperative work-up
Twelve patients (mean age of 55, range 42–66 years) having a Merendino procedure due to failed previous antireflux surgery were identified during the study period. Males dominated (10:2) and all but ten patients had a history of two or more surgical interventions and one patient had been operated on four times. The most common indication for the Merendino procedure was chronic or intermittent pain with the majority taking daily morphine derivatives to control pain (Table 1). All patients were investigated with a CT-scan and upper GI endoscopy, which revealed miscellaneous abnormalities and some of the patients were also investigated with 24 h pH measurement, esophageal manometry or esophageal barium swallow (Table 2).

Intra-operative data, postoperative complications, length of stay, follow-up time, weight loss
The median operating time was 338 (range 197–418) minutes and the median perioperative bleeding was 500 (range 250–2000) ml. Postoperative complications were common and surgical complications occurred in 7 patients (Table 3). The postoperative course was graded according to Clavien Dindo grading system for the classification of surgical complications [29, 30]. Five patients had grade 0-I, two patients grade II, three patients grade IIIb, one patient grade IVa and one patient grade IVb. Three patients needed an acute re-operation, two because of bleeding and one because of rupture of the hiatal closure with herniation of the left colon and small bowel into the left thorax. Two patients had an anastomotic leak in the esophagojejunal anastomosis that was successfully treated with covered self-expanding metal stents. Five patients developed pneumonia and four severe septicaemia, which were successfully treated with

i.v. antibiotics. Three patients developed pleural effusion that was treated conservatively ($n = 1$) or with thoracocentesis ($n = 2$). The median postoperative hospital stay was 11 days (range 6–70) and follow-up ranged from 20 to 61 months (median 35). All patients had lost weight at follow-up compared to preoperative levels, 63.5 (46–90) vs. 72.5 (50–100) kg, $p < 0.001$.

Endoscopic reinterventions and redo surgery
Dysphagia was common and resulted in re-endoscopy in five patients (Table 4). In one patient a clear stricture was found in the proximal anastomosis 26 months after surgery, which was dilated. A re-endoscopy was combined with endoscopic dilatation of the esophagojejunostomy in three of these patients and in the jejunogastrostomy in two of the patients even though the macroscopic picture of the respective anastomotic areas revealed a patent lumen and no clear stricture. Symptoms suggestive of gastric outlet obstruction, possibly due to vagal damage, occurred in three patients who subsequently underwent a dilatation of the pylorus to 35 mm using a pneumatic balloon with a temporary positive effect. Five patients developed severe symptoms including dysphagia, vomiting and weight loss postoperatively, which occurred after an essentially uneventful postoperative recovery period. These complaints could not be managed conservatively or via endoscopic interventions and therefore another reoperation was considered indicated. Four patients underwent a conversion to a RNY esophagojejunostomy without resection of the distal stomach and one patient was re-operated with resection of the blind segment in the esophagojejunal anastomosis due to a presumed pseudodiverticulum formation. However, symptoms persisted in this patient, who finally received a percutaneous endoscopic gastrostomy for nutrition. These patients have not undergone any further surgical or

Table 1 Demographic data, indication for the first fundoplication and the subsequent Merendino procedure

patient	Age	sex	number of previous fundoplications	Indication for the first fundoplication	indication for merendino
1	55	M	4	Gastroesophageal reflux	Dysphagia and pain
2	61	M	2	Gastroesophageal reflux	Dysphagia and pain
3	42	M	2	Gastroesophageal reflux	Recurrent Reflux
4	65	F	2	Gastroesophageal reflux	Recurrent reflux and dysphagia
5	46	M	1	Gastroesophageal reflux	Dysphagia and pain
6	61	M	2	Paraesophageal hernia	Dysphagia and pain
7	66	M	2	Gastroesophageal reflux	Dysphagia and pain
8	42	M	2	Gastroesophageal reflux	Dysphagia and pain
9	57	M	1	Paraesophageal hernia	Recurrent reflux and dysphagia
10	49	M	2	Gastroesophageal reflux	Dysphagia and pain
11	51	M	3	Paraesophageal hernia	Dysphagia and pain
12	56	F	3	Paraesophageal hernia	Dysphagia and pain

Table 2 Preoperative workup for patients who underwent a Merendino procedure

patient	Ph monitoring	manometry	gastroscopy	CT	esophageal Barium swallow
1	ND	ND	Paraesophageal hernia	Paraesophageal hernia	ND
2	ND	ND	Normal	Normal	Esophageal dyskinesia
3	Pathological reflux	Dyschinesia	Sliding hernia	Paraesophageal hernia	ND
4	Pathological reflux	Normal	Normal	Normal	Paraesophageal hernia
5	Normal	Normal	Normal	Paraesophageal hernia	ND
6	ND	ND	ND	Normal	Esophageal dyskinesia
7	ND	Dyschinesia	ND	Other	ND
8	ND	ND	Esophageal diverticulum	Esophageal diverticulum	Esophageal diverticulum
9	Normal	ND	Normal	Paraesophageal hernia	Paraesophageal hernia
10	ND	ND	ND	Other	ND
11	ND	ND	ND	Paraesophageal hernia	Paraesophageal hernia
12	ND	Dyschinesia	ND	Paraesophageal hernia	ND

ND = No Data available

endoscopic interventions of the upper gastrointestinal tract.

QoL and symptom score at long-term follow up

QOLRAD, GSRS and DSRS were obtained from 6 patients who still had a Merendino reconstruction and are presented in Table 5. Scores in all dimensions were generally poor. Physical/social functioning and vitality were the dimensions with the worst scores in QOLRAD, while abdominal pain and indigestion were the most intense symptoms in GSRS. Fatigue, nausea and vomiting/stomach cramps were the dimensions with the worst scores in DSRS both regarding severity and frequency. All patients except one were on an oral diet at follow-up. Four of the patients used proton-pump inhibitors (PPI) on an everyday basis due to reflux- like symptoms and one patient was treated on demand.

Investigations of the esophagus and the interposed jejunal segment at follow-up

Four of the patients with Merendino reconstruction had a HRM after surgery. Two were examined due to weight loss and dysphagia and regurgitation and 2 patients as a part of the follow-up of this study. HRM was normal in three patients (peristalsis and motility in esophagus and jejunal segment) whereas in one patient the manometry revealed a totally aperistaltic jejunal segment. This patient and one of those with a normal HRM underwent conversion to Roux-en-Y esophagojejunostomy.

Six of the patients were investigated postoperatively with esophageal barium swallow, due to dysphagia and regurgitation. In 3 patients there were signs of stenosis

Table 3 Postoperative complications and Clavien-Dindo grade

Patient	Complication	Treatment	Clavien-Dindo grade
1	Pneumonia, pleural effusion	antibiotics, thoracocentesis	II
2	None		0
3	Artial fibrilation, septicaemia, bleeding, wound rupture, abdominal abscess, pneumonia, anastomotic leak	reoperation × 3, stent, drainage and antibiotics	IIIb
4	bleeding, septicaemia, pulmonary septic embolism	Reoperation, antibiotics	IIIb
5	pneumonia, small bowel paralysis	Antibiotics	II
6	None		0
7	anastomotic leak, pneumonia, septicaemia, respiratory failure, mediastinitis, pleural effusion	Reoperation, stent, antibiotics, ventilator support,	IVa
8	bleeding, pneumonia	Reoperation, antibiotics	IIIb
9	none		0
10	none		0
11	none		0
12	respiratory failure, pleural effusion, septicaemia	Ventilator support, thoracocentesis, antibiotics	IVb

Table 4 Weight before surgery and at follow-up, postoperative endoscopic interventions, redo-surgery and follow-up time among patients who underwent a Merendino reconstruction

Patient	Weight preoperatively (kg)	Weight at follow up (kg)	Endoscopic Interventions	Reoperations	Follow up (months)
1	100	90	Proximal anastomosis ×3	RNY with J-pouch	65
2	100	83	Proximal anastomosis ×2 and pylorus ×2	RNY	46
3	104	85			29
4	90	68			20
5	50	46	Proximal anastomosis ×1, distal anastomosis ×1	resection of the blind segment in the esophagojejunal anastomosis	36
6	64	52			48
7	82	65			35
8	72	73			61
9	53	50			31
10	66	62	Distal anastomosis ×1 and pylorus ×2	RNY with J-pouch	44
11	73	61		RNY	33
12	72	49	Pylorus ×2		30
	72,5 (49,6–100)[a]	63,5 (46–89,9)[a]*			35(20–61) [a]

[a]Median (range), * = $p < 0.001$ compared to preoperative weight

in the esophagojejunal anastomosis area and in 5 patients there was a significant prolongation of barium passage through the interposed small intestinal segment. In 4 patients there were signs of reflux into the esophagus from the contrast dye accumulated in the interposed segment.

Discussion

To our knowledge the series of cases presented herein is the first describing the results of a Merendino reconstruction, i.e. jejunal interposition between the esophagus and stomach, in patients with previously failed redo-fundoplication. We found that the rate of postoperative complications was high and at least in the same range as in previous case series of RNY reconstruction in similar patients [16, 17]. In addition, re-interventions for postoperative symptoms were frequent. Alleged anastomotic narrowing were managed by endoscopic dilatations and some patients also presented with gastric

outlet obstruction symptoms suggesting pyloric dysfunction as a result of vagal damage, which may occur after repeated surgery in the hiatus area. Dilatation of the pylorus was performed in these cases, but symptoms typically persisted. As many as 4 of the 12 patients, developed postoperative symptoms of intolerable severity and therefore a redo operation and conversion to RNY esophagojejunostomy was performed. Among the patients where a questionnaire-based follow-up was available, QoL was generally poor and gastrointestinal symptoms were common. Even dumping symptoms, the risk of which, from a theoretical point, should be minimized, given the preservation of the duodenal passage and maintenance of the gastric reservoir, were also frequently reported. Taken together these data, even though the number of patients is limited, suggests that the Merendino procedure is unsuitable for the complex group of patients where redo surgery after repeat fundoplication is considered. This is important to bear in

Table 5 QOLRAD, GSRS and DSRS scores from 6 patients with Merendino reconstruction presented as median (range)

QOLRAD	median (range)	GSRS	median (range)	DSRS	median (range)
Emotional distress	2.9 (2.5–5.3)	Reflux	3.8 (1.7–5.0)	Severity score	4.0 (3.0–5.4)
Sleep disturbance	2.7 (2.2–3.8)	Abdominal Pain	5.2 (3.0–5.3)	Frequency score	3.9 (3.0–5.3)
Food/drink problems	2.8 (1.7–4.2)	Indigestion	4.3 (3.0–4.3)	Total Score	15.3 (9.7–28.8)
Physical/social functioning	3.1 (1.8–5.0)	Diarrhoea	3.3 (1.0–5.0)		
Vitality	1.7 (1.0–3.3)	Constipation	3.7 (1.3–5.0)		

In QOLRAD a score of 1 represents the lowest possible quality of life and 7 the highest. In GSRS 1 corresponds to absence of symptoms and 7 very intense symptoms. In the DSRS severity score each dumping symptom during the past week is graded from "no trouble at all" [1] to "very severe problems" [7]. In the DSRS frequency score the frequency of the symptoms during the last 2 weeks is graded from "no trouble at all" [1] to "several times a day" [6]. The mean of all severity items is the severity score and the mean of all frequency items is the frequency score. Each severity item is multiplied by the respective frequency item to a DSRS total score (maximum score 42)

mind, especially since an additional aspect in favour of resection of the gastroesophageal junction area, was the severe pain hypothetically related to the extensive scarring of the hiatal region. Redo surgery after fundoplication using other approaches than yet another fundoplication are rarely performed and there is no evidence supporting the use of any specific reconstruction method over the other. RNY reconstruction has been proposed as an alternative and more effective method in patients with obesity or esophageal dysmotility [31, 32]. In addition to this, resection of the distal esophagus, cardia and proximal stomach may be indicated if symptoms of the patient include dysphagia and pain. From a theoretical point, preservation of the duodenal passage by performing a Merendino procedure could reduce post gastrectomy symptoms as compared to RNY, but the data presented here are not supportive of this.

Previous studies of the Merendino reconstruction after resection for early Barrett cancer have shown varying short- and long-term results. In one of the largest series, Stein et al. [20] reported less postoperative complications compared to Ivor-Lewis esophagectomy and excellent long-term outcome as measured by the GIQLI (gastro-intestinal quality of life index) instrument. In a more recent publication, where the EORTC QoL questionnaires were used, both short-term and functional results were similar after a Merendino reconstruction as compared to Ivor-Lewis procedure [33]. On the other hand, proximal gastrectomy with jejunal interposition in patients with non-advanced gastric cancer, which is a procedure similar to the Merendino, seems to have a superior functional outcome compared to total gastrectomy with RNY reconstruction [23, 24]. Obviously the importance of objectively assessing long-term data also in corresponding patient cohorts is warranted to assess the clinical place of the Merendino procedure. It is therefore particularly important to try to understand our experience of the poor results of the Merendino reconstruction among patients with a failed fundoplication. The high frequency of postoperative complications was expected, since this is frequent after most reconstructive procedure in the gastrointestinal tract. Objective findings of anatomical abnormalities among the patients were not always obvious. This may suggest that a general underlying pathology of gastrointestinal motility may have been present. Manometry of the esophagus and the interposed jejunal segment was available in 4 patients and in one of these cases aperistalsis of the jejunal segment was recorded. Barium swallow was performed postoperatively in 6 patients and showed a prolonged emptying of the jejunal segment or reflux in 5 and 4 cases respectively. The underlying mechanism for the poor function of the jejunal segment regardless of objective findings is obscure, but it can be hypothesized that the partial fundoplication that was performed may

have contributed to the distal obstruction. However, also one patient with normal manometry findings had symptoms so severe, that a redo to RNY was performed. Thus, routine diagnostic methods may be inefficient in detecting possible motor disturbances of the gastrointestinal tract in this group of patients.

Finally, limitation of this study is that investigations done on a small sample of the group. Only four patients were investigated with HRM postoperatively and six patients with esophageal barium swallow. QOL data preoperatively don't exist for these 12 patients and postoperatively were obtained from 6 patients. As a result it might be difficult to interpret the severity of the symptoms at the follow up.

Conclusions
The conclusion to be drawn from this case series is that the Merendino procedure is, until proven otherwise, unsuitable for patients who undergo redo surgery after previously failed re-fundoplications.

Abbreviations
DSRS: Dumping Syndrome; GERD: Gastroesophageal Reflux Disease; GIQLI: Gastrointestinal Quality Of Life; GSRS: Gastrointestinal Symptom Rating Scale; HRM: High Resolution Manometry; PPI: Proton-Pump Inhibitors; QoL: Quality Of Life; Qolrad: Quality Of Life in Reflux And Dyspepsia

Funding
Not applicable.

Authors' contributions
AA acquired, analysed and interpreted the patient data and wrote the manuscript. ML, IR, PE, LL, MN, AT, JAT interpreted the patient data, made the statistical analysis and were major contributors in writing the manuscript. All the above authors made substantial contributions to conception and design and been involved in drafting the manuscript and revising it critically for important intellectual content. All authors read and approved the final manuscript.

Competing interests
The authors declare that they have no competing interests.

Author details
[1]Centre for Digestive Diseases, Karolinska University Hospital and Division of Surgery, Department of Clinical Intervention and Technology (CLINTEC), Karolinska Institutet, Stockhom, Sweden. [2]Department of Surgery, Nyköping Hospital, Nyköping, Sweden. [3]Centre for Clinical Research Sörmland, Uppsala University, Uppsala, Sweden.

References

1. Anvari M, Allen C. Five-year comprehensive outcomes evaluation in 181 patients after laparoscopic Nissen fundoplication. J Am Coll Surg. 2003;196:51–7.
2. Broeders JA, Rijnhart-de Jong HG, Draaisma WA, et al. Ten-year outcome of laparoscopic and conventional nissen fundoplication: randomized clinical trial. Ann Surg. 2009;250:698–706.
3. DeMeester TR, Bonavina L, Albertucci M. Nissen fundoplication for gastroesophageal reflux disease. Evaluation of primary repair in 100 consecutive patients. Ann Surg. 1986;204:9–20.
4. Catarci M, Gentileschi P, Papi C, et al. Evidence-based appraisal of antireflux fundoplication. Annals Surg. 2004;239:325–37.
5. Dassinger MS, Torquati A, Houston HL, et al. Laparoscopic fundoplication: 5-year follow-up. Am Surg. 2004;70:691–4.
6. Lundell L. Complications after anti-reflux surgery. Best Pract Clin Res Gastroenterol. 2004;18:935–45.
7. Horgan S, Pohl D, Bogetti D, et al. Failed antireflux surgery: what have we learned from reoperations? Arch Surg. 1999;134:809–15.
8. Juhasz A, Sundaram A, Hoshino M, et al. Outcomes of surgical management of symptomatic large recurrent hiatus hernia. Surg Endosc. 2012;26:1501–8.
9. Smith CD, McClusky DA, Rajad MA, et al. When fundoplication fails: redo? Ann Surg. 2005;241:861–9.
10. Iqbal A, Awad Z, Simkins J, et al. Repair of 104 failed anti-reflux operations. Ann Surg. 2006;244:42–51.
11. Funch-Jensen P, Bendixen A, Iversen MG, et al. Complications and frequency of redo antireflux surgery in Denmark: a nationwide study, 1997-2005. Surg Endosc. 2008;22:627–30.
12. Furnee EJ, Draaisma WA, Broeders IA, et al. Surgical reintervention after failed antireflux surgery: a systematic review of the literature. J Gastrointest Surg. 2009;13:1539–49.
13. Wykypiel H, Kamolz T, Steiner P, et al. Austrian experiences with redo antireflux surgery. Surg Endosc. 2005;19:1315–9.
14. Khaitan L, Bhatt P, Richards W, et al. Comparison of patient satisfaction after redo and primary fundoplications. Surg Endosc. 2003;17:1042–5.
15. Spechler SJ. The management of patients who have "failed" antireflux surgery. The. Am J Gastroenterol. 2004;99:552–61.
16. Makris KI, Lee T, Mittal SK. Roux-en-Y reconstruction for failed fundoplication. J Gastrointest Surg. 2009;13:2226–32.
17. Awais O, Luketich JD, Tam J, et al. Roux-en-Y near esophagojejunostomy for intractable gastroesophageal reflux after antireflux surgery. Ann Thorac Surg. 2008;85:1954–9.
18. Lundell LR. The knife or the pill in the long-term treatment of gastroesophageal reflux disease? Yale J Biol Med. 1994;67:233–46.
19. Wright C. Jejunal interposition for benign esophageal disease. Ann Surg. 1987;205:54–60.
20. Stein HJ, Feith M, Mueller J, et al. Limited resection for early adenocarcinoma in Barrett's esophagus. Ann Surg. 2000;232:733–42.
21. Linke GR, Borovicka J, et al. Altered esophageal motility and gastroesophageal barrier in patients with jejunal interposition after distal esophageal resection for early stage adenocarcinoma. J Gastrointest Surg. 2007;11:1262–7.
22. Pring C, Dexter S. A laparoscopic vagus-preserving Merendino procedure for early esophageal adenocarcinoma. Surg Endosc. 2010;24:1195–9.
23. Yoo CH, Sohn BH, Han WK, et al. Proximal gastrectomy reconstructed by jejunal pouch interposition for upper third gastric cancer: prospective randomized study. World J Surg. 2005;29:1592–9.
24. Takagawa R, Kunisaki C, Kimura J, et al. A pilot study comparing jejunal pouch and jejunal interposition reconstruction after proximal gastrectomy. Dig Surg. 2010;27:502–8.
25. Svedlund J, Sjodin I, Dotevall G. GSRS--a clinical rating scale for gastrointestinal symptoms in patients with irritable bowel syndrome and peptic ulcer disease. Dig Dis Sci. 1988;33:129–34.
26. Kulich KR, Madisch A, Pacini F, et al. Reliability and validity of the gastrointestinal symptom rating scale (GSRS) and quality of life in reflux and dyspepsia (QOLRAD) questionnaire in dyspepsia: a six-country study. Health Qual Life Outcomes. 2008;6:12.
27. Laurenius A, Olbers T, Naslund I, et al. Dumping syndrome following gastric bypass: validation of the dumping symptom rating scale. Obes Surg. 2013;23:740–55.
28. Wang A, Pleskow DK, Banerjee S, et al. Esophageal function testing. Gastrointest Endosc. 2012;76:231–43.
29. Dindo D, Demartines N, Clavien PA. Classification of surgical complications: a new proposal with evaluation in a cohort of 6336 patients and results of a survey. Ann Surg. 2004;240:205–13.
30. Clavien PA, Barkun J, de Oliveira ML, et al. The Clavien-Dindo classification of surgical complications: five-year experience. Ann Surg. 2009;250:187–96.
31. Mittal SK, Legner A, Tsuboi K, et al. Roux-en-Y reconstruction is superior to redo fundoplication in a subset of patients with failed antireflux surgery. Surg Endosc. 2013;27:927–35.
32. Yamamoto SR, Hoshino M, Nandipati KC, et al. Long-term outcomes of reintervention for failed fundoplication: redo fundoplication versus roux-en-Y reconstruction. Surg Endosc. 2014;28:42–8.
33. Zapletal C, Heesen C, Origer J, et al. Quality of life after surgical treatment of early Barrett's Cancer: a prospective comparison of the Ivor-Lewis resection versus the modified Merendino resection. World J Surg. 2014;38:1444–52.

18

Wide excision and reconstruction surgery for recurrent sweat gland umbilical adenocarcinoma followed by chemotherapy can prevent the risk of recurrences

Adeodatus Yuda Handaya[1]* ⓘ, Nova Yuli Prasetyo Budi[2], Guntur Marganing Adi Nugroho[2] and Aditya Rifqi Fauzi[2]

Abstract

Background: Adenocarcinoma derived from umbilicus is very rare. Most adenocarcinomas in umbilicus are secondary events. Carcinoma derived from sweat glands is sporadic, highly radioresistant and has a clinical appearance that is difficult to predict.

Case presentation: A 37-year-old woman presented with recurrent umbilicus adenocarcinoma after a history of umbilicus tumor surgery 14 months earlier and Capecitabine chemotherapy six times. Malignant cells were found in Fine Needle Aspiration Biopsy (FNAB) examination. A colonoscopy examination found pathological colitis without any colonic mass. The patient underwent wide excision and reconstruction surgery using a composite attachment visceral mesh with a size of 30 × 30 cm. Histopathologic examination of the surgery diagnosed adenocarcinoma of the sudoriferous gland with adjacent tissue free of tumor cells. Six months post operation, Positron Emission Tomography (PET) scan was performed and found neither residue nor recurrence.

Conclusions: Wide excision and reconstruction surgery for recurrent sweat gland umbilical adenocarcinoma followed by chemotherapy can be an alternative to prevent recurrences.

Keywords: Umbilical tumor, Sudoriferous adenocarcinoma, Cancer recurrence, Radical excision, Reconstruction

Background

Primary umbilical tumors are a sporadic case, with only a few cases being reported in today's era of modern medicine. Although rarely found, umbilical tumors events ranging from one-sixth to one-fourth of all malignancy events in this location. Metastasis of the umbilicus tumor is more common. Umbilical adenocarcinoma primary tumors can grow from different tissues, from pre-existing endometriomas, coelomic mesothelium or the embryological remains of the umbilicus, both from the vitello-intestinal (omphalo-mesenteric) and urachus tracts [1, 2].

Sweat gland carcinoma has local destruction capability and local tissue infiltration, and also distant metastasis which primarily occurs in adult patients with peak incidence in the fifth and sixth decades of life. The predilection of this tumor is in the genital skin and perineum (34.5%), trunk (26.4%), head and neck (18.3%) and lower extremities (13.9%) [3]. Adenocarcinoma of sweat glands appears as moderate to poor adenocarcinoma with regional variations, ranging from true ductile form to infiltrative anaplastic form. Histologic view of malignancy is similar to most epithelial tumors. The distinction between metastatic adenocarcinoma and primary adenocarcinoma of the sweat glands can be challenging [4].

* Correspondence: yudahandaya@ugm.ac.id
[1]Digestive Surgery Division, Department of Surgery, Faculty of Medicine, Universitas Gadjah Mada/Dr. Sardjito Hospital, Jl. Kesehatan No. 1, Yogyakarta 55281, Indonesia
Full list of author information is available at the end of the article

Case presentation

A 37-year-old woman presented with a painless nodule in her umbilicus which histopathology examination suggested to be a malignant umbilical tumor. Fourteen months before admission, the patient had a history of umbilical tumor surgery, with histopathology examination suggesting moderately-differentiated adenocarcinoma. The patient also had additional oral chemotherapy six times, using Capecitabine 2×1500 mg. The patient complained about a recurrent mass in her umbilicus at the surgical scar site.

On examination, cytology examination using Fine Needle Aspiration Biopsy (FNAB) results identified some malignant cells (+). As seen in Figs. 1 and 2, the adenocarcinoma of the sudoriferous gland is arranged into tubular and papillary patterns consisting of polymorphic cells, scanty cytoplasm, irregular nuclei, and coarse chromatin. Colonoscopy examination was performed to ascertain whether the tumor was primary or secondary colonic metastasis. Results were in the normal range, without intraluminal mass or stricture, and subsequent colon mucosa biopsy showed chronic colitis. CT (Computed tomography) scan was also performed, and the results showed no metastasis.

A recurrent tumor mass of adenocarcinoma with the diameter of 7 cm had been excised with the tumor margin of 5 cm. Wide excision surgery was performed leaving a 17 cm surgical defect on the anterior abdominal wall (Fig. 3). The reconstruction was performed using anti-adhesive *Parietex polyester* mesh. Reasonable collagen barrier on one side to limit visceral attachment was sized 30×30 cm. Histopathology examination of the excised tissue suggested sudoriferous gland adenocarcinoma with adjacent tissue free of tumor cells. Treatment was continued with additional chemotherapy using Capecitabine 500 mg dose 3–0-2 mg and Bevacizumab (Avastin) 400 mg 12 times. Follow up PET (Positron

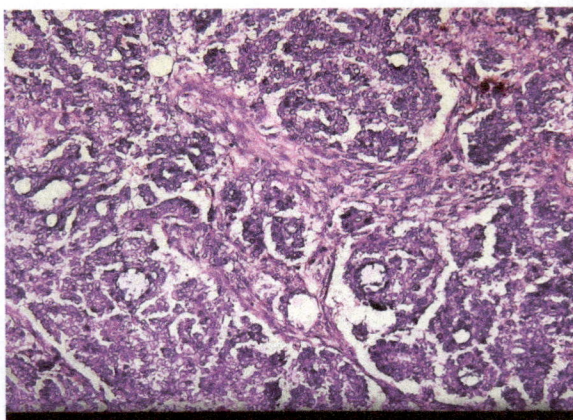

Fig. 2 Pathological anatomy view at 200× magnification

Emission Tomography) scan six months post-surgery was performed and showed no residual tumor in the umbilical region, and no apparent paraaortic nor mesenteric lymphadenopathy. Postoperative follow-up after 2 years is shown in Fig. 4.

Wide excision and reconstructive surgical technique

- Surgical technique decisions were based on pathologic review from prior umbilical tumor resections
- Our goal was excision of the tumor with negative gross and microscopic margins of resection after the previous recurrence.
- During surgery, we attempted to achieve a gross margin after recurrence with the excision distance

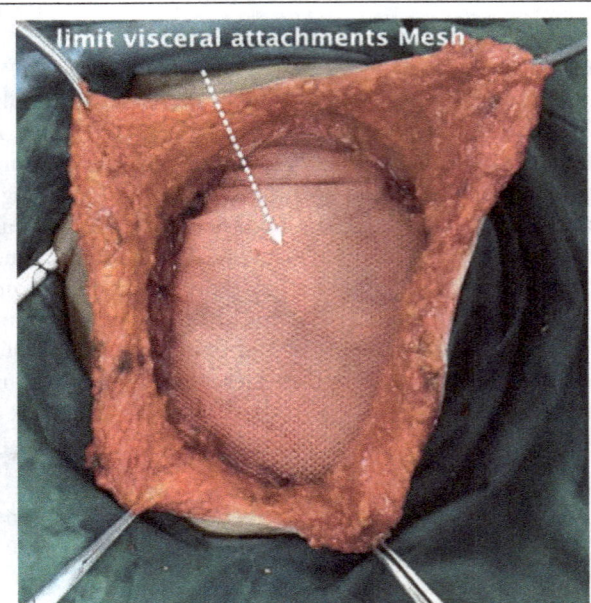

Fig. 1 Pathological anatomy view at 100× magnification

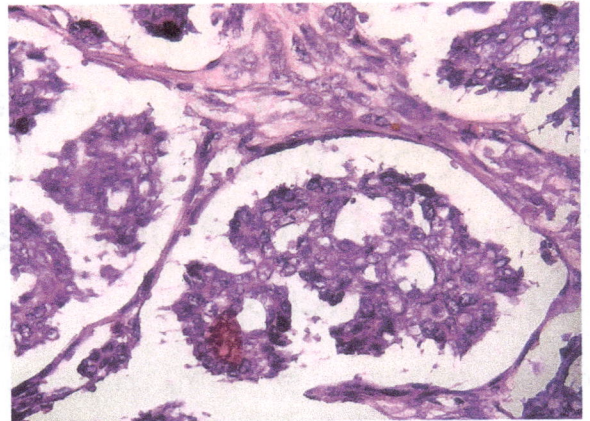

Fig. 3 Wide excision dan abdominal reconstruction using mesh

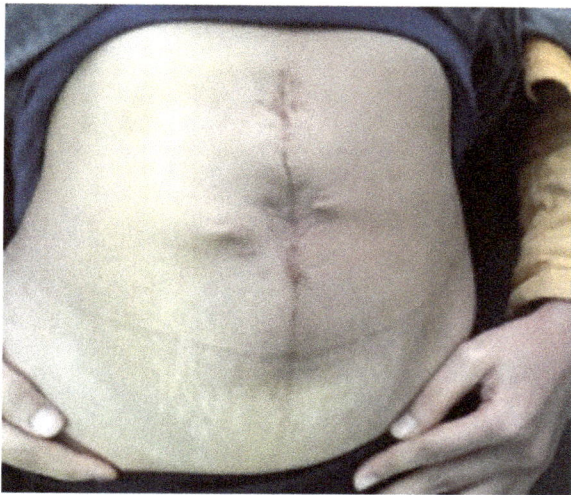

Fig. 4 Two years after surgery

from the grossly palpable lesion greater than 5 cm, while normally in first surgery we can performed with the margin 1–2 cm.

- We performed full-thickness resection of the tumor-containing abdominal wall continued with exploratory laparotomy to evaluate the intraperitoneal extent of the umbilical tumor.
- Residual defect of abdominal wall reconstruction was performed using prosthetic mesh
- The mesh in a tension-free manner was sutured with combined multiple anchors and continuous running suture to the edges of the fascial defect.
- Wound closure was performed following placement of subcutaneous vacuum drainage.

Discussion and Conclusions

Umbilical cancer has a reasonably high incidence, about 10% of all malignant tumors present on the abdominal wall. Most of umbilical tumors (80%) are from visceral organ metastases (Sister Mary Joseph Nodule) because they have adjacent vascularization and embryonic connections, while the remainder are primary tumors [1]. In our case, as in the case of primary tumors, no primary tumor was found based on colonoscopy and CT scan. Clinical symptoms that can arise include pain, ulceration and necrosis, and sometimes it can also discharge mucous or blood. Other signs such as irregular bumps can appear that enlarge progressively ranging in size from 0.5–2 cm [2, 5, 6].

The diagnostic tests used to diagnose this tumor are usually using radiologic modalities, such as cystogram, ultrasonography (USG), magnetic resonance imaging (MRI), computed tomography scan (CT-scan), and positron emission tomography (PET). Abdominal sonography usually produces the normal result [7]. In some cases, an irregular hypoechoic mass can be found with microcalcification in the umbilical region, but not extending into the peritoneal cavity [1]. Doppler imaging sometimes can show internal vascularity [8]. Local staging and evaluation of distant metastases of the tumor often uses CT scan and MRI. On the CT scan images, the tumor appears as a mixed solid and cystic mass. Differential diagnosis of the umbilical nodule includes neoplastic or non-neoplastic lesions such as Paget's disease, angioma, umbilical adenoma (raspberry tumor), umbilical hernia, endometriosis, hypertrophic scar, and umbilical granuloma. Tissue diagnosis using fine-needle aspiration biopsy (FNAB) is acceptable to establish the diagnosis [9].

The recommendation of management of primary umbilical tumors after the excisional biopsy is extensive surgery with a 1–2 cm tumor-free margin along with lymph node removal when clinically positive. A broader excision may prevent recurrence [3, 7]. The main reason we did surgery with a 5.0 cm margin was that our case is a recurrent sweat gland umbilical adenocarcinoma, and needed a wider excision to prevent its recurrence. In our case, we also used an anti-adhesive mesh, and neither a rejection nor a postoperative hernia occurred.

In surgical management, the greatest difficulty lies in the reconstruction of the umbilicus because its depth should be sufficient, especially when the patient presents a scarce panniculus adipose. By ensuring an adjacent fatty tissue is included, this technique solves this problem. Maintaining a curve in the base of the flap rather than a right angle to the approach avoids the formation of edges, thereby achieving a more rounded umbilicus and avoiding one that is elongated and closed [10]. Several studies recommend adjuvant chemotherapy and local radiotherapy as well as lymph node dissection as prophylaxis in highly undifferentiated tumors. The cutaneous sweat gland carcinomas are radioresistant, and chemotherapy has been infrequently employed.

In some cases, a more aggressive approach is used, because when metastasis occurs then the prognosis will worsen. Primary adenocarcinoma of the umbilicus from cutaneous sudoriferous glands is an uncommon neoplasm that may behave more aggressively than most tumors. Management of primary umbilical tumor involves surgical excision. Radical local umbilical surgery and reconstruction with limit visceral attachments is indicated [1]. In conclusion, wide excision and reconstruction surgery for recurrent sweat gland umbilical adenocarcinoma followed by chemotherapy can be an alternative to prevent recurrences.

Abbreviations
CT: Computed tomography; FNAB: Fine needle aspiration biopsy; MRI: Magnetic resonance imaging; PET: Positron emission tomography; USG: Ultrasonography

Acknowledgments
We thank the surgical staff and nursing team who were involved in the patient's care.

Authors' contributions
AYH conceived the study and was a major contributor in writing the manuscript. NYPB, GMAN, ARF critically revised the manuscript for important intellectual content. All authors read and approved the final manuscript.

Competing interests
The authors declare that they have no competing interests.

Author details
[1]Digestive Surgery Division, Department of Surgery, Faculty of Medicine, Universitas Gadjah Mada/Dr. Sardjito Hospital, Jl. Kesehatan No. 1, Yogyakarta 55281, Indonesia. [2]Faculty of Medicine, Universitas Gadjah Mada/Dr. Sardjito Hospital, Yogyakarta 55281, Indonesia.

References
1. Atri R, Dhull A, Kaur P, Singh G, Chauhan A. Primary Umbilical Adenocarcinoma - A Case Report. Internet J Third World Med. 2009;9:1.
2. Alnaqbi KAY, Joshi S, Ghazal-Aswad S, Abu Zidan FM. Primary umbilical adenocarcinoma. Singap Med J. 2007;48:e308–10.
3. Sharma RD, Badran R, Singhal V, Saxena S, Bansal A. Metastatic sweat gland adenocarcinoma: a clinico-pathological dilemma. World J Surg Oncol. 2003; 1(1):13.
4. Nair P, Rathod K, Chaudhary A, Pilani A. Sweat gland adenocarcinoma of scalp. Int J Trichology. 2013;5:208–10.
5. Psarras K, Symeonidis N, Baltatzis M, Notopoulos A, Nikolaidou C. Umbilical metastasis as primary manifestation of Cancer: a small series and review of the literature. J Clin Diagn Res. 2014;8:17–9.
6. Raimondo G, Conte M, Egidi F, Borghese F. Umbilical metastases: current viewpoint. World J Surg Oncol. 2005;3:13.
7. Çiçek T, Gonulalan U, Coban G, Erinannc H, Kosan M. A rare cause of urachal adenocarcinoma: urachal Diverticle. Case Rep Urol. 2013. https://doi.org/10. 1155/2013/571395.
8. Bao B, Hatem M, Wong JK. Urachal adenocarcinoma: a rare case report. Radiol Case Rep. 2016. https://doi.org/10.1016/j.radcr.2016.10.019.
9. Altaf S, Dev K, Gurawalia J, Kumar S. Umbilical metastasis as a primary presentation in carcinoma rectum: a case report. Int J Case Rep Images. 2017;8:201–4.
10. Donnabella A. Anatomical reconstruction of the umbilicus. Rev Bras Cir Plást. 2013;28:119–23.

19

Treatment of deep cavities using a perforator-based island flap with partial de-epithelization

Jung Woo Chang[1], Se Won Oh[2], Jeongseok Oh[2] and M. Seung Suk Choi[1]*

Abstract

Background: The perforator-based island flap is a popular option for defect coverage. In cases with deep cavities, however, the classical island flap may not be a suitable option. By de-epithelization of the peripheral portion of a perforator-based island flap, the distal part of the flap can be used to fill deep spaces, as the flap can be folded and inserted into the spaces.

Methods: From June 2015 to April 2017, 21 cases of deep internal defects were reconstructed with perforator-based island flaps with peripheral de-epithelization. A fasciocutaneous flap was elevated and rotated with the pivot point on the perforator. After performing de-epithelization on the periphery of the flap, the de-epithelized portion of the flap was inserted and anchored into the internal defect. Demographic information about the patients, the size of the defects, the perforators that were used, and complications were recorded.

Results: During the follow-up period (mean, 14.2 months) of total 21 cases, no major complications such as flap loss occurred. In 2 cases, a minor complication was observed. Temporary flap congestion was seen in 1 case, and was treated with a short period of leech therapy, and the other case was partial necrosis on the flap margin, which was cured with minimal debridement and conservative treatment. No major problems have occurred, especially on the de-epithelized part of the flap and in the occupied space.

Conclusions: With performing careful procedure, a perforator-based island flap with partial de-epithelization can be a useful option for the surgical treatment of deep cavities.

Trial registration: This study was retrospectively registered in the institutional review board on human subjects research and the ethics committee, Hanyang University Guri Hospital (Institutional Review Board File No. 2018–01–003-002 https://www.e-irb.com:3443/devlpg/nlpgS200.jsp).

Keywords: Deep cavity, Pressure sore, Fistula, Perforator flap, De-epithelization

Background

Deep cavities are difficult wounds to treat. Generally, deep cavities have a cutaneous opening, and a space with considerable depth from the opening is present [1]. The direction of the space is variable, and can be horizontal, vertical or oblique [2]. Iceberg-type pressure sores and cutaneous fistulae are typical examples. To treat these deep cavity wounds, surgical methods are preferred, as

conservative treatment such as negative pressure wound therapy requires a long period of treatment.

The perforator–based island flap is currently a popular surgical option for the treatment of defect wounds [3–7]. Especially in cases with pressure sore defects, it is the most popular option, as it can be transferred with less morbidity on the donor site [8–10]. However, the perforator-based island flap is usually a simple fasciocutaneous flap, meaning that it is not suitable for complex wound coverage. As deep cavities are complex wounds which easily remain seroma or bacterial colonization [11], the options for deep cavity treatment should also be complex. To fill the complex morphology of a deep cavity wound, the morphology of the flap must be modified [12].

* Correspondence: msschoi1@gmail.com
[1]Department of Plastic and Reconstructive Surgery, Hanyang University Guri Hospital, Hanyang University College of Medicine, 249-1, Gyomun-dong, Guri-si, Gyeonggi-do 471-701, Korea
Full list of author information is available at the end of the article

The modification of the flap in this study, is peripheral de-epithelization of the perforator–based island flap. As the de-epithelized portion of the flap can be folded and inserted into the deep space, it can provide a cavity-occupying effect [13, 14].

Methods

This study was conducted in conformity with the World Medical Association Declaration of Helsinki. From June 2015 to April 2017, 21 cases of deep cavities were treated using the modified perforator-based island flaps. Patient demographics, the size of the defect including the cavity, the perforators that were used, and postoperative complications, were recorded.

The operative procedure was performed under general anesthesia. For complete debridement of the affected tissues, all surface areas in the defect, including the deep cavity, were painted with gentian violet. The painted areas were completely excised to avoid recurrence after surgery. After the complete excision of the surface areas, perforator detection was performed with hand-held Doppler. When a healthy perforator was detected near the defect opening, the island flap was designed. The point where the perforator emerged was marked as the pivot point, and the distance from this point to the end of the deep cavity was measured. The flap was designed by applying the measured distance to the length from the pivot point to the end of the flap. The width of the flap was same as the width of the cavity, and the direction of the flap was decided by considering the arc of rotation and possibility of donor site closure. The ratio, length to width, was limited not to exceed 3:1, as a narrow flap can result in blood supply limit. The width of flap was also limited to 10 cm, for ensured primary closure on donor site. The arc of rotation should be less than 180° to prevent excessive twisting of the perforator.

After designing the flap, fasciocutaneous flap elevation was performed in a distal-to-proximal fashion. When dissecting near the pivot point, careful handling is needed to avoid perforator injury. Excessively fine dissection, such as skeletonization of the perforator should be avoided. After complete islanding of the flap, the flap was rotated toward the wound. When rotating the flap, there should be no tension on the perforator. If the flap can be rotated toward the wound without tension, the flap should be set according to the morphology of the wound by inserting the distal portion of the flap into the deep cavity. The inserted portion was then marked on the surface of the flap. The flap was taken out, and the marked portion was de-epithelized with the scalpel. The de-epithelized portion was inserted into the space again, and anchored with sutures to be fixed into the space. After confirming that the flap was positioned with the de-epithelized portion in the space and the intact portion on the cavity opening, both donor and flap sites were closed with sutures.

Results

The 21 cases included in this study consisted of 16 pressure sores, 2 meningomyelocele defects, and 3 cutaneous fistulae (Table 1). There were 12 males and 9 females, and their mean age was 60.4 years (range, 31–81 years). Among the 21 cases, 9 superior gluteal artery perforators (SGAPs), 3 inferior gluteal artery perforators (IGAPs), 3 deep inferior epigastric artery perforators (DIEPs), 3 deep femoral artery perforators, and 3 tensor fascia lata perforator, were used as the pedicle of the island flap. During the follow-up period, which lasted for a mean of 14.2 months (range, 7–25 months), no major complications, such as flap loss, were observed.

In 2 cases (9.5%), a minor complication was observed. Temporary flap congestion after the operation was observed in 1 case. The congestion was observed on the second postoperative day, but it was treated with a short period of leech therapy. The other case involved partial necrosis at the flap margin. After observing the demarcation, it was cured with minimal debridement and conservative treatment. Of particular note, no problems occurred in the de-epithelized part of the flap and the space it occupied. No cavity-related complications like recurrence of infection, were observed. All cases with deep cavities were completely treated using the perforator-based island flap with partial de-epithelization.

Case 1

A patient (age range 50–59 years) presented with a stage IV sacral sore. The patient was paraplegic, which led him to his chronic bedridden state. The wound measured 9 × 5 cm with its internal cavity. After complete debridement, a deep cavity was still present on cephalic side of the defect. An IGAP-based perforator flap was elevated to cover the defect, and de-epithelization was performed on the periphery to fill the cavity. After complete inset of the flap on the wound, both donor and recipient sites were closed primarily, with negative-suction drains inserted. No postoperative complications or recurrence took place during the follow-up period (Fig. 1).

Case 2

A patient (age range 50–59 years) presented with a meningomyelocele defect in the lumbar region. The patient had undergone surgery twice in another clinic. As the patient suffered from recurrent meningomyelocele, flap coverage was needed immediately after complete excision of the recurrent mass. The size of the defect after the complete excision, was 10 × 4 cm, and the depth of the cavity was 4 cm. To cover the vertically oriented cavity, an SGAP-based island flap with peripheral de-epithelization

Table 1 Patient demographics and characteristics of the flaps

No.	Age range (years)	Defect	Size, (cm²)	Depth of cavity (cm)	Size of de-epithelization (cm²)	Perforator	Follow-up (months)	Complication
1	70–79	Sacral sore	10 × 6	3	6 × 3	SGAP	25	None
2	80–89	Sacral sore	17 × 10	5	10 × 5	SGAP	20	None
3	60–69	Ischial sore	8 × 5	2	5 × 2	DFP	18	None
4	50–59	Meningomyelocele	10 × 4	4	5 × 4	SGAP	18	None
5	60–69	Sacral sore	15 × 13	3	10 × 3	SGAP	18	None
6	80–89	Sacral sore	11 × 7	4	6 × 4	IGAP	17	None
7	70–79	Ischial sore	12 × 10	3	8 × 3	DFP	15	None
8	60–69	Sacral sore	12 × 10	4	10 × 4	SGAP	15	None
9	50–59	Meningomyelocele	7 × 3	4	4 × 3	SGAP	15	None
10	30–39	Cutaneous fistula	4 × 4	9	9 × 4	DIEP	13	Congestion
11	30–39	Sacral sore	10 × 10	2	10 × 2	SGAP	13	None
12	30–39	Cutaneous fistula	4 × 4	9	9 × 4	DIEP	13	Partial necrosis
13	60–69	Trochanter sore	9 × 7	3	7 × 3	TFLP	13	None
14	50–59	Sacral sore	9 × 5	3	5 × 3	IGAP	13	None
15	60–69	Sacral sore	10 × 11	4	8 × 4	SGAP	12	None
16	40–49	Sacral sore	4 × 2	3	3 × 2	IGAP	12	None
17	40–49	Ischial sore	12 × 6	4	6 × 4	DFP	12	None
18	70–79	Cutaneous fistula	3 × 4	4	4 × 4	DIEP	10	None
19	80–89	Trochanter sore	8 × 6	2	6 × 2	TFLP	10	None
20	80–89	Trochanter sore	6 × 5	1	4 × 1	TFLP	10	None
21	60–69	Sacral	15 × 8	4	8 × 4	SGAP	7	None

Abbreviations: *SGAP* Superior gluteal artery perforator, *DFP* Deep femoral artery perforator, *IGAP* Inferior gluteal artery perforator, *DIEP* Deep inferior epigastric artery perforator, *TFLP* Tensor fascia lata perforator

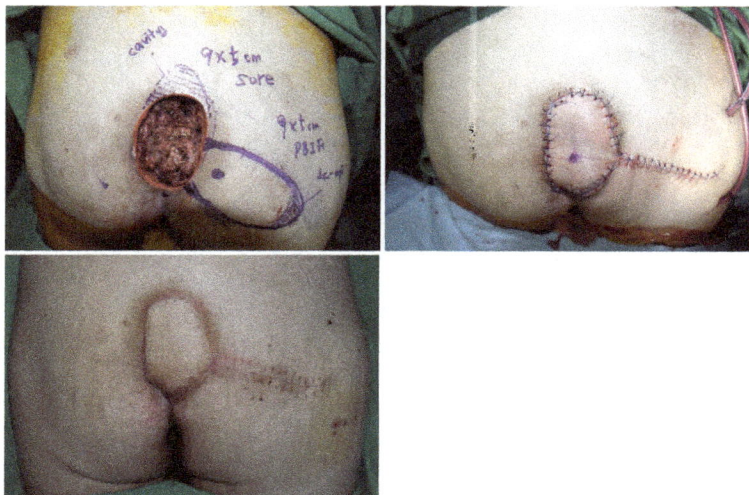

Fig. 1 A patient (age range 50–59 years) with a stage IV sacral sore. (Upper left) After complete debridement, a 9 × 5 cm wound with a horizontally oriented cavity in cephalad, was seen. The marked area on the distal portion of the flap was de-epithelized. (Upper right) After transposing the flap and filling the cavity with the de-epithelized portion, both the recipient and the donor wounds were closed with sutures. (Below) The wound healed without any problems

was elevated. The de-epithelized portion of the flap completely filled the cavity, and no complications or recurrence were observed during the follow-up period (Fig. 2).

Case 3

A patient (age range 30–39 years) presented with a cutaneous fistula on the lower abdomen. The patient had experienced a severe pelvic bone fracture and bladder rupture, which resulted in the formation of massive adhesion tissues between the pelvic bone and bladder. The cutaneous fistula was formed in the adhesion tissue. The size of the fistula was found to be 4 × 4 cm of opening and 9 cm length of tract after a complete fistulectomy. The cavity started from the cutaneous opening, and the direction was oblique to connect with the anterior portion of the bladder. After reconstructing the bladder opening by a urologic surgeon, a DIEP-based island flap with peripheral de-epithelization was elevated to fill the obliquely oriented cavity. The flap showed temporary congestion, but the congestion was straightforwardly controlled with a short period of leech therapy (Fig. 3).

Discussion

Deep cavity wounds are difficult to treat, because they are usually vulnerable to infection which prolongs healing time [15, 16]. Incomplete treatment of dead space within the wound often induces recurrence and chronicity. The rapid and complete solution for deep cavity wound is obliterating dead space with well vascularized tissue through surgical intervention [17, 18]. To provide obliteration of dead space, using muscle flap around the wound can be considered at first [19–24]. However,

using muscle flap leaves a potential of huge donor site morbidity, and requires additional skin flap to cover the cutaneous opening of the wound.

Since the perforator-based island flap was introduced by Koshima et al. [25] in 1993, it has been widely used for defect coverage. When comparing the perforator-based island flap with the musculocutaneous local flap introduced by Mathes and Nahai in 1979 [26], its advantages are, low donor site morbidity and the possibility of future reconstruction in cases of recurrence. As perforator-based island flap preserves underlying muscle, its donor site morbidity is lower than that of musculocutaneous flap which sacrifices both skin and muscle layer. Furthermore, preserved muscle contains additional perforators which enable future reconstruction with another perforator-based island flap in cases of recurrence. These advantages led this option to become popular. However, the classical form of the perforator-based island flap is not perfect for deep cavity filling. Deep cavity wounds, such as fistulae and iceberg-type pressure sores, typically have morphology with a deep internal space combined with a cave-like cutaneous opening. The classical island flap can cover only the cutaneous opening, but not the internal space. However, if the skin layer of the island flap is removed, it can be inserted into this space [27–30]. The modification of the flap in this study, was peripheral de-epithelization. The proximal portion with an intact skin layer was placed on cutaneous opening of the wound, and the distal portion that underwent de-epithelization was folded and inserted into the deep space to fill the cavity. As the proximal portion with the intact skin layer was exposed on the outside, it served as a monitoring flap. Since the distal portion, which is buried in the deep space, cannot be

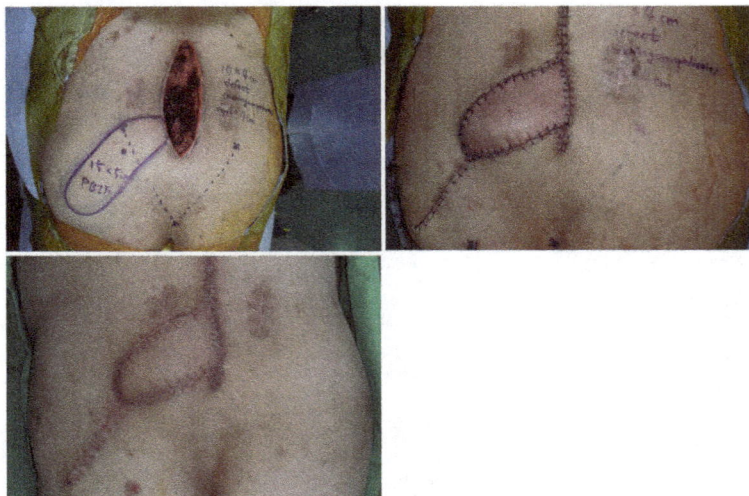

Fig. 2 A patient (age range 50–59 years) with a meningomyelocele defect on the lumbar region. (Upper left) A 10 × 4 cm wound with a vertically oriented cavity, was observed after complete excision of the meningomyelocele. The distal half of the flap was de-epithelized, and inserted into the cavity. (Upper right) After complete inset of the flap, both the recipient and the donor wounds were closed with sutures. (Below) The wound healed without any problems

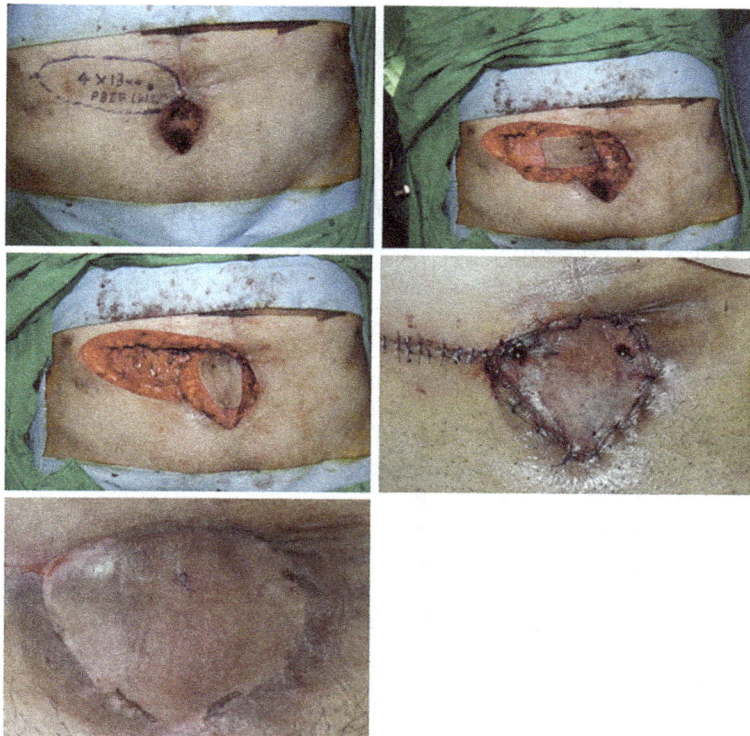

Fig. 3 A patient (age range 30–39 years) with a cutaneous fistula on the lower abdomen. (Upper left) A 4 × 4 cm cutaneous opening with a 9 cm length deep cavity obliquely oriented beneath the pelvic bone, was seen. An island flap was designed near the wound. (Upper right) The portion that would be inserted into the cavity, was de-epithelized. (Center left) The flap was transposed with its intact portion on the opening of the wound, while the de-epithelized portion was placed into the cavity. (Center right) The flap showed temporary congestion, and leech therapy was applied for a short duration. (Below) The wound healed without any problems

monitored directly, its circulatory condition should be assessed based on the monitoring flap.

Deep cavity wounds can be classified into 2 types by their orientation (Fig. 4). The first type is a horizontally oriented cavity. A typical example of this type is an iceberg-shaped pressure sores. The direction of the deep space is horizontal, and its roof is usually covered with a skin layer. If the classical perforator-based island flap is used to reconstruct this type of wound, the skin and soft tissue layer covering the roof of the cavity should be excised. Excision of the healthy skin layer of the wound is tissue-wasting. However, using the modified form of the perforator-based island flap described in this study provides the possibility of saving the tissue on the wound. The second type involves a vertically or obliquely oriented cavity. This type includes cutaneous fistulae and meningomyelocele defects. As the direction of the deep space is vertical or oblique, the de-epithelized portion of the flap

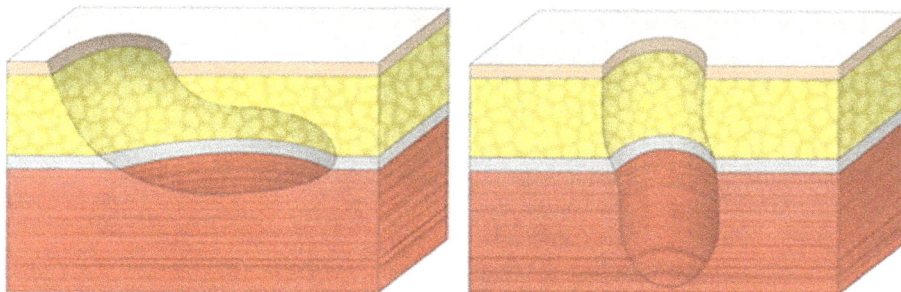

Fig. 4 Classification of deep cavity wounds according to their orientation. (Left) Schematic image of type I wounds, with a horizontally oriented cavity. (Right) Schematic image of type II wounds, with a vertically or obliquely oriented cavity

should be folded more. The proximal intact portion is usually placed horizontally on the opening of the wound, but the distal de-epithelized portion should be placed vertically or obliquely in the space. For this reason, the flap in the second type, sometimes, needs to be folded excessively, whereas the flap in the first type only requires minimal folding. As excessive folding of the flap can lead to circulatory problems in the flap, reconstruction of the second type wound requires more intensive care.

In this study, 2 circulatory problems were observed. They were venous congestion and marginal necrosis on the proximal portion, which plays a role as a monitoring flap. These problems, fortunately, were solved with conservative treatment and did not affect the distally buried component of the flap. In these 2 cases, a perforator that may have been injured, was used. In fact, these 2 problem cases belonged to the same patient, who previously underwent pelvic bone injury and bladder rupture. When the first fistulectomy and flap surgery were performed, the patient experienced temporary congestion on the flap, but it was cured completely. After complete healing, the patient experienced another event of bladder rupture, which resulted in the formation of new fistula on the other site. As the authors did not notice that the problem in the first operation resulted from using an injured deep inferior epigastric artery perforator, another similar perforator near the first flap was used for the second surgery. This time, the patient experienced marginal necrosis on the flap. After observing 2 problems on the same patient, the authors concluded that the perforators used in both operations may have been injured when the patient experienced pelvic bone fracture, resulting in circulatory problems in the flaps. If the cause of the problem has been noticed at first, another flap such as a distant pedicled flap or a free flap, would have been selected for the second operation rather than an island flap with an injured perforator.

Conclusions

The perforator-based island flap with partial de-epithelization is a modified flap for the treatment of deep cavity wounds with maintaining the benefits of classical perforator-based island flaps. However, the weak point of this flap is that the de-epithelized portion of the flap, which may be most vulnerable in terms of circulation, cannot be monitored directly, as the de-epithelized portion is buried in the cavity. For this reason, the factors that can result in poor circulatory conditions on the flap should be avoided. Excessive folding of the flap is dangerous. In trauma cases, using injured perforators from the zone of the injury also should be avoided. With careful procedures, the flap can be transferred without anxiety regarding the buried portion. As it has been proved in this study, the perforator-based island flap with partial de-epithelization is a useful option for the treatment of deep cavity wounds.

Abbreviations

DFP: Deep femoral artery perforator; DIEP: Deep inferior epigastric artery perforator; IGAP: Inferior gluteal artery perforator; SGAP: Superior gluteal artery perforator; TFLP: Tensor fascia lata perforator

Acknowledgements

There is no acknowledgment for the present study.

Funding

There is no funding for the present study.

Authors' contributions

All the authors were involved in the preparation of this manuscript. MSSC and JWC made substantial contributions to design, interpretation of data, and wrote the manuscript. OSW and JSO assisted in preparing and editing the manuscript. All the authors read and approved the final manuscript.

Competing interests

The authors declare that they have no competing interests.

Author details

[1]Department of Plastic and Reconstructive Surgery, Hanyang University Guri Hospital, Hanyang University College of Medicine, 249-1, Gyomun-dong, Guri-si, Gyeonggi-do 471-701, Korea. [2]Department of Plastic and Reconstructive Surgery, Hanyang University College of Medicine, 17 Haengdang-Dong, 133-792 Seongdong-Gu, Seoul, Korea.

References

1. Atiyeh BS, Ioannovich J, Al-Amm CA, et al. Management of acute and chronic open wounds: the importance of moist environment in optimal wound healing. Curr Pharm Biotechnol. 2002;3(3):179–95.
2. Liu Y, Zhang X, Xiao B, et al. Clinical characteristics and surgical management of 17 patients with pressure of sinus type. Zhongguo Xiu Fu Chong Jian Wai Ke Za Zhi. 2014;28(8):981–4.
3. Kocak OF, Demir CY. An ideal flap alternative for closure of myelomeningocele defects: dorsal intercostal artery perforator flap. J Craniofac Surg. 2016;27(8):1951–5.
4. Duffy FJ Jr, Weprin BE, Swift DM. A new approach to closure of large lumbosacral myelomeningoceles: the superior gluteal artery perforator flap. Plast Reconstr Surg. 2004;114(7):1864–8.
5. Pirgousis P, Fernandes R. Use of the internal mammary artery perforator flap for repair of pharyngocutaneous fistulas in the vessel-depleted neck. J Oral Maxillofac Surg. 2011;69(4):1225–8.
6. Khalil HH, Malahias MN, Karandikar S, et al. Internal pudendal artery perforator island flap for management of recurrent benign rectovaginal fistula. Plast Reconstr Surg Glob Open. 2016;4(8):e841.
7. Pignatti M, Ogawa R, Hallock GG, et al. The "Tokyo" consensus on propeller flaps. Plast Reconstr Surg. 2011;127(2):716–22.

8. Meltem C, Esra C, Hasan F, et al. The gluteal perforator-based flap in repair of pressure sores. Br J Plast Surg. 2004;57(4):342–7.

9. Leow M, Lim J, Lim TC. The superior gluteal artery perforator flap for the closure of sacral sores. Singap Med J. 2004;45(1):37–9.

10. Verpaele AM, Blondeel PN, Van Landuyt K, et al. The superior gluteal artery perforator flap: an additional tool in the treatment of sacral pressure sores. Br J Plast Surg. 1999;52(5):385–91.

11. Oliver RA, Lovric V, Yu Y, et al. Development of a novel model for the assessment of dead-space management in soft tissue. PLoS One. 2015;10(8):e0136514.

12. Türker T, Gonzalez JP, Capdarest-Arest N. Deepithelized posterior interosseous artery flap for 3-dimensional defect coverage in the hand. Tech Hand Up Extrem Surg. 2015;19(2):51–4.

13. Mehrotra ON. De-epithelialization and over-flapping in plastic surgery. Aust N Z J Surg. 1978;48(6):653–6.

14. Draf W. Possibilities of reconstruction by de-epithelization (author's transl). Laryngol Rhinol Otol (Stuttg). 1981;60(11):564–70.

15. Rispoli DM, Horne BR, Kryzak TJ, et al. Description of a technique for vacuum-assisted deep drains in the management of cavitary defects and deep infections in devastating military and civilian trauma. J Trauma. 2010;68(5):1247–52.

16. Webb LX. New techniques in wound management: vacuum-assisted wound closure. J Am Acad Orthop Surg. 2002;10(5):303–11.

17. Datli A, Suh H, Kim YC, et al. Free-style deepithelialized propeller flaps: an ideal local flap to obliterate wounds with dead space. Plast Reconstr Surg Glob Open. 2017;5(3):e1249.

18. Oh TS, Hallock G, Hong JP. Freestyle propeller flaps to reconstruct defects of the posterior trunk: a simple approach to a difficult problem. Ann Plast Surg. 2012;68(1):79–82.

19. Mathes DW, Thornton JF, Rohrich RJ. Management of posterior trunk defects. Plast Reconstr Surg. 2006;118(3):73e–83e.

20. Harry BL, Deleyiannis FW. Posterior trunk reconstruction using an anteromedial thigh free flap and arteriovenous loop. Microsurgery. 2013;33(5):416–7.

21. Guelinckx PJ, Sinsel NK. Refinements in the one-stage procedure for management of chronic osteomyelitis. Microsurgery. 1995;16(9):606–11.

22. Auregan JC, Begue T, Tomeno B, et al. Distally-based vastus lateralis muscle flap: a salvage alternative to address complex soft tissue defects around the knee. Orthop Traumatol Surg Res. 2010;96(2):180–4.

23. Manoso MW, Boland PJ, Healey JH, et al. Limb salvage of infected knee reconstructions for cancer with staged revision and free tissue transfer. Ann Plast Surg. 2006;56(5):532–5.

24. Whiteside LA. Surgical technique: vastus medialis and vastus lateralis as flap transfer for knee extensor mechanism deficiency. Clin Orthop Relat Res. 2013;471(1):221–30.

25. Koshima I, Moriguchi T, Soeda S, et al. The gluteal perforator-based flap for repair of sacral pressure sores. Plast Reconstr Surg. 1993;91(4):678–83.

26. Mathes SJ, Nahai F, editors. Clinical atlas of muscle and musculocutaneous flaps. St. Luis: Mosby; 1979.

27. Musters GD, Lapid O, Bemelman WA, et al. Surgery for complex perineal fistula following rectal cancer treatment using biological mesh combined with gluteal perforator flap. Tech Coloproctol. 2014;18(10):955–9.

28. Masuoka T, Sugita A, Sekiya S, et al. Breast reconstruction with perforator-based inframammary de-epithelized flap: a case report. Aesthet Plast Surg. 2002;26(3):211–4.

29. Mohan AT, Rammos CK, Akhavan AA, et al. Evolving concepts of keystone perforator island flaps (KPIF): principles of perforator anatomy, design modifications, and extended clinical applications. Plast Reconstr Surg. 2016; 137(6):1909–20.

30. Mericli AF, Martin JP, Campbell CA. An algorithmic anatomical subunit approach to pelvic wound reconstruction. Plast Reconstr Surg. 2016;137(3):1004–17.

20

Effect on the tensile strength of human acellular dermis (Epiflex®) of in-vitro incubation simulating an open abdomen setting

Mario Vitacolonna[1], Michael Mularczyk[2], Florian Herrle[1], Torsten J Schulze[3], Hans Haupt[2], Matthias Oechsner[2], Lothar R Pilz[4], Peter Hohenberger[1] and Eric Dominic Rössner[1*]

Abstract

Background: The use of human acellular dermis (hAD) to close open abdomen in the treatment process of severe peritonitis might be an alternative to standard care. This paper describes an investigation of the effects of fluids simulating an open abdomen environment on the biomechanical properties of Epiflex® a cell-free human dermis transplant.

Methods: hAD was incubated in Ringers solution, blood, urine, upper gastrointestinal (upper GI) secretion and a peritonitis-like bacterial solution in-vitro for 3 weeks. At day 0, 7, 14 and 21 breaking strength was measured, tensile strength was calculated and standard fluorescence microscopy was performed.

Results: hAD incubated in all five of the five fluids showed a decrease in mean breaking strength at day 21 when compared to day 0. However, upper GI secretion was the only incubation fluid that significantly reduced the mechanical strength of Epiflex after 21days of incubation when compared to incubation in Ringer's solution.

Conclusion: hAD may be a suitable material for closure of the open abdomen in the absence of upper GI leakage and pancreatic fistulae.

Keywords: Acellular dermis, Open abdomen, Breaking strength, Biologicals

Background

Acellular dermal products and transplants are starting to play a significant role in reconstructive surgery [1-3]. Human acellular dermis (hAD) may offer some advantages over xenogeneic material, such as reduced immunogenicity and increased safety with regard to potential prion infections [4]. Although the hAD Alloderm® has been extensively used outside of Europe and in particular in the USA [5-9], it is not approved for use in Germany where tissue transplants are required to meet the stringent safety requirements of the German drug law. Epiflex® is currently the only hAD approved for use as a medicinal product in Europe [4].

Dermis is rich in collagen of various subtypes [10] and its biomechanical strength is principally a function of the density and degree of hydration [11] and crosslinking [12] of the collagen fibers. These factors will also influence the extent to which a hAD retains its mechanical strength when incubated in aggressive fluids akin to those present in an infected open abdomen.

An open abdomen is defined as an abdominal wall fascial defect persisting after laparotomy. This condition may be induced, or accepted in case of a planned second look, for prevention of abdominal compartment syndrome or during "damage control surgery", or it may simply be impossible to close the abdomen due to loss of domain, extensive abdominal wall resection or insufficient fascial stability in the case of peritonitis [13]. Due to the success of commercial and non-commercial vacuum therapy regimes in open abdomen management, fascial closure rates of up to 100% in young damage control trauma patients can be achieved [13,14]. Closure rates in multi-

* Correspondence: eric.roessner@umm.de
[1]Division of Surgical Oncology and Thoracic Surgery, Department of Surgery, University Medical Centre Mannheim, Heidelberg University, Theodor Kutzer Ufer 1-3, 68167 Mannheim, Germany
Full list of author information is available at the end of the article

morbid septic abdominal populations are approximately only 30%. In cases where fascial closure fails or vacuum therapy is not available the abdomen is traditionally closed with a synthetic mesh [15]. Since the abdominal compartment is usually contaminated in such patients, a resorbable mesh (e.g. Vicryl) is used. These meshes resorb in the time taken for the abdominal defect to be filled by granulation tissue and a planned ventral hernia is developing. This hernia will then be repaired after 6–12 months, when secondary wound healing finished and an aseptic condition is achieved, with non-resorbable, synthetic meshes and/or component separation techniques [16]. Application of a biological mesh such as hAD in the initial phase could be a novel approach in such patients. To function in this setting, a hAD must be sufficiently structurally resistant to the hostile environment of an open abdomen containing blood, urine or stool from fistulas and typical bacteria found in peritonitis patients. If such a treatment regime could obviate planned ventral hernias, this could reduce morbidity, and the requirement for revisions. Manufactures of these biological meshes are heavily advertising these for the closure of a septic open abdomen, claiming their biostability without a proper proof. The intention was the proof of principle and to identify conditions not suitable for a repair with acellular dermis.

The present study focuses on an *in-vitro* examination of the effect of incubation in Ringer's solution (physiological solution serving as a control group), urine, blood, a bacteria mixture and upper gastrointestinal (upper GI) secretion on the mechanical strength of hAD.

Methods

All of our research was carried out in compliance to the Helsinki declaration. The blood donation was approved by the local ethics committee (Ethic Approval 87/04 of the Ethik Kommission II der Medizinischen Fakultät Mannheim).

Human acellular dermis

Epiflex® (German Institute for Cell and Tissue Replacement, Berlin, Germany) was used as hAD. The transplant material used in the study originated from five screened and consenting human cadaveric donors. The mechanical processing, decellularization, sterilization and preservation methods [4] and collagen content [10] are described in detail elsewhere. All samples were derived from same body region. Each donor was randomized into one of the five groups (control, blood, urine, upper GI secretion and bacterial solution).

Incubation fluids and culture conditions

The hAD were incubated in Ringer's solution, in 1 of 3 different human body fluids; whole blood, duodenal

secretion, urine or in a bacteria mixture consisting of enterococcus faecalis (gram+; streptococci), staphylococcus aureus (gram+; staphylococci), e.coli (gram-; enterobacteriaceae) and pseudomonas aeruginosa (gram-; nonfermenter). The bacterial strains were provided by the Institute for Medical Microbiology and Hygiene, (University Medical Center Mannheim) and added at a concentration of $1 \times 10^5 ml^{-1}$ in Dulbecco's Modified Eagle Medium (DMEM) with high glucose (4.5 g/l) and no additives (PAA, Germany), aliquoted and frozen at −80°C (mixed 1:1 with glycerol) for later use. Upper gastro intestinal secretion was collected from consenting patients during upper gastrointestinal endoscopy procedures. In all cases it was necessary to evacuate the upper GI in order to examine the intestinal mucosa. Upper GI pathology could be ruled out in all patients and none had been taking anti-acid medication. The secretions were pooled into volumes of 5 litres, aliquoted into 15 ml tubes and stored at −80°C. Urine was collected daily from healthy voluntary donors.

Blood was retrieved from the Institute of Transfusion Medicine and Immunology, German Red Cross Blood Service. Centrifugation of whole blood separates the samples into erythrocyte concentrate, plasma and a thrombocyte and leucocyte rich buffy coat. The latter are further used to create pooled thrombocyte concentrates. Due to use of mainly - antihypertensive - medication, the buffy coats and plasma were not permitted for use in patients. To simulate cellular blood composition, especially of leucocytes that are mainly regarded responsible for digestion of foreign bodies, the blood used in these experiments was composed of both buffy coat and plasma of volunteer blood donors.

Culture conditions

The transplant samples were rehydrated in Ringer´s solution for 30 minutes at room temperature and then incubated at 37°C in 10 ml of one of the test fluids. The test fluid completely covered the hAD sample. Nine samples were incubated in each of the fluids. The incubation fluids were replaced on a daily basis. With the exception of the bacteria mixture, the dishes were supplemented with a 1:100 dilution of a Penicillin/ Streptomycin mixture (PAA, Germany) to give a final concentration of 100 U/ml Penicillin and 0,1 mg/ml Strepavidin. Samples were incubated for 0 (briefly rinsed), 7, 14 and 21 days.

Measurement of mechanical properties

Samples for mechanical testing were punched out of the transplants with a die cutter (Figure 1). The cut samples were submersed in Ringer´s solution for about 30 minutes prior to testing. The thickness of the mechanical test samples was measured at 5 points using a digital micrometer

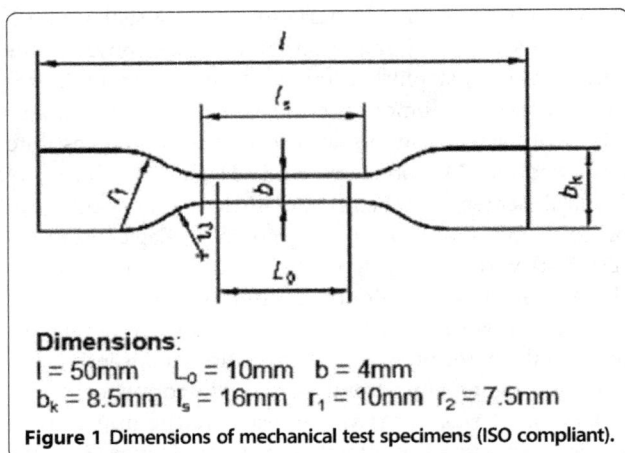

Dimensions:
l = 50mm L_0 = 10mm   b = 4mm
b_k = 8.5mm l_s = 16mm r_1 = 10mm r_2 = 7.5mm

Figure 1 Dimensions of mechanical test specimens (ISO compliant).

and the mean was calculated (JD200, Kaefer, Germany). The samples were evaluated in a tensile testing apparatus (H10KM, Richard Hess MBV GmbH, Sonsbeck, Germany) for ultimate load-at-failure according to EN ISO 527 (Figure 2). The test was carried out with a 100 N load cell at a constant strain rate of 50 mm/min.

Histology

At the end of the respective incubation period, transplant samples were fixed in 10% formalin for 24 hours, sliced into 3 equal parts, embedded in paraffin and sectioned (7 μm) with a microtome (Microm, Germany) for a complete edge-to-edge cross- sectional view. Samples were mounted onto glass slides, dried overnight at 37°C, de- paraffinized with 3 washes of 5 minutes in a xylene bath followed by 3 washes of 2 minutes each through a dilution series of 100%, 96% and 80% ethanol. The autofluorescence of the samples was observed with a 488 nm excitation filter and a 514 nm emission filter in a fluorescence microscope (Zeiss, Germany) and stitched with ICE (Image Composite Editor, V1.4.4, Microsoft, USA).

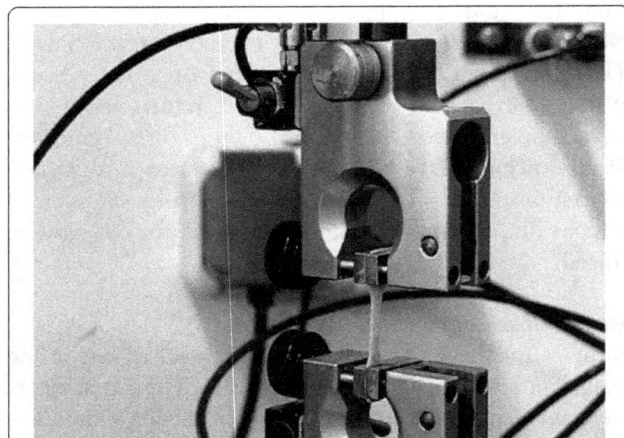

Figure 2 Sample clamped in the tensile testing machine.

Statistics

For data collection and handling Excel 2010 was used (Microsoft, Redmond). Data was analyzed for normal distribution. A two-sided multiple Wilcoxon rank test with a correction according to Bonferroni- Holm for multiple testing was used. Tests were considered significant when $\alpha \leq 0.05$. For all statistics SAS (SAS Institute Inc., Carry, NC, USA) and StatXact 9 (Statcon, Witzenhausen, Germany) software was used. For the Koziol test the statistic system ADAM version 2.54 (DKFZ, Heidelberg, Germany) was used. Statistical analyses were conducted by a statistician of the Medical Faculty Mannheim, Heidelberg University, Germany.

Results

Results are show in Figure 3. The breaking strength of hAD in Ringer's Solution decreases over time. At day 21 the hAD has lost approximately 30% of its breaking strength. Although there is a continuous decrease of the mean breaking strength the differences between day 0 (35.28 ± 3.12 N/mm^2) and day 7 (34.19 ± 3.50 N/mm^2) and between day 14 (29.32 ± 2.67 N/mm^2) and day 21 (24.69 ± 3.27 N/mm^2) were not significant. In blood the breaking strength declines as well over time about 32%, although only the comparison between day 0 (34.14 ± 5.46 N/mm^2) and 21 (23.38 ± 2.97 N/mm^2) and between day 7 (30.0 ± 3.3 N/mm^2) and day 21 were significant. A 40% decrease in breaking strength was measured for hAD incubated in urine for 21 days. The decrease was not significant between day 0 (34.3 ± 4.48 N/mm^2) and day 7 (32.2 ± 4.215 N/mm^2) and between day 7 and day 14 (27.29 ± 3.49 N/mm^2). Incubation in a bacterial solution decreased the hAD breaking strength by 51% over a period of 21 days. Although the decrease from day 0 (32.42 ± 1.99 N/mm^2) to 21 (16.06 ± 6.87 N/mm^2) was significant the intervals from day 0 to 7 (29.01 ± 4.77 N/mm^2), from day 7 to 14 (21.33 ± 2.54 N/mm^2) and from day 14 to 21 were not significant. Breaking strength of hAD incubated in upper GI secretion showed the most distinct decrease of 78% over 21 days. All intervals showed a significant decrease in breaking strength. Mean breaking strength at day 0 was 33.42 ± 4.79 N/mm^2, at day7: 25.19 ± 2.94 N/mm^2, at day 14: 12.14 ± 2.045 N/mm^2 and at day 21: 7.157 ± 2.84 N/mm^2 (Table 1).

Comparing the breaking strengths of hAD in the different mediums at day 0 there were no significant differences. At day 7 the only significantly different treatment incubation in upper GI secretion. At day 14 both incubation in upper GI secretion and incubation in the bacteria solution resulted in mechanical strength being lower at the same time point than in the other 3 treatment groups. At this time point, hAD incubated in upper GI was significantly weaker than that incubated in the bacteria solution. At day 21 material incubated in upper GI secretion was again

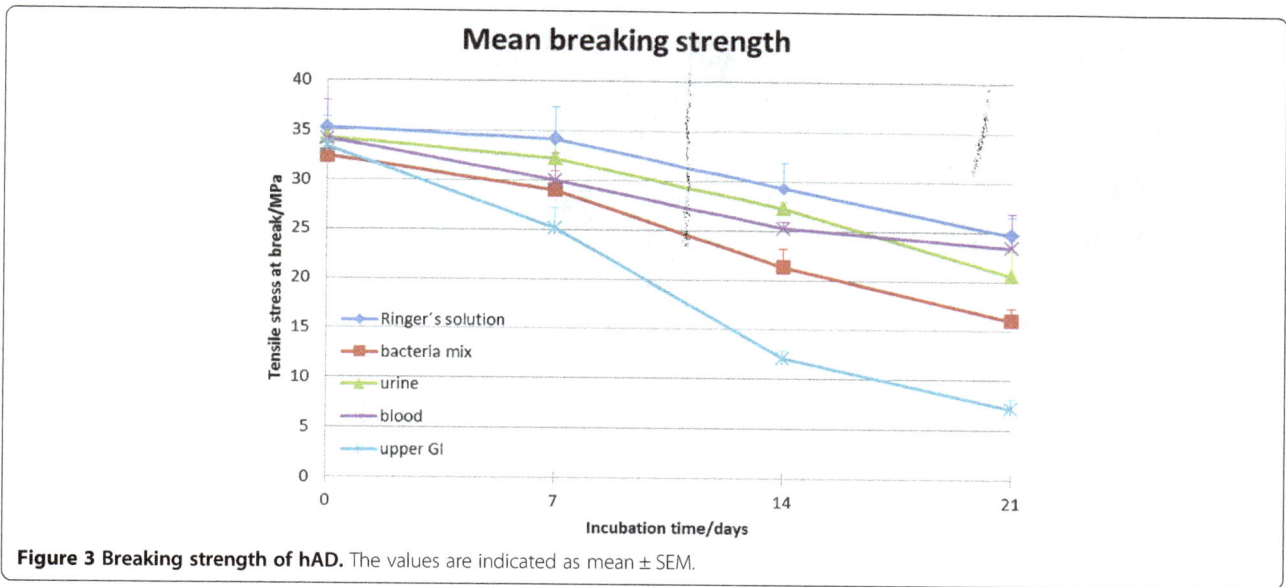

Figure 3 Breaking strength of hAD. The values are indicated as mean ± SEM.

mechanically weaker than that in all other treatments. However, there were no longer any significantly differences amongst the samples incubated in Ringer's solution, blood, urine and bacteria solution (Table 2).

In the non-parametric analysis of the curves over time according to Koziol et al. the curve of the hAD incubated upper GI secretion is significantly (p = 0.0001) lower than the other curves.

The microscopy analysis of the hAD specimens showed disaggregation of the collagen fibers in all groups over time. In the bacterial and upper GI secretion group, disaggregation seems to occur more rapidly and more distinct when compared over time (Figure 4).

Discussion

Since open abdomen is a therapeutic option in the treatment of traumatized abdomen or severe peritonitis there is a need for minimizing sequelae [17]. The well-established method of closure with a synthetic resorbable mesh prevents evisceration and chronic foreign body infection, although complication such as massive adhesions and

small bowel fistulae are well known [18,19]. The need for major surgery to reconstruct the abdominal wall and for programmed ventral hernia raises the possibility of further morbidity, increased costs and mortality [20]. With introduction of intra-abdominal negative pressure dressings, delayed primary closure became an option in a high percentage of young trauma patients [21]. Delayed primary closure might be the best option in such patients, but in a majority of older patients with severe peritonitis due to septic focuses this is not feasible [22]. Closure with a tissue transplant could be helpful if adequate mechanical stability could be retained in an open abdomen environment.

Hollinsky and co-workers [23] measured the tensile strength of healthy human abdominal wall using specimens excised from fresh cadaver tissue. They were able to show that the linea alba fails in longitudinal and transversal direction at 39 N. This was calculated to be equivalent to a tensile strength of 10 N/mm^2 and this may be regarded as the maximum strength required in a healthy human under extreme loads. The mean tensile strength of the transplants in the control group was 35 N/mm^2 at day 0. Even 25 N/mm^2, which was the mean strength after 21

Table 1 Comparison of measured strength between paired time points within treatment groups ((+) significant difference) ((−) no significant difference)

	Day 0 vs. 7	Day 7 vs. 14	Day 14 vs. 21	Day 0 vs. 21
Ringer's solution	-	+	-	+
Blood	-	-	-	+
Urine	-	-	+	+
Bacteria	-	-	-	+
Upper GI secretion	+	+	+	+

Table 2 Comparison of measured strength at individual time points between treatment groups ((+) significant difference) ((−) no significant difference)

	Day 0	Day 7	Day 14	Day 21
Ringer's solution vs. blood	-	-	-	-
Ringer's solution vs. urine	-	-	-	-
Ringer's solution vs. bacteria	-	-	+	-
Ringer's solution vs. GI secretion	-	+	+	+

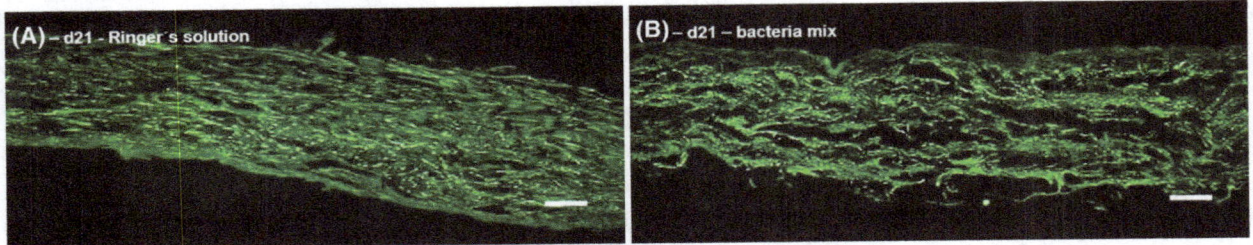

Figure 4 Representatice fluorescence photomicrographs of hAD specimens incubated in (A) Ringer´s solution at day 21 and (B) in bacteria mix (collagen autofluorescence excitation 488 nm, emission 514 nm). The figure shows a qualitative comparison of the matrix disaggregation incubated in control solution and bacteria mix. It can be seen, that matrix disaggregation in the bacteria group was more pronounced than in Ringer´s solution, presumably due to enzymatic cleavage (e.g. collagenases). Scale bars equal 50 µm.

days of incubation should be sufficient for Epiflex® to be able to withstand the maximum anticipated force, more so since the *in-vitro* test disregards adhesion and integration phenomena.

The breaking strength of hAD samples incubated in blood was not significantly different to that of transplants incubated in Ringer's solution. Epiflex® should therefore be strong enough to reconstruct ventral hernias in an uninfected situation.

Epiflex® incubated in urine had similar properties. It should therefore be suitable for ventral reconstruction in the presence of an urinoma or urinary tract leakage.

Incubation in a bacteria solution resulted in no significant loss of strength at day 0 and 7 when compared to incubation in Ringer's solution, but there was a significant difference at day 14. At day 21 there was no longer a significant difference. Typical intestinal flora may be capable of reducing the mechanical strength of Epiflex® within the time frame under investigation to a greater extent than blood or urine, although the residual mechanical strength of 16 N/mm^2 still exceeds the calculated requirement.

The study has limitations with regard to the composition of the bacteria solution. Although the solution represents a common mixture of bacteria found in peritonitic patients, different bacteria mixtures could well have significantly different effects on hAD, since different bacteria strains and species excrete different concentrations of active agents such as collagenase.

The samples were incubated in high concentrations of bacteria that would only arise in an uncontrolled septic focus in the open abdomen. In such cases, an attempt at a primary closure would not normally be indicated. The combined effect of bacterial secretions and the inflammatory host response on the mechanical strength of candidate materials for abdominal wall closure cannot be simulated *in-vitro*.

Upper GI tract secretion had a powerful effect on the mechanical strength of Epiflex®. Loss of mechanical strength was continuous and when compared to the effects of the

other incubation fluids, significantly increased at day 7, 14 and 21. The presence of an upper GI leakage, the closure of an open abdomen with Epiflex® might be compromised. At this stage of an open abdomen therapy, a definite closure is rarely indicated. It is unclear whether a pure pancreatic secretion from a pancreas fistula would have the same impact on the mechanical strength of Epiflex®.

The decrease in mechanical strength in the different liquids might be caused by various factors. Upper GI secretion is a mixture of gastric fluid, bile and pancreatic fluid and contains a heterogeneous mixture of digestive enzymes including proteases, lipases and amylases [24,25]. The upper GI secretion was frozen shortly after collection at −80°C to retard reduction of enzyme activity. Since the extracellular matrix consists of various proteins, glycoproteins and polysaccharides, enzymatic hydrolysis would seem to be a likely contributor to loss of tensile strength [26,27]. Bacteria also secrete hydrolytic enzymes such as collagenases, whereby the extent and the composition depends on species and strain. Furthermore, microbial organisms can modify the pH of the environment [28-30]. This may influence the degradation of bioresorbable materials [31-33]. It is known that superoxide ions from leukocytes and macrophages accelerate the degradation of absorbable materials [34]. The mechanism leading to loss of mechanical strength in Ringer's solution after 21 days is unclear. Temperature may affect biodegradation [35,36], however the incubation temperature in our study (37°C) seems unlikely to have exacerbated hydrolysis. Numerous studies demonstrated a significant loss in strength of biodegradable materials in aqueous solutions, presumably by cumulative low-level irreversible hydrolysis [33,36,37].

Limitations of the studyy

In the clinical situation wound healing processes such adhesions to the transplant and integration, remodeling, vascularization, inflammation and scaring will have an effect on the mechanical strength of the transplant and the forming abdominal wall. This limits our findings especially after 21 days of incubation. Some of these effects are likely to be positive, although it cannot be ruled out that the remodeling process in itself results periods during healing during which mechanical strength is reduced, if resorption processes advance more rapidly than synthetic processes. The uniaxial tensile stresses applied to the transplants in our study do not ideally represent the stresses that occur in vivo. The latter are dynamic and multidirectional and can best be analyzed in a clinical setting.

Conclusion

Epiflex® exhibits reduced mechanical strength after 3 weeks of incubation in Ringer's solution, in body fluids (blood, urine, upper GI secretion) and in a bacteria solution. It seems unlikely that the loss of mechanical strength arising from incubation in Ringer's solution, blood and urine would be clinically significant in the setting of a primary closure of an open abdomen. The loss of mechanical strength arising from incubation in a bacteria solution suggests that this might be clinically significant in an infected open abdomen situation, depending on the concentration, species and strain of the contaminating organisms. Incubation of Epiflex® in upper GI secretion caused a more pronounced loss of mechanical strength. Use of hAD for open abdomen closure in the presence of upper GI leakage or of a pancreatic fistula may be inappropriate. The authors intend to proceed with a phase I clinical study. The superiority of hAD in regards to the development of ventral hernia must be shown in a phase III study.

Abbreviations
hAD: Human acellular dermis; Upper GI secretion (UGI): Upper gastro intestinal secretion; DMEM: Dulbecco's Modified Eagle Medium; SEM: Standard error of the mean.

Competing interests
The authors declare that they have no competing interests.

Authors' contributions
The study was conceived and designed by MV, ER and PH. The experiments were conducted and the results analyzed by MV, MM, FH, TJS, HH, MO and LRP. The manuscript was written by MV and ER. All authors read and approved the final manuscript.

Acknowledgements
The authors thank Dr. Mark D. Smith and Dr. Jan C. Brune from the German Institute for Cell and Tissue Replacement (DIZG) for advice relating to use of Epiflex® and for assistance with data analysis and editing of the final manuscript. We acknowledge financial support by Deutsche Forschungsgemeinschaft and Ruprecht-Karls-Universität Heidelberg within the funding programme Open Access Publishing.
We acknowledge financial support by Deutsche Forschungsgemeinschaft and Ruprecht-Karls-Universität Heidelberg within the funding programme Open Access Publishing.

Author details
[1]Division of Surgical Oncology and Thoracic Surgery, Department of Surgery, University Medical Centre Mannheim, Heidelberg University, Theodor Kutzer Ufer 1-3, 68167 Mannheim, Germany. [2]Center for structural Materials, State Material Testing Institute Darmstadt (MPA), Chair and Institute for Material Science (IfW), Technische Universität Darmstadt, Darmstadt, Germany. [3]German Red Cross Blood Service, Baden Württemberg-Hessen, Medical Faculty of Mannheim, Institute of Transfusion Medicine and Immunology, Heidelberg University, Mannheim, Germany. [4]Medical Faculty Mannheim, Heidelberg University, Heidelberg, Germany.

References
1. Losee JE, Smith DM: **Acellular dermal matrix in palatoplasty.** *Aesthet Surg J* 2011, **31**(7 Suppl):108S–115S.
2. Bengtson BP, Baxter RA: **Emerging applications for acellular dermal matrices in mastopexy.** *Clin Plast Surg* 2012, **39**(2):159–166.
3. Taner T, Cima RR, Larson DW, Dozois EJ, Pemberton JH, Wolff BG: **The use of human acellular dermal matrix for parastomal hernia repair in patients with inflammatory bowel disease: a novel technique to repair fascial defects.** *Dis Colon Rectum* 2009, **52**(2):349–354.
4. Rossner E, Smith MD, Petschke B, Schmidt K, Vitacolonna M, Syring C, von Versen R, Hohenberger P: **Epiflex((R)) a new decellularised human skin tissue transplant: manufacture and properties.** *Cell Tissue Bank* 2011, **12**(3):209–217.
5. Scott BG, Welsh FJ, Pham HQ, Carrick MM, Liscum KR, Granchi TS, Wall MJ Jr, Mattox KL, Hirshberg A: **Early aggressive closure of the open abdomen.** *J Trauma* 2006, **60**(1):17–22.
6. Adetayo OA, Salcedo SE, Bahjri K, Gupta SC: **A meta-analysis of outcomes using acellular dermal matrix in breast and abdominal wall reconstructions: event rates and risk factors predictive of complications.** *Ann Plast Sur* 2011.
7. Singh MK, Rocca JP, Rochon C, Facciuto ME, Sheiner PA, Rodriguez-Davalos MI: **Open abdomen management with human acellular dermal matrix in liver transplant recipients.** *Transplant Proceed* 2008, **40**(10):3541–3544.
8. de Moya MA, Dunham M, Inaba K, Bahouth H, Alam HB, Sultan B, Namias N: **Long-term outcome of acellular dermal matrix when used for large traumatic open abdomen.** *J Trauma* 2008, **65**(2):349–353.
9. Diaz JJ Jr, Conquest AM, Ferzoco SJ, Vargo D, Miller P, Wu YC, Donahue R: **Multi-institutional experience using human acellular dermal matrix for ventral hernia repair in a compromised surgical field.** *Archiv Surgery* 2009, **144**(3):209–215.
10. Roessner ED, Vitacolonna M, Hohenberger P: **Confocal laser scanning microscopy evaluation of an acellular dermis tissue transplant (Epiflex (R)).** *PloS One* 2012, **7**(10):e45991.
11. Ateshian GA, Wang H: **Rolling resistance of articular cartilage due to interstitial fluid flow.** *Proc Inst Mech Eng H* 1997, **211**(5):419–424.
12. Buehler MJ: **Nanomechanics of collagen fibrils under varying cross-link densities: atomistic and continuum studies.** *J Mech Behav Biomed Mater* 2008, **1**(1):59–67.
13. Vargo D, Richardson JD, Campbell A, Chang M, Fabian T, Franz M, Kaplan M, Moore F, Reed RL, Scott B, *et al*: **Management of the open abdomen: from initial operation to definitive closure.** *Am Surg* 2009, **75**(11):S1–S22.
14. Van Hensbroek Boele P, Wind J, Dijkgraaf MG, Busch OR, Carel Goslings J: **Temporary closure of the open abdomen: a systematic review on delayed primary fascial closure in patients with an open abdomen.** *World J Surg* 2009, **33**(2):199–207.
15. Regner JL, Kobayashi L, Coimbra R: **Surgical strategies for management of the open abdomen.** *World J Surg* 2012, **36**(3):497–510.
16. Jernigan TW, Fabian TC, Croce MA, Moore N, Pritchard FE, Minard G, Bee TK: **Staged management of giant abdominal wall defects: acute and long-term results.** *Annal Surg* 2003, **238**(3):349–355. discussion 355–347.
17. Demetriades D: **Total management of the open abdomen.** *Inter Wound J* 2012, **9**(Suppl 1):17–24.
18. Bee TK, Croce MA, Magnotti LJ, Zarzaur BL, Maish GO 3rd, Minard G, Schroeppel TJ, Fabian TC: **Temporary abdominal closure techniques: a prospective randomized trial comparing polyglactin 910 mesh and vacuum-assisted closure.** *J Trauma* 2008, **65**(2):337–342. discussion 342–334.
19. Prichayudh S, Sriussadaporn S, Samorn P, Pak-Art R, Kritayakirana K, Capin A: **Management of open abdomen with an absorbable mesh closure.** *Surgery Today* 2011, **41**(1):72–78.
20. DeMaria EJ, Moss JM, Sugerman HJ: **Laparoscopic intraperitoneal polytetrafluoroethylene (PTFE) prosthetic patch repair of ventral hernia. Prospective comparison to open prefascial polypropylene mesh repair.** *Surg Endos* 2000, **14**(4):326–329.

21. Wondberg D, Larusson HJ, Metzger U, Platz A, Zingg U: **Treatment of the open abdomen with the commercially available vacuum-assisted closure system in patients with abdominal sepsis: low primary closure rate.** *World J Surg* 2008, **32**(12):2724–2729.

22. Quyn AJ, Johnston C, Hall D, Chambers A, Arapova N, Ogston S, Amin AI: **The open abdomen and temporary abdominal closure systems - historical evolution and systematic review.** *Col Dis Offic J Ass Coloproctol Gr Br Irel* 2012, **14**(8):e429–e438.

23. Hollinsky C, Sandberg S: **Measurement of the tensile strength of the ventral abdominal wall in comparison with scar tissue.** *Clin Biomech (Bristol, Avon)* 2007, **22**(1):88–92.

24. Muftuoglu MA, Ozkan E, Saglam A: **Effect of human pancreatic juice and bile on the tensile strength of suture materials.** *Am J Surg* 2004, **188**(2):200–203.

25. Kalantzi L, Goumas K, Kalioras V, Abrahamsson B, Dressman JB, Reppas C: **Characterization of the human upper gastrointestinal contents under conditions simulating bioavailability/bioequivalence studies.** *Pharmaceut Res* 2006, **23**(1):165–176.

26. Tian F, Appert HE, Howard JM: **The disintegration of absorbable suture materials on exposure to human digestive juices: an update.** *Am Surg* 1994, **60**(4):287–291.

27. Sugimachi K, Sufian S, Weiss MJ, Pavlides CA, Matsumoto T: **Evaluation of absorbable suture materials in biliary tract surgery.** *Inter Surg* 1978, **63**(3):135–139.

28. Mailman ML: **The efficacy of bacterial collagenase for the digestion of gingival tissue collagen.** *J Den Res* 1979, **58**(4):1424.

29. Maclennan JD, Mandl I, Howes EL: **Bacterial digestion of collagen.** *J Clin Invest* 1953, **32**(12):1317–1322.

30. Chung E, McPherson N, Grant A: **Tensile strength of absorbable suture materials: in vitro analysis of the effects of pH and bacteria.** *J Surg Edu* 2009, **66**(4):208–211.

31. Chu CC, Moncrief G: **An in vitro evaluation of the stability of mechanical properties of surgical suture materials in various pH conditions.** *Annal Surg* 1983, **198**(2):223–228.

32. Chu CC: **A comparison of the effect of pH on the biodegradation of two synthetic absorbable sutures.** *Annal Surg* 1982, **195**(1):55–59.

33. Chu CC: **The in-vitro degradation of poly(glycolic acid) sutures–effect of pH.** *J Biomed Mat Res* 1981, **15**(6):795–804.

34. Lee KH, Chu CC: **The role of superoxide ions in the degradation of synthetic absorbable sutures.** *J Biomed Mat Res* 2000, **49**(1):25–35.

35. Tomihata K, Suzuki M, Ikada Y: **The pH dependence of monofilament sutures on hydrolytic degradation.** *J Biomed Mat Res* 2001, **58**(5):511–518.

36. Freudenberg S, Rewerk S, Kaess M, Weiss C, Dorn-Beinecke A, Post S: **Biodegradation of absorbable sutures in body fluids and pH buffers.** *Europ Res Euro Chirurg Fors Rech Chirurg Europ* 2004, **36**(6):376–385.

37. Cam D, Hyon SH, Ikada Y: **Degradation of high molecular weight poly(L-lactide) in alkaline medium.** *Biomaterials* 1995, **16**(11):833–843.

21

Subjective outcome related to donor site morbidity after sural nerve graft harvesting: a survey in 41 patients

Alexander Hallgren, Anders Björkman, Anette Chemnitz and Lars B Dahlin[*]

Abstract

Background: The sural nerve is the most commonly used nerve for grafting severe nerve defects. Our aim was to evaluate subjective outcome in the lower leg after harvesting the sural nerve for grafting nerve defects.

Methods: Forty-six patients were asked to fill in a questionnaire to describe symptoms from leg or foot, where the sural nerve has been harvested to reconstruct an injured major nerve trunk. The questionnaire, previously used in patients going through a nerve biopsy, consists of questions about loss of sensation, pain, cold intolerance, allodynia and present problems from the foot. The survey also contained questions (visual analogue scales; VAS) about disability from the reconstructed nerve trunk.

Results: Forty-one out of 46 patients replied [35 males/6 females; age at reconstruction 23.0 years (10–72); median (min-max), reconstruction done 12 (1.2-39) years ago]. In most patients [37/41 cases (90%)], the sural nerve graft was used to reconstruct an injured nerve trunk in the upper extremity, mainly the median nerve [19/41 (46%)]. In 38/41 patients, loss of sensation, to a variable extent, in the skin area innervated by the sural nerve was noted. These problems persisted at follow up, but 19/41 noted that this area of sensory deficit had decreased over time. Few patients had pain and less than 1/3 had cold intolerance. Allodynia was present in half of the patients, but the majority of them considered that they had no or only slight problems from their foot. None of the patients in the study required painkillers. Eighty eight per cent would accept an additional sural nerve graft procedure if another nerve reconstruction procedure is necessary in the future.

Conclusions: Harvesting of the sural nerve for reconstruction nerve injuries results in mild residual symptoms similar to those seen after a nerve biopsy; although nerve biopsy patients are less prone to undergo an additional biopsy.

Keywords: Sural nerve, Nerve reconstruction, Nerve injury, Cold intolerance, Allodynia, Pain

Background

The sural nerve is located on the back of the lower leg. It is formed by joining the medial sural cutaneous nerve with the peroneal branch of the lateral sural cutaneous nerve where after it runs down along the leg. It pierces the fascia in the middle of the leg and is located superficially in the fat together with the lesser saphenous vein behind the lateral malleolus. The nerve innervates the skin mainly around the heel, but in some individuals it innervates also the lateral side of the foot, including the little toe [1].

The sural nerve is used in many ways in today's medicine; it can be used in nerve biopsies to assist in diagnosing polyneuropathies of unclear origin and to detect efficiency of pharmacological substances to treat neuropathy [2,3]. It is important that the indications for a sural nerve biopsy are accurate [4] since pain and discomfort may develop following the biopsy. In addition, the sural nerve is the most common autologous donor nerve, in nerve grafting, to reconstruct severe nerve defects in both adults and children. Although the sural nerve is extensively used as a donor nerve, a limited number of studies have investigated the sequelae following harvesting of the sural nerve [5-9],

* Correspondence: lars.dahlin@med.lu.se
Department of Clinical Sciences Malmö, Hand Surgery, Lund University, Malmö, Sweden

particularly as related to the symptoms seen in subjects and patients that have undergone a sural nerve biopsy.

To be able to inform patients about possible residual symptoms and subjective outcomes when the sural nerve is used as a nerve graft or for a biopsy, knowledge about pain, sensory deficit, allodynia and other problems following harvesting of the sural nerve have to be improved. Based on such knowledge, patients can be offered more accurate and detailed information about possible sequelae following the procedure, which should be put into perspective of the expected result of the nerve reconstruction. Therefore, it is of interest to analyse to which extent the symptoms occur when the sural nerve is used as a nerve graft and also to compare this to the symptoms that are seen after a sural nerve biopsy. Thus, our aim was to evaluate subjective outcome in the lower leg after harvesting the sural nerve for nerve grafting.

Methods

Patient material

Patients, operated on with nerve reconstruction at our department between 1973 and 2010 with one or two sural nerves (harvest of the whole length of the sural nerve at reconstruction) used as nerve grafts, were identified by the hospital´s patient registration system. Exclusion criteria were reconstruction of the sciatic or tibial nerves on the same side as the sural nerve graft was harvested and follow up less than 14 months. Forty-six patients filled the criteria and were asked to fill out a questionnaire [4,10] to describe symptoms from the leg or the foot where the nerve graft was harvested. The different parameters investigated included gender, age at reconstruction, age at follow up, time since injury, type of injured nerve, cause of injury, type of incision on leg and the patient´s occupation. The Central Ethical Review Board in Lund (i.e. regional ethics committee) judged the study and found it sound. A formal approval was not necessary, since such a study is not included in the applicable law (Research in humans; law 2003:460). Thus, there were no ethical problem involved (2011/607). Therefore, no formal informed consent was needed from each patient, which was not considered to affect the results.

Questionnaire

In the autumn of 2011 a questionnaire, used previously, but slightly modified to better fit the present patients, to evaluate residual subjective symptoms following sural nerve biopsies in subjects with or without diabetes [4,10], were sent to the 46 identified patients (Additional file 1). It consists of 14 different questions where the patients have to subjectively evaluate their post-operative symptoms from the lower leg. It includes loss of sensation, pain in the operated area (and if so if the patient had to take painkillers to cope with the pain), cold intolerance, numbness and tingling sensation.

A scoring system, based on the patient´s subjective perceptions and symptoms from the questionnaire, was created to compare any symptoms and discomfort with the overall general outcome of the reconstructed nerve. The scoring system was designed as:

I.) Do you have loss of sensation in the operated foot compared to the other foot? [no = 0; yes = 1].

II.) Do you feel pain in the foot/lower leg? [no = 0; day time = 1; night time = 2].

III.) Do you have problem with cold intolerance in the operated foot/lower leg? [no = 0; rarely = 1; sometimes = 2; frequently = 3].

IV.) Have you experienced problems with increased skin sensation when the skin is touched? [no = 0; rarely = 1; sometimes = 2; frequently = 3].

V.) Do you experience discomfort or tingling along the outside of the foot? [no = 0, impacts against surgical site = 1; during walking = 2; at rest = 3].

VI.) How would you describe your problems at the moment? [none = 0; mild = 1; affecting daily living = 2; severe = 3; disturbed sleep = 4].

The survey also contained three different visual analogue scales (VAS) focusing on the outcome on the patients by the injured and reconstructed nerve. The patients were asked to rate a) at present how much does your nerve injury, i.e. the reconstructed nerve, affect you? b) what impact has your nerve injury had on leisure activities and c) how does your injury affect your work or school attendance?

For comparison, the results from a previous study, using the same questionnaire, describing the postoperative complaints after a whole, not a fascicular, sural nerve biopsy had been taken in 21 subjects without diabetes [4].

Statistics

Values are presented as median (min − max) or numbers (%). Mann Whitney U-test was used to test for any significant difference between patients with an age ≤ or > 20 years of age at injury and Kruskal-Wallis to detect any differences between the various injuries leading up to the nerve grafting procedures. Correlations were done with the Spearman correlation test. A p-value of < 0.05 was accepted as significant. Analyses were done with using StatView for windows (SAS Institute Inc, Cary, NC, USA, version 5.0.1) and IBM SPSS Statistics (Statistical Package for the Social Sciences, SPSS Inc., Chicago, Il, USA) version 20 for Mac.

Results

Patients' characteristics are shown in Table 1. Forty-one out of 46 patients responded to the questionnaire

Table 1 Patient characteristics

Gender [male/female]:		35/6 (85/15%)
Age at reconstruction [years]:		23.0 (10–72)
Time since reconstruction [months]:		144 (14–468)
Reconstructed nerve:	Nerves in lower extremity	4/41 patients
	Nerves in upper extremity	40/41 patients
	Brachial plexus	3/41 patients
Occupation:	Student	9/41 (22%)
	Non-manual labour	4/41 (10%)
	Manual labour	15/41 (37%)
	Retired	1/41 (2%)
	Unknown	12/41 (29%)

Values are numbers (%) or median (min-max).

[35 males/6 females; median age at reconstruction was 23 years (min-max 10–72)]. The nerve reconstructions were done at a median of 12 years (min-max 1.2-39 years) ago. In 22/41 (54%) of the patients multiple incisions were used and in 6/41 (15%) of the cases a single longitudinal incision was the surgical technique of choice when harvesting the sural nerve. In 13/41 (32%) of the cases the surgical notes did not say which type of incision the surgeon used. There were no reports of postoperative complications, such as infection or deep vein thrombosis, in any of the patients included in this study, where the whole length of the sural nerve was harvested.

Residual symptoms from the foot and leg

The residual symptoms following harvesting of the sural nerve did not depend on type of injury for which the nerve was harvested (p = 0.58). In most patients [37/41 cases (90%)], the sural nerve graft was used to reconstruct one or several nerve trunks in the upper extremity; mainly the median nerve [(19/41 (46%); Table 1]. Discomfort from the leg was noted in 26/41 (63%) of the patients directly following surgery (Table 2). 38/41 (93%) had loss of sensation, to a variable extent, in the skin areas innervated by the sural nerve, which persisted at follow up. However, 19/41 (46%) patients noted that this area had decreased over time. Immediately following the operation, 18/41 (44%) experienced pain in the foot, while 21 (51%) did not (no reply from two patients). The pain did not, however, presently require more potent painkillers in any of the cases. Instead, it was consistently graded as mild by the patients and only 3/41 (5%) had pain during night-time.

The patients were asked to mark the area of the skin with sensory loss after harvesting (question number five). The image (i.e. a topographic map) displayed in Figure 1 shows a combined illustration of all the patients' drawings.

The more intense red colour of certain areas, the more patients have experienced symptoms from this area. The results indicate that 93% of the patients noticed impaired sensation around the heel. In 5/41 (12%) cases, there were no drawings at all in the survey.

Less than one third of the patients had symptoms, such as cold intolerance, and of those that had; only three classified them as frequent. Instead, the most common grade was "sometimes" [6/41 (15%); Table 2]. Allodynia was present in half of the patients 21/41 (51%), and of those affected the most common occasion was "rare" [9/21 (43%)]. A similar number of patients [i.e. 22/41 (54%)] experienced discomfort or tingling sensations along the lateral side of the foot. However, they only perceived such symptoms when the area of previous incision was percussed [15/41 (37%)]; few patients [6/41 (15%)] had tingling sensations in the foot at rest.

On the question on how the symptoms from the sural nerve harvest affected the patients at the moment, 2/41 (5%) classified it as powerful; 5/41 (12%) felt that it affected their daily activities; and the majority 35/41 (85%) responded that it was mild or none at all. No patients had sleeping problems due to symptoms. If necessary in the future 36/41 (88%) patients were positive to another sural nerve graft procedure.

Disability of the reconstructed nerve injury and its impact on leisure, school and work activities

The patients considered the overall disability (VAS 0–100) from their reconstructed nerve injury as low [25 (0–100)], with little impact on their leisure activity, school or work activities [8.5 (0–100) and 11.5 (0–100), respectively].

Residual symptoms and correlation with general outcome of nerve reconstruction and age

The results of the scoring system of residual symptoms in the leg showed a low value [3.5 (0–13)]. The residual symptom score did correlate with the VAS score of the general outcome (rho-value = 0.45; p = 0.004), but did not correlate with the time of follow up (p = 0.39). Age at injury did not correlate with general outcome or residual symptoms scores (p > 0.05). In addition, there were no differences in residual symptoms (p = 0.86) or general outcome of reconstruction of the nerve injury (p = 0.43) between subjects that had their injured nerve reconstructed with a sural nerve graft at an age ≤ or > 20 years of age.

Discussion

The present study shows that symptoms in the lower leg after harvesting the sural nerve for reconstructive surgery are relatively modest and include sensory loss, tingling sensations and sensitive to cold. More than half of the patients did not experience any discomfort immediately following surgery and none of the patients in this

Table 2 Questionnaire

	Present patient (n = 41)	Healthy patients with sural nerve biopsy (Dahlin et al. 1997) [4]: (n=21)
1. Did you have any discomfort in the foot directly after the operation?		
Yes	15 (37%)	2 (10%)
No	24 (59%)	19 (90%)
No reply	2 (5%)	
2. Did you experience any loss of sensation in the operated area after the operation?		
Yes	38 (93%)	19 (90%)
No	3 (7%)	2 (10%)
3. Did you experience pain in the operated area after the operation?		
Yes	21 (51%)	7 (33%)
No	18 (44%)	14 (67%)
No reply	2 (5%)	
4. Do you have loss of sensation in the operated foot compared with the other foot?		
Yes	35 (85%)	19 (90%)
No	6 (15%)	2 (10%)
5. Mark the area of sensory deficit in the figure.	See Figure 1 for details. 5 (12%) did not draw at all.	
6. (a) Has the area with loss of sensation decreased compared with the time directly following surgery?		
Yes	19 (46%)	8 (38%)
No	22 (54%)	13 (62%)
(b) If yes, how much (%)		
0-25	3 (7%)	2 (10%)
26-50	6 (15%)	1 (5%)
51-75	7 (17%)	3 (14%)
76-100	3 (7%)	2 (10%)
7. (a) Do you feel pain in the foot/lower leg?		
Yes	8 (20%)	1 (5%)
No	33 (80%)	20 (95%)
(b) When?		
Day time	5 (12%)	0 (0%)
Night time	2 (5%)	0 (0%)
Day time and Night time	1 (2%)	1 (5%)
8. (a) Do you have problems with cold intolerance in the operated foot/lower leg?		
Yes	12 (29%)	1 (5%)
No	29 (71%)	20 (95%)
(b) If yes, how often?		
Frequently	3 (7%)	0 (0%)
Sometimes	6 (15%)	0 (0%)
Rarely	3 (7%)	1 (5%)

Table 2 Questionnaire *(Continued)*

9. (a) Have you experienced problems with increased skin sensation when the skin is touched?		
Yes	21 (51%)	7 (33%)
No	20 (49%)	14 (67%)
(b) If yes, how often?		
Frequently	7 (17%)	0 (0%)
Sometimes	5 (12%)	4 (19%)
Rarely	9 (22%)	3 (14%)
10.(a) Do you experience discomfort or tingling along the outside of the foot?		
Yes	22 (54%)	10 (48%)
No	19 (46%)	11 (52%)
(b) If so, when do these symptoms occur?		
At rest	6 (15%)	3 (14%)
During walking	4 (10%)	1 (5%)
Impact against surgical site	15 (37%)	6 (29%)
11. How would you describe your problems at the moment?		
Disturbed sleep	0 (0%)	0 (0%)
Powerful	2 (5%)	1 (5%)
Affecting daily living	5 (12%)	1 (5%)
Mild	19 (46%)	11 (52%)
None	16 (39%)	8 (38%)
12. Do you have to take painkillers often?		
Yes	0 (0%)	0 (0%)
No	37 (100%)	21 (100%)
13. (a) Do you have any disease that can affect the nervous system, for example; diabetes, vitamin deficiency or thyroid disease.		
Yes	3 (7%)	-
No	38 (93%)	-
(b) If yes, which?		
	Diabetes mellitus	-
	Thyreoiditis	
14. A theoretical question: would you be positive to have your other sural nerve harvested if you had to undergo another nerve reconstructive surgery?		
Yes	36 (88%)	7 (33%)
No	5 (12%)	14 (67%)
Right now how much does your nerve injury affect you? (VAS)	25 (0–100)	-
[0 = no impact at all; 100 = severe impact]		
What impact has your nerve injury had on leisure activities? (VAS)	8.5 (0–100)	-
[0 = no impact at all; 100 = severe impact]		
How does your injury affect your work or school attendance? (VAS)	11.5 (0–100)	-
[0 = no impact at all; 100 = severe impact]		

study had any postoperative complications from harvesting the sural nerve. With this in mind, the nerve harvest procedure can be considered a safe procedure in healthy individuals. The results correlate well with previously published studies [5-9,11], where it was concluded that the majority of patients tolerate harvest of a sural nerve well and that there are only minor persisting symptoms from the donor site, which was irrespective of the length of follow up.

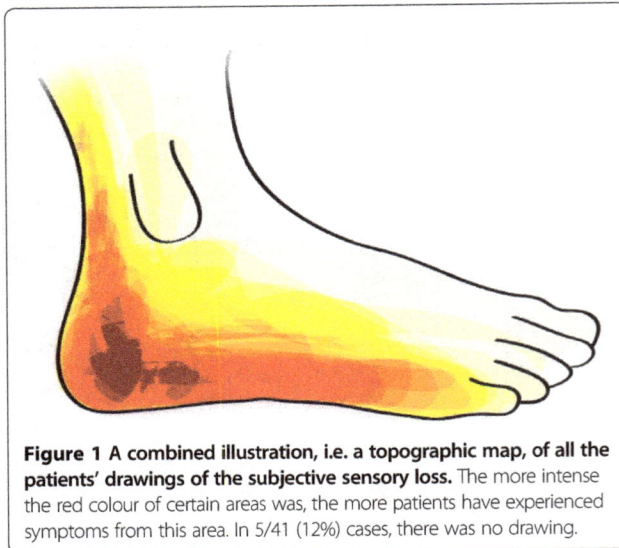

Figure 1 A combined illustration, i.e. a topographic map, of all the patients' drawings of the subjective sensory loss. The more intense the red colour of certain areas was, the more patients have experienced symptoms from this area. In 5/41 (12%) cases, there was no drawing.

Such statement has also been emphasized in paediatric patients [7].

The subjectively most common symptom, as expected [5] and experienced by over 90% of the present patients, was some degree of sensory loss at the foot most commonly in the skin around the heel (Figure 1), which correspond well with our previous results [4,7-10], where the same questionnaire was used to evaluate sequele after biopsy of the whole sural nerve. Interestingly, the patients experienced that the area of sensory loss in the skin decreased over time. In accordance, healthy subjects also notice a similar phenomenon after a sural nerve biopsy [4,9,10,12]. Previous studies, based on telephone interviews, did not focus on reduction of the sensory loss [6,11]. The gradual decrease of the area of sensory loss may depend on a combination of collateral sprouting from sensory nerves adjacent to the cutaneous area formerly innervated by the sural nerve [9,12] and brain plasticity [6,9,13]. Information, regarding the possibility for sensory loss around the heel and lateral foot and that this area may decrease over time as well as information about mild or intermittent allodynia seen in 50% of the patients, should be provided to the patients before harvesting the sural nerve. The experienced pain, both immediately and years after the sural nerve harvesting, was described mostly as mild or none at all, which is consistent with our previous study on symptoms following a sural nerve biopsy in healthy volunteers [10]. Interestingly, there was no need among our patients to presently use potent painkillers. In few patients (n = 3) the sural nerve was harvested bilateral. Thereby, it was not possible to statistically test for any differences in subjective outcome of the harvest procedure or to ask them to compare with the contralateral side. In addition, we anticipated that the patients operated on bilaterally responded on the subjective

outcome of the procedure as related to their possible worse side. This is a limitation and in future use of this questionnaire it should be clearly stated.

The overall score, how the patients experienced their general outcome of the reconstructed nerve [median = 25; highest score 100], were rather low (i.e. limited problems) and with minor problems from the donor site [median = 3; maximal score 16]; scores that correlated with each other, i.e. a worse result of the reconstruction procedure correlated positively with residual problems from the sural nerve harvest. Such a finding may be understandable, but one should also consider psychological mechanisms in this context; thus, a poor result may lead to that the patient experience more problems from the leg. A number of patients (37%) had demanding physical job, such as factory worker or auto mechanic, but the impact of the nerve injury on their work capability was surprisingly low. Two patients were unable to return to their regular work. Their work tasks included lifting of heavy objects and requirements to work manually with equal use of both arms and hands. However, the main reason that they had to change occupation was the severe nerve injury in their upper extremities requiring nerve grafting. Miloro et al. [5] described an association between an age >38 years and a worst general outcome locally in the leg after harvesting the sural nerve, but we did not see any difference in residual symptom or general outcome score in the patients with an age ≤ or > 20 years of age (i.e. injury during childhood and adolescence) at the time of reconstruction. In addition, age did not correlate with residual symptoms or general outcome score. Thus, such information should be provided to the patients that undergo a nerve reconstruction procedure. Harvest of the sural nerve for nerve reconstruction is a safe procedure also in paediatric patients [7]. Recently, it was reported that outcome of nerve repair in the forearm is worse when such a nerve injury is repaired or reconstructed after the age of 12 years [14]. Notably, most of the present patients were above 12 years of age, which may influence the results.

There are also other limitations of the study since some patients were operated on 30 years ago [8]. They may have difficulties to remember the immediate postoperative symptoms. Interestingly, the length of follow up did not correlate with the residual symptoms (i.e. value of total score). Another limitation is that the patients included had various nerve injuries, extending from a pure nerve injury to a complete amputation of their forearm or even a brachial plexus injury. Such factors may influence how the patients experience their illness and thus their answers in the questionnaire. However, according to the response, the experience of residual symptoms in the foot or leg after harvesting the sural nerve is not dependent on type of nerve injury. Notably, here we used a questionnaire sent to the patients allowing them to unbiased fill out the questions. A previous study [6] has been based on answers from a telephone questionnaire and there is a possibility that the subjects may be influenced by the person interviewing them.

As always, it is a matter of balancing benefits and risks against each other in nerve reconstruction procedures. In the case of a new nerve injury, 36 out of 41 patients would accept an additional sural nerve grafting procedure if necessary. The positive attitude to further surgery can be explained by that the majority of the patients´ injuries in their extremities affect their daily living much more than the residual symptoms that arise after harvesting the sural nerve. In contrast, a reduced willingness to perform an additional sural biopsy from the contralateral side is low among subjects with or without diabetes although they may have similar symptoms after the biopsy [4,10] (Table 2). Only 5% graded their symptoms as severe, but none of the patients in any of the studies experienced symptoms disturbing sleep [4,10]. Thus, patients, who had a whole sural biopsy, were not nearly as willing to undergo a further harvest of the sural nerve [7/21 (33%)] as the patients in the present study [36/41 (88%)], which is reasonable since the present patients would have a greater gain from their nerve graft reconstruction.

Conclusions

We conclude that harvest of a sural nerve to reconstruct an injured nerve trunk is a safe procedure with mild residual symptoms similar to those seen after a sural nerve biopsy, but such patients are less prone to undergo an additional biopsy.

Abbreviations
VAS: Visual analogue scale.

Competing interests
The authors have no competing interests related to the present study, except that LD has received reimbursements from AxoGen Inc, FL, USA.

Authors' contributions
LD and ABN designed the study. AH, together with ACZ, collected all questionnaires. AH assembled the results and wrote the manuscript together with the other authors. All authors approved the final submitted manuscript.

Acknowledgements
The research of our groups is supported by grants from the Medical Research Council (Medicine), Skåne University Hospital, Lund University, Region Skåne and HEALTH-F4-2011-278612 BIOHYBRID. We thank Lena Olsson and Tina Folker for administrative help.

References
1. de Moura W, Gilbert A: Surgical anatomy of the sural nerve. *J Reconstr Microsurg* 1984, **1**(1):31–39.
2. Dyck PJ, Karnes J, Lais A, Lofgren EP, Stevens JC: Pathologic alterations of the peripheral nervous system of human. In *Peripheral neuropathy*. 2nd edition. Edited by Dyck PJ, Thomas PK, Lambert EH, Bunge R. Philadelphia: W.B. Saunders; 1984:771–778.
3. Sima AA, Bril V, Nathaniel V, McEwen TA, Brown MB, Lattimer SA, Greene DA: Regeneration and repair of myelinated fibers in sural-nerve biopsy specimens from patients with diabetic neuropathy treated with sorbinil. *N Engl J Med* 1988, **319**(9):548–555.
4. Dahlin LB, Eriksson KF, Sundkvist G: Persistent postoperative complaints after whole sural nerve biopsies in diabetic and non-diabetic subjects. *Diabet Med* 1997, **14**(5):353–356.
5. Miloro M, Stoner JA: Subjective outcomes following sural nerve harvest. *J Oral Maxillofac Surg* 2005, **63**(8):1150–1154.
6. Ehretsman RL, Novak CB, Mackinnon SE: Subjective recovery of nerve graft donor site. *Ann Plast Surg* 1999, **43**(6):606–612.
7. Lapid O, Ho ES, Goia C, Clarke HM: Evaluation of the sensory deficit after sural nerve harvesting in pediatric patients. *Plast Reconstr Surg* 2007, **119**(2):670–674.
8. IJpma FF, Nicolai JP, Meek MF: Sural nerve donor-site morbidity: thirty-four years of follow-up. *Ann Plast Surg* 2006, **57**(4):391–395.
9. Martins RS, Barbosa RA, Siqueira MG, Soares MS, Heise CO, Foroni L, Teixeira MJ: Morbidity following sural nerve harvesting: a prospective study. *Clin Neurol Neurosurg* 2012, **114**(8):1149–1152.
10. Dahlin LB, Lithner F, Bresater LE, Thomsen NO, Eriksson KF, Sundkvist G: Sequelae following sural nerve biopsy in type 1 diabetic subjects. *Acta Neurol Scand* 2008, **118**(3):193–197.
11. Ng SS, Kwan MK, Ahmad TS: Quantitative and qualitative evaluation of sural nerve graft donor site. *Med J Malaysia* 2006, **61**:13–17.
12. Aszmann OC, Muse V, Dellon AL: Evidence in support of collateral sprouting after sensory nerve resection. *Ann Plast Surg* 1996, **37**(5):520–525.
13. Theriault M, Dort J, Sutherland G, Zochodne DW: A prospective quantitative study of sensory deficits after whole sural nerve biopsies in diabetic and nondiabetic patients. *Surgical approach and the role of collateral sprouting. Neurology* 1998, **50**(2):480–484.
14. Chemnitz A, Bjorkman A, Dahlin LB, Rosen B: Functional outcome thirty years after median and ulnar nerve repair in childhood and adolescence. *Journal of Bone and Joint Surgery (Am)* 2013, **95**(4):329–337.

22

Microvascular free-flap transfer for head and neck reconstruction in elderly patients

Francesco Turrà[1], Simone La Padula[1], Sergio Razzano[1], Paola Bonavolontà[2], Gisella Nele[1], Sergio Marlino[1], Luigi Canta[1], Pasquale Graziano[2], Giovanni Dell'Aversana Orabona[2], Fabrizio Schonauer[1*]

Abstract

Background: With the increase in life expectancy, the incidence of head and neck cancer has grown in the elderly population. Free tissue transfer has become the first choice, among all the reconstructive techniques, in these cases. The safety and success of micro vascular transfer have been well documented in the general population, but its positive results achieved in elderly patients have received less attention.

Methods: We retrospectively studied 28 patients over the age of 60 years. The aim of this paper was to study the success rate of free tissue transfer and investigate the complication incidence in this patient population.

Results: Twenty-eight free flaps were performed to reconstruct medium to large cervico-facial surgical defects in six years. No difference was noted between success and complication rates observed between general and elderly population.

Conclusion: This study indicates that free-flap technique for head and neck reconstruction could be considered a safe option in elderly patients when a good pre-operative general status is present.

Background

Microsurgical free-tissue transfer has gained a central role in plastic surgery for difficult reconstruction of head and neck defects, modifying the treatment of cancer in this region.

Although this technique has become a safe choice, complications may occur in 5-25%; these patients may require a surgical re-exploration of the free flap [1].

The proportion of elderly people with head and neck cancer is rising due to an overall increase in life expectancy.

The safety and success of free flap transfer have been well documented in the general population; positive results achieved in elderly patients have received less attention [2].

The aim of the present study is to investigate the effect of age on the outcome of such procedures, the medical impact of prolonged surgery and if it is worthy

against the functional benefits and the better life expectancy achieved by the use of microvascular reconstruction.

Methods

We retrospectively reviewed our experience with microsurgical free-tissue transfer in patients over the age of 60 whom we arbitrarily defined as "elderly".

Between January 2007 and February 2013, 28 patients with head and neck cancer were treated at the Maxillo-facial Surgical Unit and reconstructed by our Plastic Surgery team.

The patients were classified into two groups according to age: between 60 and 69 years (age group I) and between 70 and 79 years (age group II), respectively. Table 1.

The oral cavity was the most frequent site of reconstruction in all groups. All patients undergoing microsurgical free-tissue transfer were recovered in intensive care unit until their stabilization. The flap was monitored by checking paddle skin colour, bleeding and, if necessary, Doppler signal, every 2 hours for the first day, every 6h

* Correspondence: fschona@libero.it
[1]Unit of Plastic, Reconstructive and Aesthetic Surgery, Federico II University, Via S.Pansini 5, 80131, Naples, Italy
Full list of author information is available at the end of the article

Table 1 Patient series

Name	Age	Group	ASA	Type of tumour	Site	Reconstruction	Days in Intens.Care	Complications
PO	60	I	1	SCC	Cheek	Radial forearm	1	-
AR	60	I	2	Sarcoma	Mandible	Fibula osteocutaneous	1	Venous throbosis
GE	61	I	1	SCC	Mandible	Fibula osteocutaneous	2	-
AG	62	I	1	SCC	Palate	Radial forearm	1	-
MD	62	I	2	SCC	Tongue	Radial forearm	1	-
PM	63	I	2	SCC	Larynx and pharynx	Radial forearm	2	-
TD	64	I	1	BCC	Cheek (ext.)	Radial forearm	1	-
CG	65	I	2	SCC	Scalp	Latissimus dorsi	1	-
FS	65	I	1	SCC	Cheek (ext.)	Latissimus dorsi	1	-
DA	66	I	2	SCC	Tongue	Ulnar forearm	1	-
AP	66	I	2	SCC	Tongue	Ulnar forearm	1	-
DR	66	I	1	SCC	Floor and tongue	Radial forearm	1	-
DN	67	I	1	SCC	Floor and tongue	Radial forearm	1	-
SA	68	I	2	SCC	Cheek	Radial forearm	1	-
IB	69	I	1	SCC	Pharynx	Radial forearm	2	-
BM	70	II	2	SCC	Floor	Radial forearm	1	-
DC	70	II	1	SCC	Mandible	Fibula osteocutaneous	2	-
RA	71	II	1	SCC	Lips and cheek	Radial forearm	1	-
PA	72	II	3	SCC	Tongue	Radial forearm	3	Pulmonary failure
RM	72	II	2	SCC	Floor and tongue	Radial forearm	1	-
CR	72	II	1	SCC	Scalp	Latissimus dorsi	2	-
SG	73	II	2	SCC	Cheek	Radial forearm	1	Haematoma
SM	75	II	1	SCC	Tongue	Radial forearm	1	-
FS	75	II	2	SCC	Mandible	Fibula osteocutaneous	2	Partial necrosis
DM	75	II	1	SCC	Floor and tongue	Radial forearm	1	-
PI	76	II	2	SCC	Half right face	Rectum abodminis muscle	3	Venous thrombosis
GG	77	II	2	SCC	Half right face	Rectum abodminis muscle	2	-
TC	77	II	1	SCC	Floor and tongue	Radial forearm	1	-

on day 2-3 and then less frequently until patient's discharge.

Many variables were analysed for each group. Our records were reviewed searching for diagnosis, free-flap type, defect site, patient age and sex, preoperative medical problem, length of operation, complications and operative mortality. We classified complications into two main clusters: technique-related (seroma, haematoma, infection, dehiscence, thrombosis, congestion and skin or flap loss) and general conditions-related. Technique complications were classified as major, requiring surgical re-exploration, or minor, not requiring re-exploration.

Long-term functional outcomes (speech, swallowing and chewing) were assessed 6 month after surgery.

Results and discussion
A total of 28 patients (20 male, 8 female; ranging 60 to 77 years) underwent a free-tissue transfer for head and neck tumours. Fifteen patients, were aged between 60 and 69 years (age group I) and thirteen patients were aged between 70 and 79 years (age group II).

Most frequent histological diagnosis, preoperatively indicated by biopsy, was squamous cell carcinoma.

Various free flap types were used to reconstruct a variety of defects. Microvascular free flaps used were: radial forearm (n = 17), fibula (n = 4), latissimus dorsi (n = 3), ulnar forearm (n = 2), rectus abdominis (n = 2). Total success rate was 93% (26/28).

Preoperative medical problems were evaluated through American Society of Anesthesiologists (ASA) score; just one patient classified as ASA III class underwent microvascular technique.

Donor site major complications were not observed.

Total complication rate was 17,9% (5/28); complications were divided into two different groups: technique-related and systemic condition-related. Four technique-related complications were observed (14,3%): of these three were major and one minor. Major flap complications (10,7%) consisted of one venous thrombosis of the pedicle and one partial necrosis in age group II (15,4%) and one venous thrombosis in age group I (6,7%). Flap salvage was possible in the younger patient with venous thrombosis by exploring the flap and performing a new anastomosis; in the older patient with partial necrosis another local flap was needed; total flap loss occurred in another case.

A minor flap complication occurred in the age group II (7,7%): an haematoma occurred at the recipient site and was evacuated at the patient bed, with no surgical re-exploration.

One patient, in the age group II, had a systemic complication that resulted in respiratory failure soon after the transfer to the intensive care unit. This patient with COPD was an heavy smoker.

Speech, swallowing and chewing assessed in our patients 6 months after surgery resulted well preserved.

Head and neck tumours are often diagnosed late, because of their lack of symptoms in the early stage. In these cases a large demolition is needed. Because of the importance of the quality of life, surgery has to be safe and give satisfactory functional outcomes. Microvascular free-tissue transfer has gained a central role for these large reconstructions to protect important functions of this region. The success rate of this surgery at the present time is reported to be in the range of 91% to 99% in large series from major microsurgical centers [3-5].

Age has been regarded frequently as an independent risk factor for bad surgical outcomes; before the 1960s the mortality rate for elderly patients undergoing elective surgery was 2-6 times higher than in the general population [6]. The reasons that may explain this difference are well documented; the most common medical problems that affect the mortality are heart failure, or the compromise of pulmonary function [7,8].

The improvements in anaesthesia techniques explain the reduction of the mortality rate in elderly patients during these 40 years, especially for patients with cardiac disease [9].

Studies on microsurgical free flap conducted in elderly patients do not agree in defining the term "elderly", but they demonstrated that age is not an important factor influencing the success of this surgery [10-13]. Pompei et al. in a large study of pedicled and free flaps for head and neck reconstructions showed that complications were related with comorbidities more than the age [14].

A reliable predictor of postoperative morbidity could be the ASA status as suggested in a study by Serletti et al. [13].

However, these studies stress how several factors can lead to free-flap complication; most of them reported that age does not impact the free transfer success, but results are variable.

Our results are comparable to the ones showed by Shestak et al. in their small series of cases. In this study 19 patients underwent a free flap reconstruction and results showed a 16% major surgical complication rate in patients over 70 years and 13% in patients under 70 years [10].

In the present study one patient died after this surgery (mortality rate 3,5%); this fatal post-operative complication was correlated with a higher ASA class.

Conclusion

In conclusion our study shows that microsurgical free-flap transfer can be considered a safe technique for head and neck reconstruction in all age groups. Pre-existing systemic disease could influence peri- and post-operative complications, and ASA status could be a well accepted way to select patients undergoing this surgery.

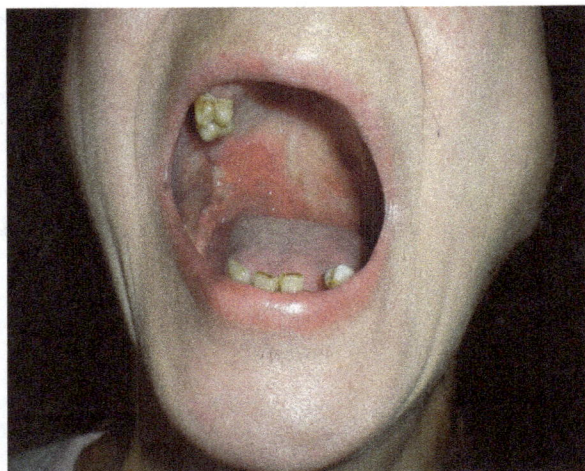

Figure 1 Squamous cell carcinoma of the right cheek and tonsillar pillar.

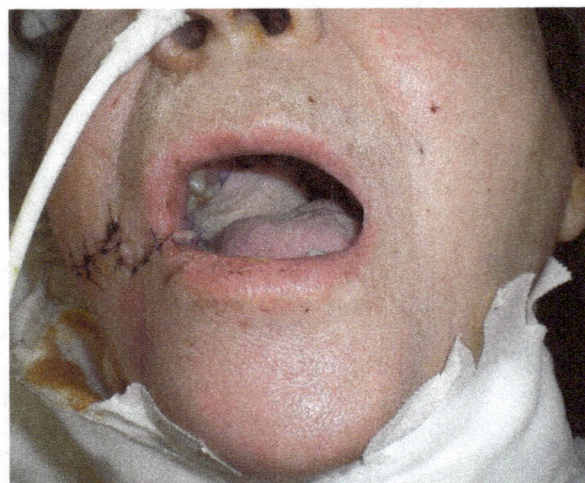

Figure 2 Transferred radial forearm free flap at two weeks.

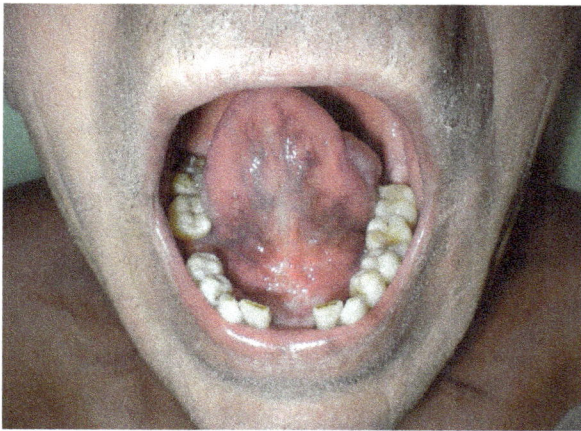

Figure 3 Squamous cell carcinoma of the floor of the mouth.

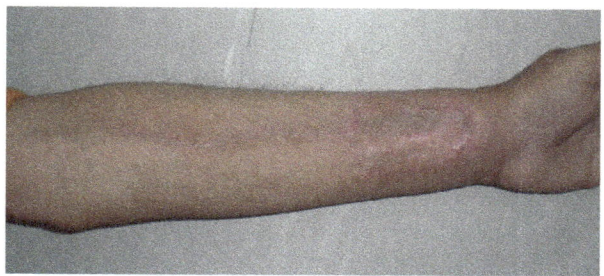

Figure 6 Healed skin grafted radial forearm free flap donor site 6 months after surgery.

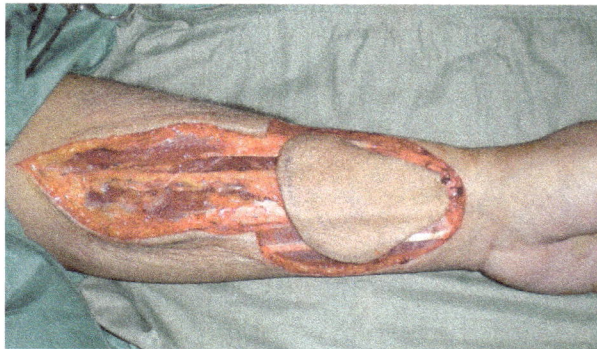

Figure 4 Radial forearm free flap harvesting and its pedicle.

List of abbreviations used
ASA= American Society of Anesthesiologists; COPD= Chronic Obstructive Pulmonary Disease; SCC= Squamous Cell Carcinoma; BCC= Basal Cell Carcinoma.

Competing interests
The authors declare that they have no competing interests.

Authors' contributions
F.T.: conception and design, acquisition and interpretation of data, drafting the manuscript, given final approval of the version to be published. S.L.P.: acquisition of data, given final approval of the version to be published. S.R.: interpretation of data, drafting the manuscript, given final approval of the version to be published. P.B, S.M, L.C, P.G: critical revision, interpretation of data, given final approval of the version to be published. G.N.: drafting the manuscript, given final approval of the version to be published. G.D.A.O.: acquisition and interpretation of data, critical revision, given final approval of the version to be published. F.S.: conception and design, acquisition and interpretation of data, drafting the manuscript, critical revision, given final approval of the version to be published.

Authors' information
FT: Medical Doctor. SLP: Resident in Plastic, Reconstructive and Aesthetic Surgery at University Federico II, Naples. SR: Resident in Plastic, Reconstructive and Aesthetic Surgery at University Federico II, Naples. PB: Resident in Maxillofacial Surgery at University Federico II, Naples. GN: Medical Student. SM: Resident in Plastic, Reconstructive and Aesthetic Surgery at University Federico II, Naples. LC: Specialist in Plastic, Reconstructive and Aesthetic Surgery at University Federico II, Naples. PG: Specialist in Maxillofacial Surgery at University Federico II, Naples. GDAO: Assistant Professor in Maxillofacial Surgery at University Federico II, Naples. FS: Assistant Professor in Plastic, Reconstructive and Aesthetic Surgery at University Federico II, Naples

Declarations
Publication of this article was funded by research university funding.
This article has been published as part of *BMC Surgery* Volume 13 Supplement 2, 2013: Proceedings from the 26th National Congress of the Italian Society of Geriatric Surgery. The full contents of the supplement are available online at http://www.biomedcentral.com/bmcsurg/supplements/13/S2.

Authors' details
[1]Unit of Plastic, Reconstructive and Aesthetic Surgery, Federico II University, Via S.Pansini 5, 80131, Naples, Italy. [2]Department of Maxillofacial Surgery, Federico II University, Via S.Pansini 5, 80131, Naples, Italy.

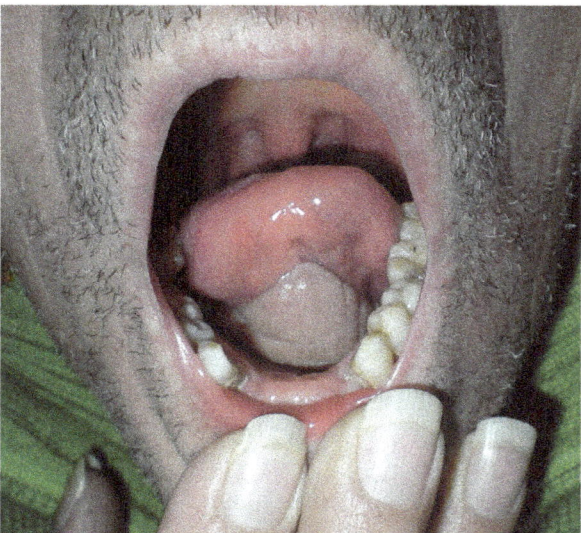

Figure 5 Settled radial forearm free flap at 6 months follow-up.

References
1. Salgado CJ, Moran SL, Mardini S: **Flap monitoring and patient management.** *Plast Reconstr Surg* 2009, **124(6 suppl)**:e295-e302.

2. Yu P, Chang DW, Miller MJ, *et al*: **Analysis of 49 cases of flap compromise in 1310 free flaps for head and neck reconstruction.** *Head Neck* 2009, **31**:45-51.

3. Shaw WW: **Microvascular free flaps: the first decade.** *Clin Plast Surg* 1983, **10**:3.

4. Khouri RK: **Free flap surgery: the second decade.** *Clin Plast Surg* 1992, **19**:757.

5. Hidalgo DA, Jones CS: **The role of emergent exploration in free-tissue transfer: A review of 150 consecutive cases.** *Plast Reconstr Surg* 1990, **86**:492.

6. Cole WH: **Prediction of operative reserve in the elderly patient.** *Ann Surg* 1968, **168**:310.

7. Guarnieri T, Filbrun CR, Zitnik G, *et al*: **Contractile and biochemical correlates of b-adrenergic stimulation of the aged heart.** *Am J Physiol* 1980, **239**:H501-8.

8. Mannino DM, Davis KJ: **Lung function decline and outcomes in elderly population.** *Thorax* 2006, **61**:472-7.

9. Foster ED, Davis KB, Carpenter JA, *et al*: **Risk of noncardiac operation in patients with defined coronary disease.** *Ann Thorac Surg* 1986, **41**:42-50.

10. Shestak KC, Jones NF: **Microsurgical free-tissue transfer in the elderly patients.** *Plast Reconstr Surg* 1991, **88**:259-63.

11. Bonawitz SC, Schnarrs RH, Rosenthal AI, *et al*: **Free tissue transfer in elderly patients.** *Plast Reconstr Surg* 1991, **87**:1074-79.

12. Ziffren SE, Hartford CE: **Comparative mortality for various surgical operations in older versus younger age group.** *J Am Geriatr Soc* 1972, **20**:485-9.

13. Classen DA, Ward H: **Complications in a consecutive series of 250 free flap operations.** *Ann Plast Surg* 2006, **56**:557-61.

14. Pompei S, Tedesco M, Pozzi M, *et al*: **Age as a risk factor in cervicofacial reconstruction.** *J Exp Clin Cancer Res* 1999, **18**:209-12.

23

Ca^{2+}-dependent nitric oxide release in the injured endothelium of excised rat aorta: a promising mechanism applying in vascular prosthetic devices in aging patients

Roberto Berra-Romani[1], José Everardo Avelino-Cruz[2], Abdul Raqeeb[3], Alessandro Della Corte[4], Mariapia Cinelli[5], Stefania Montagnani[5], Germano Guerra[6*], Francesco Moccia[2], Franco Tanzi[2]

Abstract

Background: Nitric oxide is key to endothelial regeneration, but it is still unknown whether endothelial cell (EC) loss results in an increase in NO levels at the wound edge. We have already shown that endothelial damage induces a long-lasting Ca^{2+} entry into surviving cells though connexin hemichannels (CxHcs) uncoupled from their counterparts on ruptured cells. The physiological outcome of injury-induced Ca^{2+} inflow is, however, unknown.

Methods: In this study, we sought to determine whether and how endothelial scraping induces NO production (NOP) in the endothelium of excised rat aorta by exploiting the NO-sensitive fluorochrome, DAF-FM diacetate and the Ca^{2+}-sensitive fluorescent dye, Fura-2/AM.

Results: We demonstrated that injury-induced NOP at the lesion site is prevented in presence of the endothelial NO synthase inhibitor, L-NAME, and in absence of extracellular Ca^{2+}. Unlike ATP-dependent NO liberation, the NO response to injury is insensitive to BTP-2, which selectively blocks store-operated Ca^{2+} inflow. However, injury-induced NOP is significantly reduced by classic gap junction blockers, and by connexin mimetic peptides specifically targeting Cx37Hcs, Cx40HCs, and Cx43Hcs. Moreover, disruption of caveolar integrity prevents injury-elicited NO signaling, but not the accompanying Ca^{2+} response.

Conclusions: The data presented provide the first evidence that endothelial scraping stimulates NO synthesis at the wound edge, which might both exert an immediate anti-thrombotic and anti-inflammatory action and promote the subsequent re-endothelialization.

Background

Endothelial injury is regarded as the early event that leads to the onset and progression of severe vascular disorders, such as thrombosis, hypertension, and atherosclerosis [1]. Endothelial cell (EC) loss physiologically occurs due to physiological turnover in focal areas of the inner surface of blood vessels which are adjacent to regions with low or absent replication [2,3]. When the extent of EC loss is such small, i.e. limited to a belt of cells around the whole circumference of the arterial vessel, the re-endothelization process is driven by proliferation, spreading, and migration of surviving ECs into the damaged site [4]. On the other hand, larger areas of injury may release chemical messages, such as concentration gradients of vascular endothelial growth factor (VEGF) and stromal derived factor-1α (SDF-1α), that recruit circulating endothelial progenitor cells to the wound edge in order to replace damaged endothelium [5-10]. The break

---

* Correspondence: germano.guerra@unimol.it
[6]Department of Medicine and Health Sciences, University of Molise, via F. De Sanctis, 86100, Campobasso, Italy
Full list of author information is available at the end of the article

in the anatomic integrity of vascular endothelium is significantly larger in subjects undergoing medical interventions, such as deployment of endovascular devices and percutaneous transluminal coronary angioplasty [2,11,12]. Such a heavy loss of ECs from the vascular wall dampens the beneficial effects of reconstructive surgery and prompts the quest for pharmacological treatments aiming at restoring the continuity of endothelial monolayer [2,11-13]. Accordingly, the de-endothelialisation of arterial vessels may cause thrombi formation and neointimal hyperplasia, giving raise to a process termed as "in-stent restenosis" (ISR) which renarrows the arterial lumen [2,11,12]. Drug-eluting stents (DES) may be implanted during or after angioplasty to inhibit neointimal hyperplasia and prevent ISR [2,12,14]. Unfortunately, the most commonly employed stents deliver drugs, such as sirolimus and paclixatel, that cause a long-term inhibition of endothelial proliferation and migration. These untoward off-target effects significantly delay endothelial regrowth, thereby leaving uncovered the surface of the stent and increasing the risk of late in-stent thrombosis [14,15].

Aging is accompanied by a decline in the healthy function of multiple organ systems, leading to increased incidence of mortality from many diseases. Oxidative stress and elevated ROS (Reactive oxygen species) has been implicated in the mechanism of senescence and aging; they are also involved in cancer, diabetes, neurodegenerative, cardiovascular and other diseases [16,17] Overproduction of oxidant molecules is due to several stress agents such chemicals, drugs, pollutants, high-caloric diets and exercise [18].

Nitric oxide (NO), a gasotransmitter that may be synthesized and released by ECs [1,19], might play a key role in healing injured endothelium. Accordingly, NO inhibits apoptosis and enhances EC proliferation, migration, and tubulogenesis [19]. Moreover, NO might serve as anti-inflammatory signal at the injured site by preventing local platelet activation and thrombus formation, by causing vasorelaxation, and by inhibiting the phenotypic switch of vascular smooth muscle cell (VSMC) [1,19]. Restoration of NO production at the site of vascular injury may attenuate neointimal hyperplasia and adverse the onset of the atherosclerotic process [20]. In vascular endothelium, NO may be synthesized by two different isoforms of NO synthase (NOS), namely inducible NOS (iNOS/NOS2), which mediates NO liberation during inflammatory reactions, and endothelial NOS (eNOS/NOS3), which is preferentially recruited by stimuli [19,21]. The catalytic reaction consists in the conversion of L-arginine to L-citrulline and requires several cofactors, such as NAPDH, tetrahydrobiopterin and O_2 [19]. Unlike iNOS, which is inducible and Ca^{2+}-independent, both iNOS and eNOS are constitutive and bear a calmodulin-binding site

whose binding to cytosolic Ca^{2+} is essential to stimulate NO synthesis [19]. In several types of ECs, eNOS is preferentially recruited by Ca^{2+} store-operated Ca^{2+} entry (SOCE), which is gated by depletion of the inositol-1,4,5-trisphosphate ($InsP_3$)-sensitive stores within the endoplasmic reticulum (ER) [8,22]. This feature is due to the close proximity between eNOS and SOC channels at the caveolae, cholesterol-enriched surface microdomains that compartmentalize signal transduction molecules [23]. Cholesterol-binding drugs, such as methyl-β-cyclodextrin (MβCD), have been used to disrupt caveolae and impair NO signalling in vascular endothelium [24]. That NO is involved in EC response to injury has been suggested by the elevation in both eNOS protein and enzyme activity in the regenerating endothelium of rat aorta [25]. Moreover, a recent study carried out on this preparation reported an increase in $[Ca^{2+}]_i$ in ECs nearby the lesion site [2,9,26,27]. The Ca^{2+} response to injury comprises an initial peak, mainly due to Ca^{2+} release from $InsP_3$-sensitive receptors ($InsP_3Rs$), which is followed by a long-lasting decay phase mediated by Ca^{2+} entry across the plasma membrane [27]. $InsP_3$ synthesis requires phospholipase C (PLC) activation by ATP (or ATP-derived nucleotides) released from ruptured cells [27]. Ca^{2+} inflow is supported by connexin (Cx) hemichannels (CxHcs), which have recently been described as alternative Ca^{2+} entry routes in vascular ECs as well as other non-excitable cell types [26-31]. Cxs may be classified on the basis of the molecular weight with three main isoforms (Cx37, Cx40, and Cx43) being found in ECs from several vascular beds, including rat aorta [32,33]. Despite the available evidences show an increase both in eNOS activity and in $[Ca^{2+}]_i$ within lesioned endothelium, there is no report of injury-induce NO release in blood vessels. Understanding the signal transduction machinery leading to endothelial activation and NO synthesis might be clinically relevant to design alternative strategies to restore endothelial integrity and prevent ISR.

In the present investigation, we sought to determine whether NO synthesis occurs in ECs facing the injury site of excised rat aorta. We further aimed at elucidating the signal transduction pathway responsible for NO release by lesioned endothelium. These goals were accomplished by loading ECs with Fura-2/AM, a Ca^{2+}-sensitive fluorochrome, and DAF-FM diacetate, a NO-sensitive fluorescent dye. We provided, for the first time, the evidence that mechanical injury induces a long lasting NO production (NOP) in cells nearby the lesion site which requires Ca^{2+} entry through uncoupled Cx37Hcs, Cx40Hcs, and Cx43Hc. These results might aid in developing novel pharmacological treatments devoted to restore endothelial integrity upon invasive medical interventions.

Methods

Dissection of the aorta

Wistar rats aged 2-3 months were sacrificed with an overdose of diethyl ether. The thoracic and abdominal aorta were dissected out and perfused with physiological salt solution (PSS). The vessel was cleaned of the surrounding connective tissue, cut in ~5 mm long rings, stored in PSS at room temperature (22-24 °C) and used within 5 hours. All the animal protocols were approved by the East Tennessee State University's Animal Care and Use Committee. All experiments conform to the Guide for the Care and Use of Laboratory Animals published by the US National Institutes of Health (NIH Publication No. 85-23, revised 1996). The animal handling was under the continuous control of the Veterinary Surgeon of the University of Pavia.

Solutions

PSS had the following composition (in mM): 150 NaCl, 6 KCl, 1.5 $CaCl_2$, 1 $MgCl_2$, 10 Glucose, 10 Hepes. In Ca^{2+}-free solution (0 Ca^{2+}), Ca^{2+} was substituted with 2 mM NaCl, and 0.5 mM EGTA was added. Solutions were titrated to pH 7.4 with NaOH. Aortic rings were bathed in 0 Ca^{2+} for no longer than 90 sec before inducing the injury. Control experiments have demonstrated that such a short pre-incubation period is not able deplete intracellular Ca^{2+} stores [27].

$[Ca^{2+}]_i$ and NO measurements.

The technique used to evaluate changes in $[Ca^{2+}]_i$ in intact endothelium has been previously described [26,27,34-37]. The aortic ring was opened and loaded with 16 μmol Fura-2/AM for 60 min at room temperature, washed and fixed by small pins with the luminal face up. In situ ECs were visualized by an upright epifluorescence Axiolab microscope (Carl Zeiss, Oberkochen, Germany), equipped with a Zeiss ×63 Achroplan objective (water-immersion, 2.0 mm working distance, 0.9 numerical aperture). ECs were excited alternately at 340 and 380 nm, and the emitted light was detected at 510 nm. The exciting filters were mounted on a filter wheel (Lambda 10, Sutter Instrument, Novato, CA, USA). Custom software, working in the LINUX environment, was used to drive the camera (Extended-ISIS Camera, Photonic Science, Millham, UK) and the filter wheel, and to measure and plot on-line the fluorescence from 10-15 rectangular "regions of interest" (ROI) enclosing one single cell. $[Ca^{2+}]_i$ was monitored by measuring, for each ROI, the ratio of the mean fluorescence emitted at 510 nm when exciting alternatively at 340 and 380 nm (shortly termed "ratio"). An increase in $[Ca^{2+}]_i$ causes an increase in the ratio. Ratio measurements were performed and plotted on-line every 5 s. The experiments were performed at room temperature (21-23 °C).

NO production in ECs in intact rat aorta was monitored with the membrane permeant 4-Amino-5-methylamino-2',7'-difluorofluorescein (DAF-FM) diacetate. Once open, the aortic ring was fixed by small pins with the luminal side facing up, loaded with 10 μM DAF-FM for 60 min at room temperature and washed in PSS for one hour. DAF-FM fluorescence was measured by using the same equipment described for Ca^{2+} recordings but with a different filter set, i.e. excitation at 480 nm and emission at 535 nm wavelength (emission intensity was shortly termed "NO_i"). NO measurements were performed and plotted on-line every 5 s. Again, off-line analysis was performed by using custom-made macros developed by Microsoft Office Excel software. The experiments were performed at room temperature. DAF-FM is essentially non-fluorescent until it irreversibly reacts with the nitrosonium cation produced by spontaneous oxidation of newly synthesized NO. The resulting fluorescent compound is trapped in the cytoplasm, so that DAF-FM fluorescence summates with continual NO production. As also found in bovine aortic ECs [38], DAF-FM fluorescence in rat aortic ECs underwent a persistent and linear increase likely due to the basal NO synthesis [19]. Accordingly, the change in baseline fluorescence was dramatically reduced when aortic rings were pre-incubated with L-NAME (5 mM), which inhibits eNOS by competing with its natural substrate, L-arginine (data not shown), or in 0Ca (data not shown). This observation was somehow expected since aortic endothelium has long been known to regulate vascular tone by basal release of NO [19]. Therefore, for each experiment, the basal DAF-FM signal was recorded for at least 20 minutes and the resulting curve fitted off-line by a linear regression equation in order to calculate the slope (i.e. the rate) of basal fluorescence increase. The slope was subtracted from the recorded trace, thus enabling to measure S-Nitroso-N-acetylpenicillamine (SNAP)-, ATP- and injury-induced NOP independently on basal eNOS activity [39] (see below). NO synthesis was evaluated by subtracting the baseline level (1 min before the increase in DAF-FM fluorescence) to the average value of the plateau phase (1 min before the end of the recording) recorded upon either ATP administration or endothelial scraping.

In order to assess the ability of the fluorimetric set up to detect evoked changes in intracellular NO levels, aortic rings were exposed to the NO donor, SNAP, and ATP, which has been shown to elicit NO production in a variety of ECs from different vascular districts [38,40]. As shown in Figure 1A and Figure 1B, respectively, SNAP (500 μM) and ATP (300 μM) caused an increase in the intensity of DAF-FM fluorescence in 19 out of 19 cells and in 170 out of 170 cells, respectively.

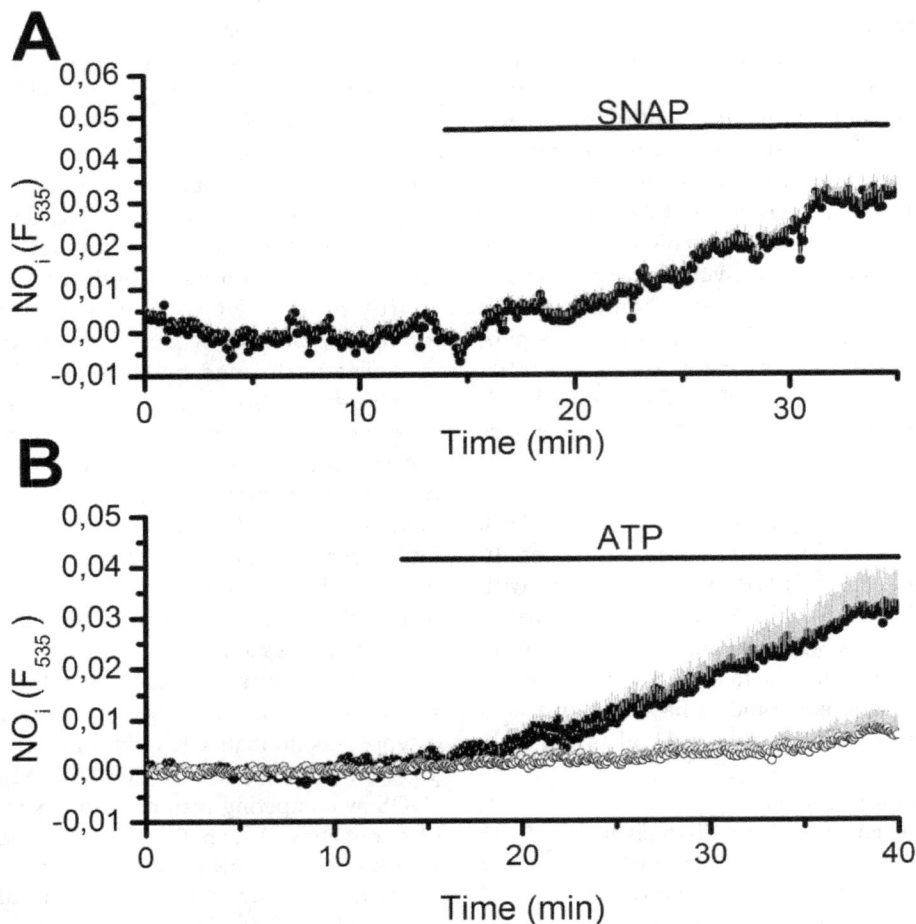

Figure 1 NO production in rat aortic endothelium. A, exposition to SNAP (500 µM) caused an increase in DAF-FM fluorescence in native rat aortic endothelium *in situ*. The trace is the mean±SE of 11 cells from the same visual field. B, ATP (300 µM) induced an elevation in intracellular NO (closed circles) that was dramatically hampered when the rings were pre-treated with L-NAME (5 mM) for 40 min (white circles). The traces are the mean±SE, respectively, of 10 (PSS) and 8 (L-NAME) cells from two aortic rings harvested from the same animal on the same day.

On average, L-NAME (5 mM) reduced by 86% ATP-induced NO production (0.025 ± 0.001, $n = 170$, vs. 0.0041 ± 0.0009, $n = 192$, p < 0.001) (Figure 1B).

Mechanical disruption of ECs

As shown in [26,27], aortic endothelium was injured under microscopic control by means of a glass microelectrode with a broken tip of about 30 µm diameter, driven by an XYZ hydraulic micromanipulator (Narishige, Japan). Images of either Fura-2 or DAF-FM/Fura-2 loaded ECs, together with numbered ROIs, were taken before the lesion, in order to identify the cells facing the injury site. As aforementioned, the dissection procedure could itself damage the intimal layer and cause SMCs to be loaded with Fura-2. These rings were, therefore, discarded. The microelectrode was first positioned almost parallel and very near to the endothelium surface. It was then moved downward, along the Z-axis, until the electrode tip gently touched the endothelium, and moved horizontally across the visual field to scrape 1-3 consecutive rows of ECs along the whole diameter of the aortic ring. The following lesion was 170 µm long and 20 µm wide. This procedure, which allowed monitoring of NO signals in ECs adjacent to the lesion, mimics the ablation of the endothelial lining achieved in pre-clinical studies addressing the cellular mechanisms of intimal regrowth upon stent deployment [41-43]. The scraping of the endothelial monolayer imposed a physical stretching on the underlying SMCs which resembles the condition occurring during clinical interventions. Ethidium bromide (EB), a fluorescent molecule unable to cross an intact plasma membrane and therefore indicative of damaged/dead cells, was used to check the viability of both ECs nearby the injury and underlying SMCs [27]. When smooth muscle fibers were lesioned by mechanical scratching and stained by EB, the experiments were discarded.

Data analysis

For each protocol, data were collected from at least three rats. The amplitude of the peak Ca^{2+} response was measured as the difference between the ratio at the peak and the mean ratio of 1 min baseline before the peak. The details of NO measurements have been reported above. Only cells residing in the first row nearby the wound were used to elaborate the average value. For Ca^{2+} and NO measurements, statistical comparisons were made by Student's t-test for unpaired observations.

Chemicals

Fura-2/AM and DAF-FM was obtained from Molecular Probes (Molecular Probes Europe BV, Leiden, The Netherlands). N-(4-[3,5-bis(trifluoromethyl)-1H-pyrazol-1-yl]phenyl)-4-methyl-1,2,3-thiadiazole-5-carboxamide (BTP-2) was purchased from Calbiochem (La Jolla, CA, USA). All other chemicals were purchased from Sigma. Cx-mimetic peptides, including [37,43]Gap27 and [40]Gap27, were synthesized by Severn Biotech (Kidderminster, UK); purity was >95%. In more detail, [37,43]Gap27 and [40]Gap27 mimic a highly conserved SRPTEK sequence present in the second extracellular loop of Cxs 37 and 43 and of Cx 40, respectively [15,19]. Their scrambled versions were also synthesized by Severn Biotech. All other chemicals were of analytical grade and obtained from Sigma.

Results

Injury augments intracellular NO levels in the intact endothelium of rat aorta

Figure 2A depicts the injury-induced increase in $[Ca^{2+}]_i$ occurring within the ECs adjacent to the lesion site and which have lost their contact with the scraped cells. The Ca^{2+} signal consisted in an initial transient peak, mainly due to $InsP_3$-dependent Ca^{2+} release, followed by a prolonged decay phase caused by Ca^{2+} entry from the extracellular milieu [27]. When the damage was performed on an aortic ring loaded with DAF-FM, it induced a gradual increase in fluorescence that reached a plateau after about 20 min (Figure 2B). This feature is consistent with the concomitant long-lasting Ca^{2+} inflow [27], which might sustain NO synthesis [19,38]. In the presence of the eNOS inhibitor, L-NAME (5 mM), mechanical damage failed to augment intracellular NO (Figure 2B). The statistical analysis is reported in Figure 3A. Similar to the intercellular Ca^{2+} wave, which did not spread farther than the 4th raw of cells, the amplitude of the NO signal significantly ($p < 0.05$) decayed at this location (Figure 2C). This feature hints at a strong correlation between the increase in $[Ca^{2+}]_i$ triggered by the injury and the accompanying NO synthesis.

Injury-induced NOP depends on extracellular Ca^{2+} entry

It has long been known that, in vascular endothelium, eNOS is selectively activated by Ca^{2+} inflow rather than intracellular Ca^{2+} release [8,22,40]. When mechanical damage was carried out in absence of extracellular Ca^{2+}, a maneuver which abolished the prolonged decay-phase of the Ca^{2+} signal, the injury did not result in a detectable NOP (Figure 3A). The involvement of intracellular Ca^{2+} mobilization was investigated with the aid of thapsigargin (2 μM), an inhibitor of the endoplasmic reticulum Ca^{2+}-ATPase, which prevents Ca^{2+} re-uptake into the stores and leads to their depletion. Preliminary experiments showed that pre-incubating the rings for 30 min with 2 μM thapsigargin abolished the intracellular Ca^{2+} mobilization triggered by supramaximal concentrations of ATP (300 μM) ($n = 79$; data not shown). Therefore, such a treatment causes the depletion of the Ca^{2+} reservoir underlying the initial Ca^{2+} response to injury [27]. The NO signal induced by endothelial scraping, however, was not significantly affected by thapsigargin (Figure 3A). Overall, these results strongly suggest that injury-promoted NOP in surviving ECs is sustained by Ca^{2+} entry, while is insensitive to Ca^{2+} release from ER. SOCE represents the preferential route for extracellular Ca^{2+} to engage eNOS in ECs [8,22,40]. However, BTP-2 (20 μM), a widely employed blocker of store-dependent Ca^{2+} inflow [6,8], does not significantly affect injury-induced NO synthesis (Figure 3A). We subsequently focused on the response to ATP, which elicits a BTP-2-sensitive SOCE in rat aortic endothelium [27]. ATP-induced NO synthesis was strongly inhibited in 0 Ca^{2+} (Figure 3B) and in the presence BTP-2 (Figure 3B). Collectively, these data concur with our previous findings on injury-induced Ca^{2+} inflow and rule out a detectable role for SOCE in NO release by lesioned endothelium.

Gap junction inhibitors reduce NO synthesis induced by Ca^{2+} entry in injured endothelium

The long-lasting decay phase of injury-induced Ca^{2+} elevation in rat aortic rings is dramatically diminished by gap junction blockers, such as octanol, palmitoleic acid and oleamide [26,27,44,45]. In agreement with the Ca^{2+} measurements [27], octanol (4 mM), oleamide (200 μM), and palmitoleic acid (50 μM) dramatically affected NO synthesis elicited by endothelial scraping (Figure 3C). In the light of our previous observations [27], these findings hint at a role for Ca^{2+} inflow through CxHcs in mediating NOP in injured endothelium. We assessed the specificity of gap junction blockers by measuring the Ca^{2+} response to ATP (20 μM) in the presence of octanol. At this dose, ATP evokes an $InsP_3$-dependent Ca^{2+} release, which is subsequently buffered by the combined action of SERCA and Na^+/Ca^{2+} exchanger [27,34,46]. As shown in Figure 4, pre-incubating rat aortic rings with 4 mM octanol for 20 min did not significantly affect either the magnitude of the $[Ca^{2+}]_i$ elevation or the rate of its decay phase to the baseline. This result concurs with previous evidence

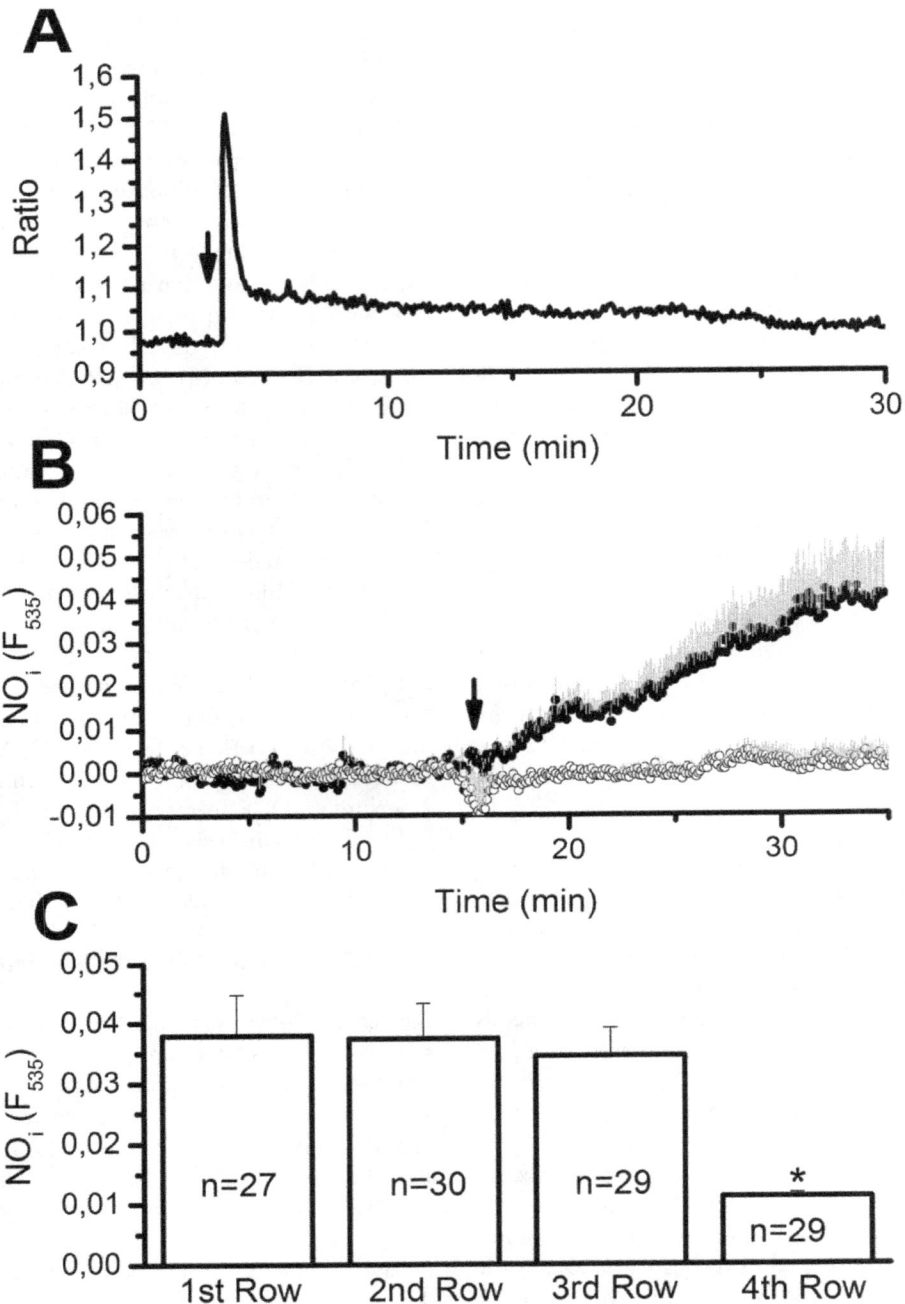

Figure 2 NO synthesis induced by mechanical injury rat aortic endothelium. A, Ca^{2+} signal elicited by lesioning rat aorta in PSS. The trace, recorded from a single cell, is representative of 10 cells from the same visual field. B, injury induced an elevation in intracellular NO levels that was abolished when the cells were pre-treated with the eNOS inhibitor, L-NAME (5 mM), for 40 min. The traces are the mean±SE, respectively, of 10 (PSS, closed circles) and 5 (L-NAME, open circles) cells from two aortic rings harvested from the same animal on the same day. C, mean±SE of the NO signal recorded at increasing distance from the lesion site. In this and the following figures, the arrow indicates when injury is performed. Asterisk indicates a level of significant difference <0.05.

about the efficacy of gap junction blockers as selective uncoupling drugs in rat aortic rings [47,48], and further support the role of CxHcs in mediating NO synthesis in injured endothelium.

Effect of Cx-mimetic peptides on injury-induced Ca^{2+} elevation and NO production

Rat aortic endothelium may express three Cx isoforms, namely Cx37, Cx40, and Cx43 [32,49], albeit a recent

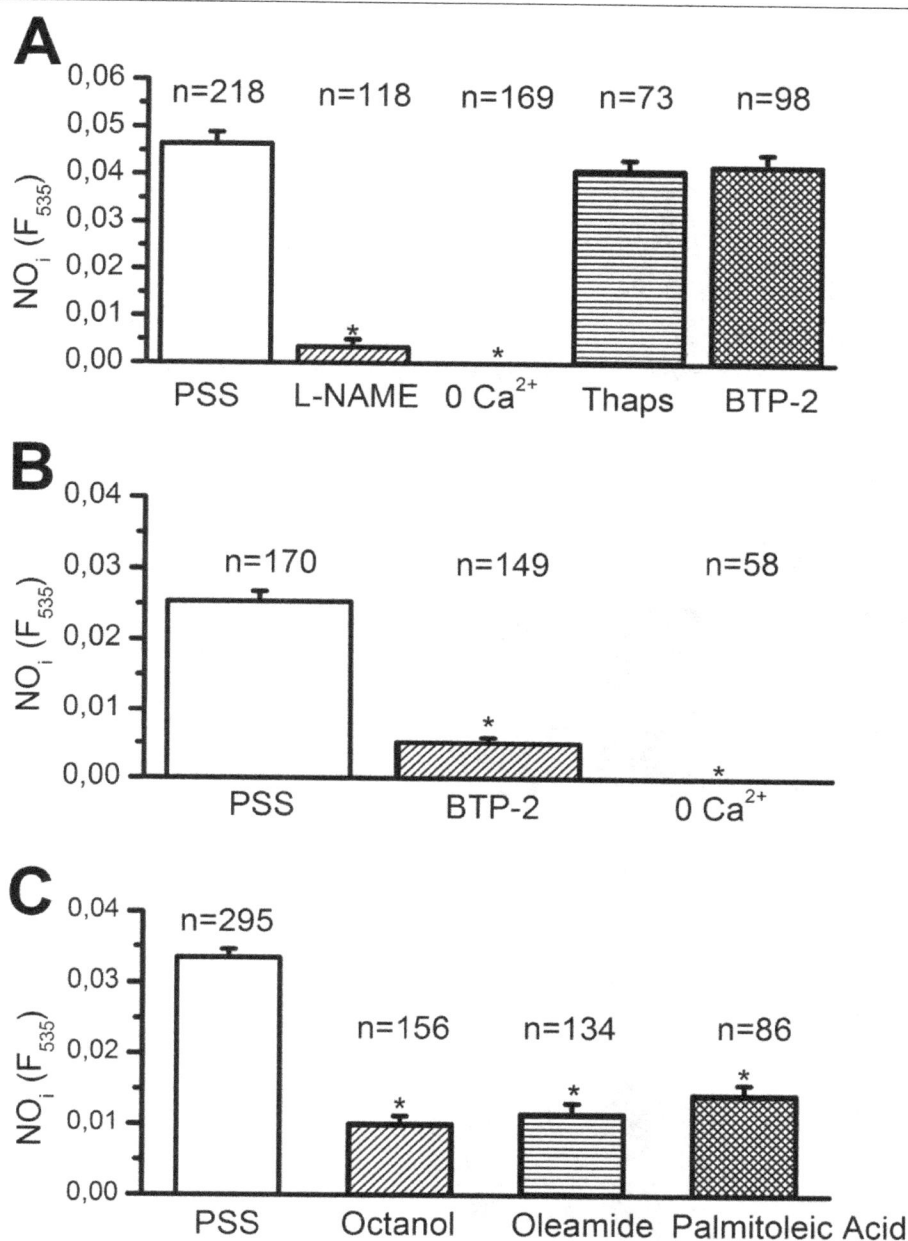

Figure 3 Amplitude of the NO response to injury (A and C) and ATP (B) following the designated treatments. The asterisk indicates a level of significant difference <0.05. The number of ECs analyzed in each condition, harvested from 3-9 animals, is indicated above the bars. See the text for drug concentrations.

work reported the presence of Cx32 in various cultured human ECs [50]. The contribution of each Cx isotype to injury-evoked NO liberation was examined by exploiting Cx-mimetic peptides containing amino acid sequences corresponding to the Gap27 extracellular domain of Cx37 and Cx43 ([37,43]Gap27) and to the Gap27 extracellular domain of Cx40 ([40]Gap27). Although initially designed to impair gap junctional communication, the primary target of these compounds is provided by CxHcs. The extracellular-loop sequence that interacts with the peptides is freely available in the CxHc form [51], so that full blockade of the unpaired hemichannel requires a much shorter pre-incubation (minutes vs. hours or longer) and much lower doses (micromolar vs. millimolar range) than inhibition of gap junctional coupling [51]. These compounds have been found to selectively inhibit Cx-dependent signalling in a variety of cell types, including rat aortic ECs [49,52], when the genetic

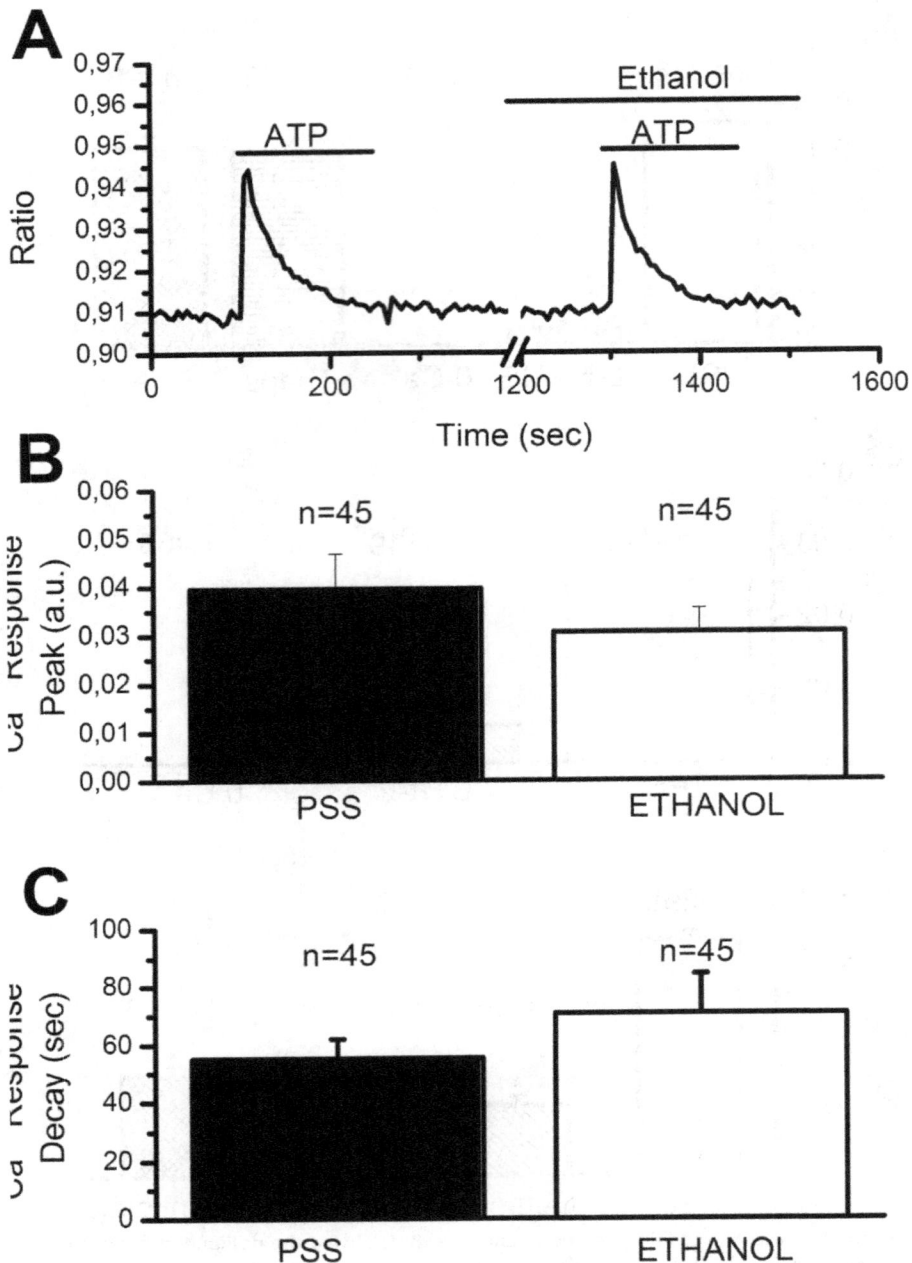

Figure 4 Ethanol does not significantly affect the Ca^{2+} response to ATP. A, 20 min pre-incubation with octanol (4 mM) does not remarkably affect either the amplitude or the kinetics of the Ca^{2+} response to ATP (20 µM). The trace is the average of 16 cells from the same microscopic field of view. B, mean±SE of the peak of ATP-induced elevation in [Ca^{2+}]$_i$. The asterisk indicates a level of significant difference <0.05. The number of ECs analyzed in each condition is indicated above the bars. C, B, mean±SE of the rate of decay of ATP-induced Ca^{2+} signal. The decay was measured by fitting the Ca^{2+} tracings with a first order exponential equation (OriginPro 7, OriginLab Corp, Northampton MA). The asterisk indicates a level of significant difference <0.05. The number of ECs analyzed in each condition is indicated above the bars.

suppression of specific Cx isoforms is not feasible, such as in rat endothelium [33,45]. In addition, Cx-mimetic peptides do not present the drawbacks reported in Cx-deficient mice [53]. For instance, Cx40-/- mice manifest either higher [54] or lower [55] levels of Cx37 as well as a

significant decrease in Cx43 expression [56]. This feature makes the interpretation of the physiological data collected from these animals difficult. Incubating the aortic rings for 1 hour with either [37,43]Gap27 (300 µM) or [40]Gap27 (300 µM) significantly (p < 0.05) reduced injury-evoked NOP (Figure 5A and Figure 5B). The statistical analysis of these experiments has been reported in Figure 5C and Figure 5D. NO signalling was unaffected by peptides corresponding to scrambled sequences in Gap27, indicating that the inhibition resulted from specific sequence recognition on the selected Cx isotypes (Figure 5C and Figure 5D). Therefore, it is reasonable to conclude that Ca^{2+} entry driving eNOS activity and NO liberation at the wound edge is supported by Cx37Hcs, Cx40Hcs, and Cx43Hcs. As discussed elsewhere [57], eNOS activation requires a sub-plasmalemmal Ca^{2+} increase rather a bulk increase in cytosolic Ca^{2+} levels. Such a localized Ca^{2+} event may not even be detected by conventional epifluorescence microscopy [58]. As a consequence, we went on in assessing whether Cx-mimetic peptides targeting Cx37, Cx40, and Cx43 were also able to reduce the long-lasting decay phase of the Ca^{2+}

response to mechanical damage. Figures 6A to 6D depict that neither ^{37,43}Gap27 (300 µM) nor ^{40}Gap27 (300 µM) significantly reduce either the initial Ca^{2+} peak or the subsequent decay phase. Rather, both Cx-mimetic peptides increased the amplitude of the initial Ca^{2+} response (Figure 6A-6C). Consistently, acute application of both peptides during recovery of the Ca^{2+} signal towards the baseline did not decreased the $[Ca^{2+}]_i$ ($n = 31$, ^{40}Gap27; $n = 52$, ^{37,43}Gap27) (not shown). The same results were found by extending the pre-incubation period with both ^{37,43}Gap27 and ^{40}Gap27 up to 2 hours (Figure 6B-6D) [49]. Taken as a whole, these results suggest that Cx37Hcs, Cx40Hcs, and Cx43Hcs mediate the submembranal Ca^{2+} elevation responsible for eNOS activation, but not the bulk increase in $[Ca^{2+}]_i$ caused by mechanical damage in surviving ECs. As the pharmacological profile of the decay phase is consistent with a CxHc

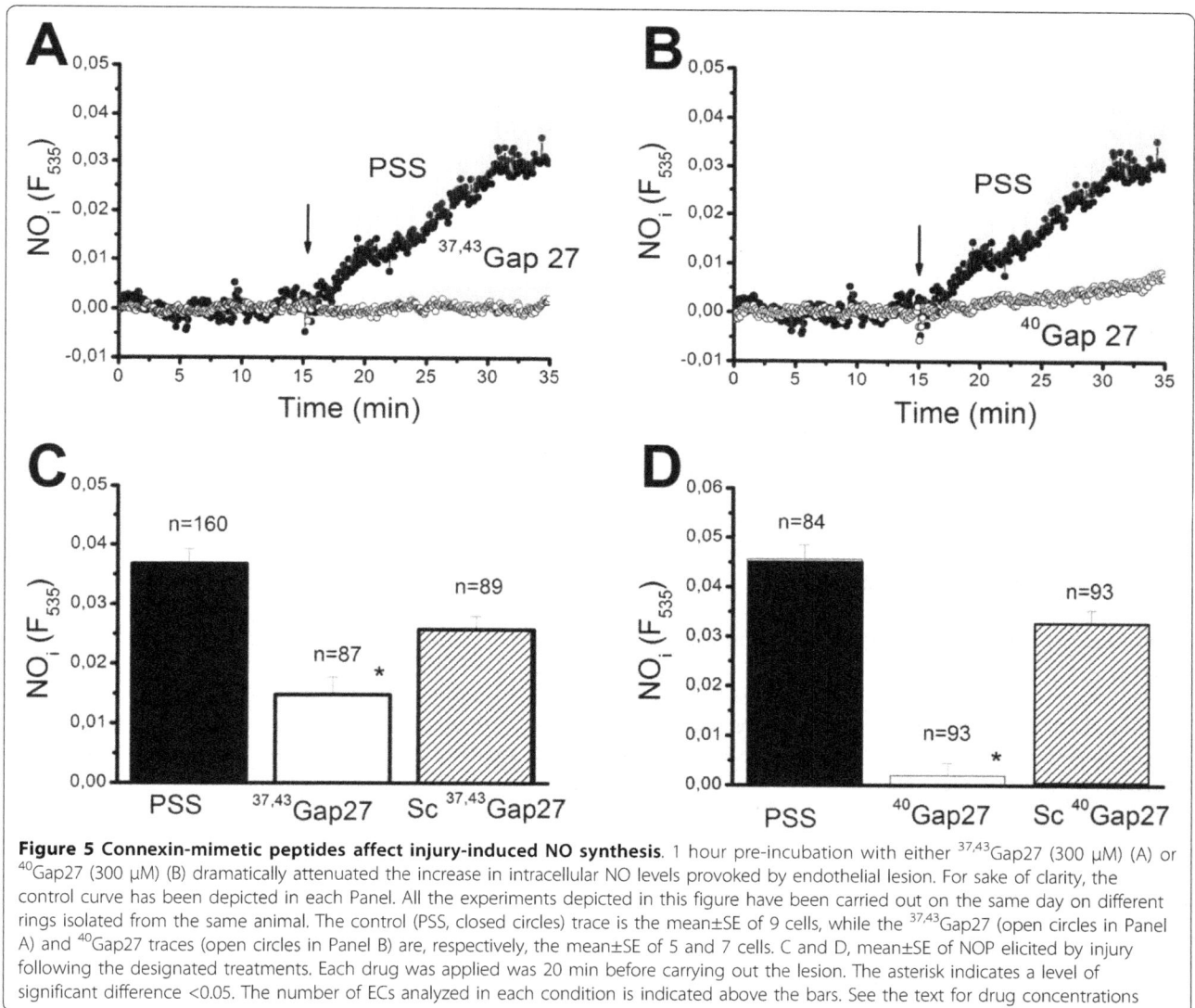

Figure 5 Connexin-mimetic peptides affect injury-induced NO synthesis. 1 hour pre-incubation with either ^{37,43}Gap27 (300 µM) (A) or ^{40}Gap27 (300 µM) (B) dramatically attenuated the increase in intracellular NO levels provoked by endothelial lesion. For sake of clarity, the control curve has been depicted in each Panel. All the experiments depicted in this figure have been carried out on the same day on different rings isolated from the same animal. The control (PSS, closed circles) trace is the mean±SE of 9 cells, while the ^{37,43}Gap27 (open circles in Panel A) and ^{40}Gap27 traces (open circles in Panel B) are, respectively, the mean±SE of 5 and 7 cells. C and D, mean±SE of NOP elicited by injury following the designated treatments. Each drug was applied was 20 min before carrying out the lesion. The asterisk indicates a level of significant difference <0.05. The number of ECs analyzed in each condition is indicated above the bars. See the text for drug concentrations

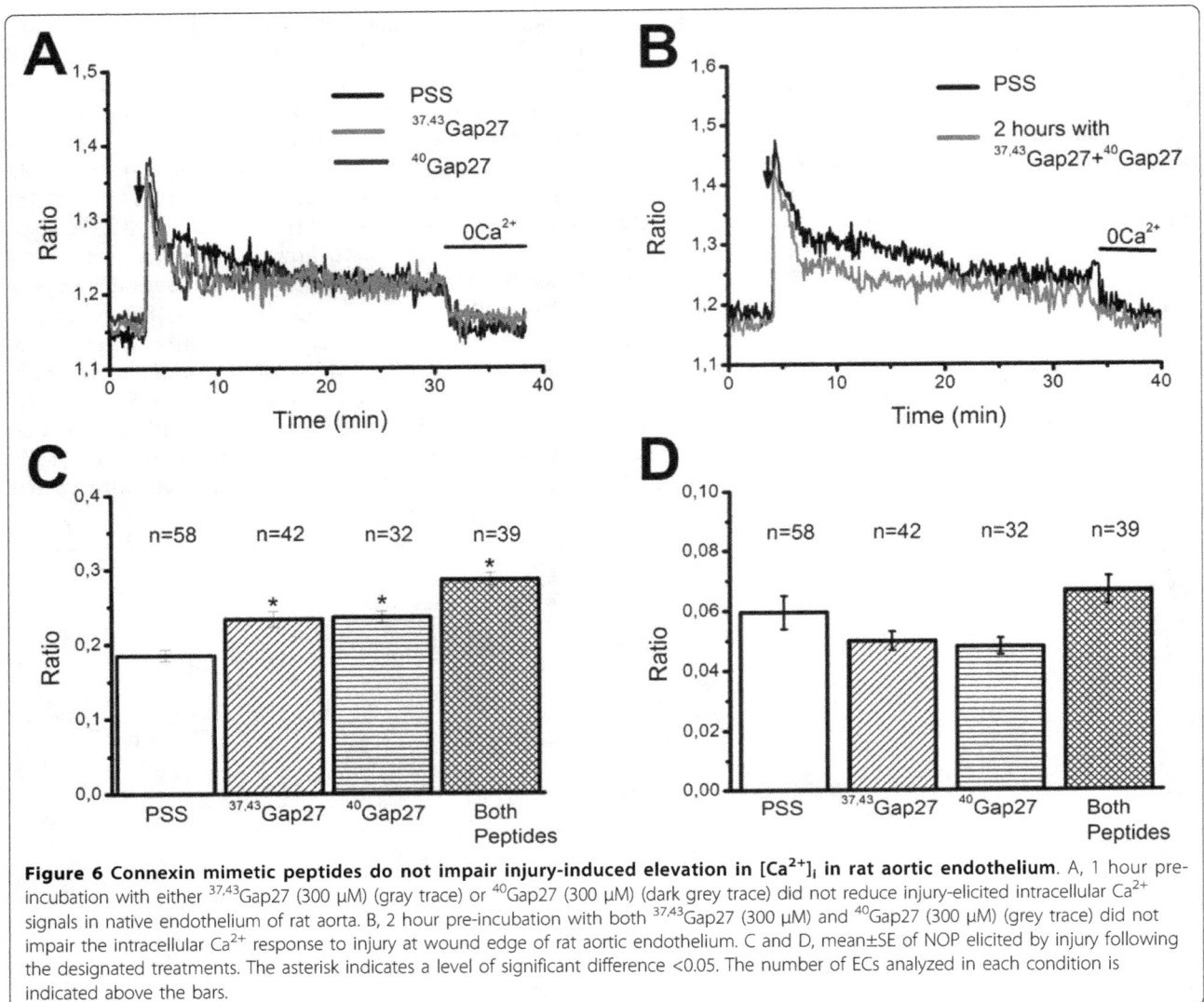

Figure 6 Connexin mimetic peptides do not impair injury-induced elevation in [Ca²⁺]ᵢ in rat aortic endothelium. A, 1 hour pre-incubation with either ^{37,43}Gap27 (300 μM) (gray trace) or ^{40}Gap27 (300 μM) (dark grey trace) did not reduce injury-elicited intracellular Ca²⁺ signals in native endothelium of rat aorta. B, 2 hour pre-incubation with both ^{37,43}Gap27 (300 μM) and ^{40}Gap27 (300 μM) (grey trace) did not impair the intracellular Ca²⁺ response to injury at wound edge of rat aortic endothelium. C and D, mean±SE of NOP elicited by injury following the designated treatments. The asterisk indicates a level of significant difference <0.05. The number of ECs analyzed in each condition is indicated above the bars.

pathway [2,26,27], it is conceivable that one or more additional Cx isoforms are expressed in rat aortic endothelium.

NO synthesis is abolished by caveolar disruption with MβCD

NO production by a highly localized Ca²⁺ signal sneaking beneath the plasma membrane requires the spatial proximity between the Ca²⁺ source and eNOS [57,58]. Caveolae represent a signalling platform responsible for translating Ca²⁺ entry into specific signal transduction pathways [24,57]. MβCD is a cholesterol-binding agent which has been widely employed to disrupt caveolar integrity in a variety of cell types, including ECs [24]. We first probed MβCD (10 mM) efficacy in impairing caveolae-dependent signalling by testing its effect on SOCE. As shown elsewhere [27,35], SOCE sustains the

Ca²⁺ response to high concentrations of ATP (300 μM) in the endothelium of excised rat aorta. As shown in Figure 7A, MβCD significantly reduced the amplitudes of both the initial Ca²⁺ peak and the subsequent plateau, which are both supported by SOCE [27]. Consistently, MβCD inhibited ATP-dependent NOP in 85 out of 85 cells, whereas 93 out of 93 untreated cells liberated NO when exposed to ATP (Figure 7B). Then, to assess the role of caveolae in coupling CxHcs-mediated Ca²⁺ inflow with eNOS activation, rat aortic rings were pre-incubated (30 min) in the presence of MβCD (10 mM). Exposition to MβCD did not significantly affect the Ca²⁺ response to injury (Figure 8A and Figure 8B), but prevented the downstream NO synthesis (Figure 8C and Figure 8D). Collectively, these data indicate that the proximity between CxHcs and eNOS is maintained by the caveolar

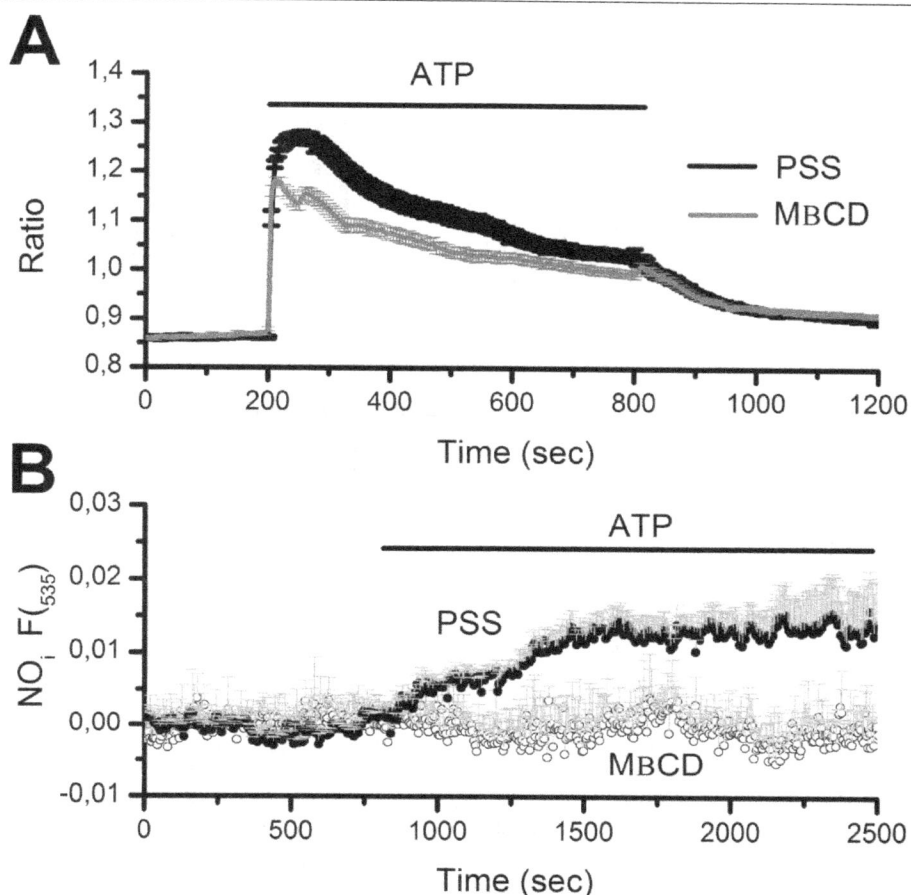

Figure 7 Caveolar impairment impairs both the Ca^{2+} response to ATP and the accompanying NO production in rat aortic endothelium. A, pre-treatment with 10 mM MβCD to disrupt caveolae significantly hinders both the magnitude and the plateau of the Ca^{2+} response to ATP (300 μM). Both phases depend on store-dependent Ca^{2+} inflow when ATP is administered at this dose. The traces are the mean ±SE of 220 (PSS, black trace) and 186 cells (MβCD, red trace), respectively, from no less than three different animals. B, MβCD (10 mM) suppresses ATP-induced NO synthesis. The traces are the mean±SE, respectively, of 150 (PSS, closed circles) and 4 (MβCD, open circles) cells from no less than three different animals.

signalling platform within the plasma membrane. This feature is consistent with the highly localized nature of the Ca^{2+} signal driving NO synthesis.

Discussion

Endothelial-derived NO drives a number of processes which protects the vessel wall by pro-atherosclerotic events and maintain vascular homeostasis. NO exerts both an anti-aggregating and anti-inflammatory action, promotes endothelial survival, proliferation and migration, and prevents the phenotypic remodeling of the underlying layer of SMCs [2,19,59]. The present investigation provides the first evidence that endothelial ablation similar to that induced *in vivo* by stent deployment causes a local increase in NO levels by activating the ECs immediately adjacent to the lesion site. We further elucidated the molecular machinery responsible for

eNOS recruitment and showed that injury-induced NOP is triggered by Ca^{2+} entry though Cx37Hcs, Cx40Hcs, and Cx43Hcs. The coupling between Ca^{2+} inflow and eNOS activation might be provided by cholesterol enriched membrane microdomains, such as caveolae. These data shed novel light on the endothelial reaction to mechanical scraping and hint at the Ca^{2+} machinery as a novel target to restore endothelial integrity after reconstructive surgery and to treat vascular diseases [2,12].

NO synthesis in the injured endothelium of rat aorta is supported by CxHcs-mediated Ca^{2+} entry

The procedure that we adopted for mechanical scraping mimics the partial denudation of the endothelial monolayer that has been described upon stent deployment in a number of pre-clinical models [41-43]. The extent of the lesion we inferred is smaller as compared to the degree

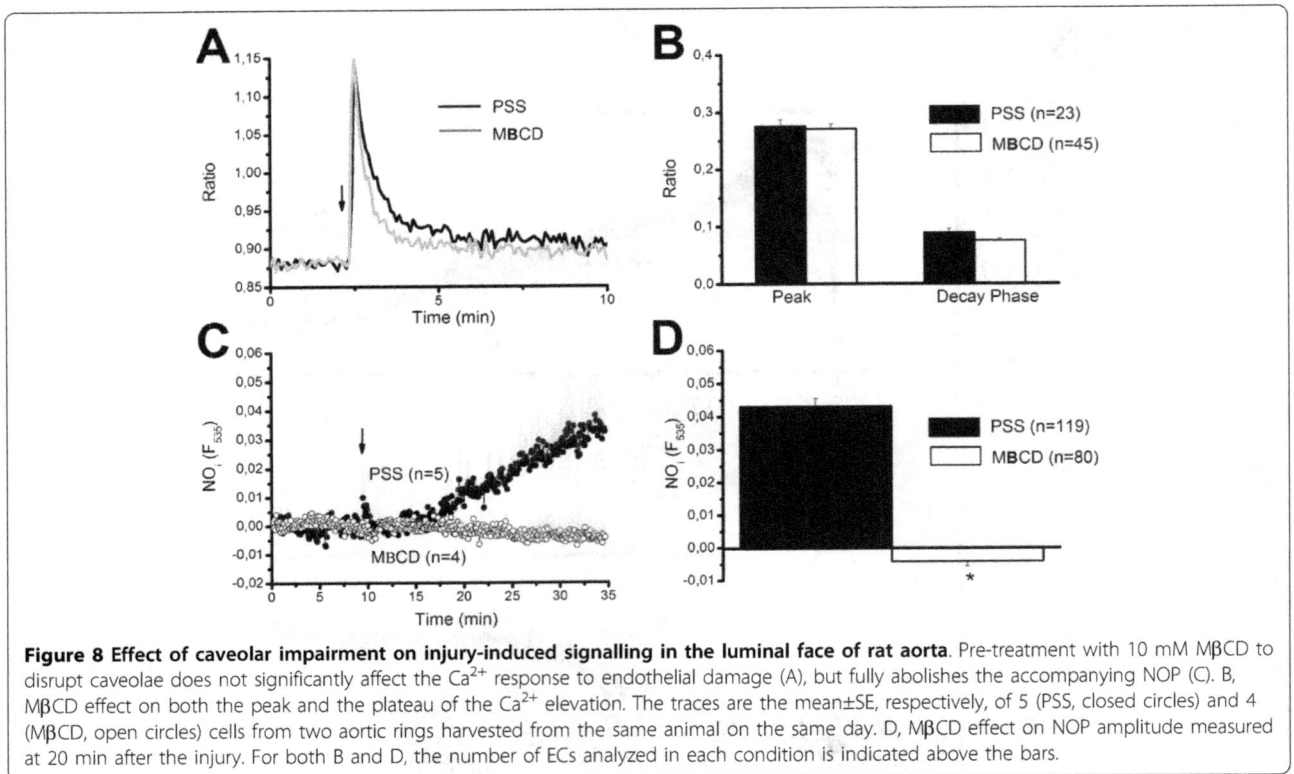

Figure 8 Effect of caveolar impairment on injury-induced signalling in the luminal face of rat aorta. Pre-treatment with 10 mM MβCD to disrupt caveolae does not significantly affect the Ca^{2+} response to endothelial damage (A), but fully abolishes the accompanying NOP (C). B, MβCD effect on both the peak and the plateau of the Ca^{2+} elevation. The traces are the mean±SE, respectively, of 5 (PSS, closed circles) and 4 (MβCD, open circles) cells from two aortic rings harvested from the same animal on the same day. D, MβCD effect on NOP amplitude measured at 20 min after the injury. For both B and D, the number of ECs analyzed in each condition is indicated above the bars.

of endothelial ablation observed after coronary stenting in humans in patients [60], albeit it is in the same range as that described in previous studies addressing the role of Ca^{2+} signals in the regeneration of wounded monolayers [2,12]. However, a focal region devoid of the EC covering is rapidly repaired by neighbouring ECs, which spread into the lesioned area and undergo mitosis [61]. Accordingly, the daily rate of EC replication is increased by 50% at these sites in the rat aorta [62]. Therefore, the approach we utilized to perform the endothelial injury is useful to: 1) get insights into the acute response to the arterial damage in terms of Ca^{2+} response and accompanying NO synthesis and 2) elucidate the molecular machinery driving the subsequent process of endothelial regeneration Three pieces of evidences suggest that injury-induced NO synthesis is mainly driven by Ca^{2+} influx. First, there is no detectable NOP when the endothelium is scraped in absence of extracellular Ca^{2+}. Second, injury-elicited NOP is not significantly affected by depletion of the InsP$_3$-sensitive Ca^{2+} stores with thapsigargin, although we cannot rule out the possibility that InsP$_3$-sensitive NOP falls below the resolution of our fluorimetric system. Third, blockade of Ca^{2+} entry by classic gap junction blockers, but not by BTP-2, dampen NO synthesis. These observations are consistent with the Fura-2 data and strongly suggest that CxHcs, rather than SOCE, provide the Ca^{2+} source driving NO liberation in

damaged endothelium. Rat aortic endothelium has been found to express three main Cx isoforms, namely Cx37, Cx40, and Cx43 [32,49]. In order to elucidate which of them underpins NO synthesis, we exploited the reported selectivity of Cx-mimetic peptides [33,45]. Both [37,43]Gap27 and [40]Gap27 significantly attenuated NOP triggered by Ca^{2+} entry at the lesion site. The following lines of evidence confirm the specificity of [37,43]Gap27 and [40]Gap27: 1) pre-treatment with scrambled peptides did not detectably alter injury-induced NO synthesis (present study); and 2) [37,43]Gap27 and [40]Gap27 do not alter endogenous expression of Cx40 and Cx43 in the smooth muscle cell line A7r5, as well as connexin trafficking and *de novo* formation of gap plaques in A7r5 cells expressing Cx43-GFP [49]. These data strongly suggest that injury-elicited NOP at the wound edge of the aortic surface is sustained by Ca^{2+} influx through Cx37Hcs, Cx40Hcs, and Cx43Hcs. These results are further supported by previous studies, which showed that Cx43-containing gap junctions mediate the spreading of pro-inflammatory Ca^{2+} waves in lung capillaries [36] and sustain ATP-promoted Ca^{2+} bursts in uterine artery ECs [63]. Consistent with the role served by CxHc as Ca^{2+} entry pathways in vascular endothelium, Cx37Hc and Cx43Hc were recently shown to maintain bradykinin-induced intracellular Ca^{2+} oscillations in rat brain endothelial cells [29], while Cx32Hc- and Cx43Hc-mediated Ca^{2+} inflow supports the spiking response to bradykinin in Madin-Darby canine kidney cells [30]. Similarly, Cx43Hcs has already been shown to mediate Ca^{2+} influx and activate Ca^{2+}-dependent downstream targets in a variety of cell types other than endothelial cells [31,64].

Caveolar integrity is required to support injury-dependent NO synthesis in rat aortic endothelium

The subcellular analysis of the Ca^{2+} signal driving eNOS activation has shown that Ca^{2+} entry results in a highly localized Ca^{2+} microdomain which is restricted to the inner leaflet of the plasma membrane [57,58]. Therefore, CxHcs and eNOS are likely to tightly interact in order for Ca^{2+} inflow to stimulate NOP in injured endothelium. This hypothesis is supported by a number of recent studies. First, eNOS physically interacts with both Cx37 and Cx40 in *in situ* ECs of mouse aorta [65]. Second, Cx43 colocalizes with eNOS in native ECs covering the lumen of mice thoracodorsal arteries [66]. Third, Cx37 coimmunoprecipitates with eNOS in a number of human primary ECs [67]. The physical coupling between CxHcs and eNOS might be provided by cholesterol enriched membrane domains, such as caveolae. Indeed, MβCD abrogated injury-triggered NOP without affecting the underpinning Ca^{2+} signal. This feature suggests that disruption of caveolae does not modify CxHs gating, but physically displaces eNOS from the local source of Ca^{2+} responsible for its engagement. Consistently, caveolin-1 regulates the correct trafficking and localization to the plasma membrane of several Cx isoforms, including Cx 37, 40, and 43 [66,68,69]. Moreover, the expression of Cx37, Cx40 and Cx43 is decreased in caveolin-1 knock out arteries as compared to wild-type mice [70]. On the other hand, eNOS is targeted to caveolae by cotranslational N-myristoylation and posttranslational palmitoylation and interacts with the scaffolding domain of caveolin-1 [23]. It this, therefore, likely that caveolae maintain CxHcs in close proximity to eNOS and, perhaps, to other relevant signalling proteins, as recently suggested in [70]. Interestingly, while ineffective in regulating the Ca^{2+}-mobilizing properties of CxHcs, caveolar integrity is key to SOCE recruitment in vascular ECs [57]. In line with these evidences, cholesterol depletion with MβCD prevents store-operated Ca^{2+} inflow and NOP triggered by ATP in native rat aortic endothelium.

The putative role of NO in lesioned endothelium

The increase in NO levels at the wound edge represents an immediate, localized self-protecting response of the vessel wall to EC loss. Indeed, the NO signal is confined within the area experiencing the elevation in $[Ca^{2+}]_i$ induced by the injury and does not spread farther away (see Figure 2C). EC detachment due to physiological turnover or pathological events causes the exposition of patches of sub-endothelial matrix which may activate platelets, a process known to promote an inflammatory reaction which favours the onset of atherosclerosis [71].

However, increased local NO synthesis inhibits both platelet aggregation and VSMC proliferation and migration, thus adversing both neointima formation and inflammation [1,19]. NO might play a key role also in subsequent healing [19,59]. Accordingly, NO inhibits apoptosis and stimulates proliferation and migration, which are an essential pre-requisite for ECs to spread and cover the de-endothelized area [19,59]. In injured rat aortic rings, both eNOS protein and enzyme activity have been shown to augment at the proliferating wound edge, but not in ECs distant from the lesion [25]. Moreover, aortic segments obtained from eNOS knock-out (KO) mice and cultured in Matrigel displayed a dramatic reduction in EC sprouting and proliferation as compared to wild-type animals [72]. Consistent with these *in vitro* observations, intravenous infusion of a NO donor accelerated *in vivo* regeneration of the endothelium lining the lumen of injured rat carotid artery [73]. In addition, neo-vascularization of ischemic hindlimbs, which depends on EC proliferation and migration, is significantly reduced in eNOS KO mice [74] and enhanced in eNOS overexpressing mice [75]. Finally, NO liberated by cells at the wound edge might recruit circulating endothelial progenitor cells and speed up the healing process [76].

The changes in DAF-FM fluorescence measured from the endothelial layer could also reflect some NOP occurring within the underlying SMCs, which generate a Ca^{2+} wave in response to mechanical injury [48]. This Ca^{2+} signal might, in turn, activate SMC eNOS and contribute to the increase in DAF-FM fluorescence we recorded from ECs at the wound edge [77]. However, injury-induced Ca^{2+} waves in SMCs entirely depend on intracellular Ca^{2+} release, rather than Ca^{2+} influx [48]. As a consequence, the fact that all the protocols impairing injury-elicited Ca^{2+} inflow into ECs nearby the lesion site (i.e. removal of external Ca^{2+} and exposition to gap junction blockers) affected the accompanying increase in DAF-FM fluorescence strongly hint at the endothelial origin of the NO signal. Nevertheless, the possibility that NO synthesis also takes place within the tunica media of damaged rat aortic rings cannot be ruled out.

Evidence for the expression of additional Cx isoforms in the endothelium of rat aorta

The results presented in the current investigation support a role for Cx37Hcs, Cx40Hcs, and Cx43Hcs in driving the Ca^{2+}-dependent eNOS activation at the wound edge of rat aortic endothelium. However, the decay phase of the Ca^{2+} response to injury is not significantly affected by 1 hour pre-treatment with Cx-mimetic peptides. This feature concurs with the highly localized, sub-membranal nature of the Ca^{2+} signal engaging eNOS in vascular ECs [57,58], which are detected by genetically-encoded Ca^{2+} fluorophores selectively targeting the caveolae, but not the bulk cytoplasm [58]. This finding raises us to wonder about the molecular nature of the membrane pathway(s) responsible for the massive Ca^{2+} influx observed during the decay phase. As widely discussed elsewhere [2,12], the pharmacological profile of such a route is typical of a CxHc. The lack of effect of Cx-mimetic peptides on the bulk increase in $[Ca^{2+}]_i$ that features the decay phase of the Ca^{2+} response to injury, therefore, suggests that Cx isoforms other than Cx 37, 40, and 43 are expressed in the native endothelium of rat aorta. This hypothesis is strongly supported by the recent discovery of Cx32 mRNA and protein in both cultured and blood vessel ECs [50]. Cx32Hcs, in particular, has recently been shown to mediate Ca^{2+} influx when transfected in HeLa cells [78] and in Madin-Darby canine kidney cells [30]. Additional Cx isoforms that have been implicated in Ca^{2+} entry across the plasmalemma are Cx26 [79] and Cx45 [80]. That Cx isoforms other than Cx37, Cx40, and Cx43 are expressed in the vessel wall has also been proposed by Tang and Vanhoutte [52] and by Sorensen et al. [81]. Both groups reached the same conclusion upon the finding that connexin mimetic peptides failed to reproduce the effects of classic gap junction blockers in the vasculature. Recent evidence hinted at pannexins (Pxs), which are hexameric channels structurally unrelated to Cxs, as the molecular substrates for the hemichannels (the so-called pannexons) present in the nonjunctional area of cell membrane [82]. However, to the best of our knowledge, Px expression has hitherto been reported only in microvascular beds rather than in macrovessels, such as aorta [82]. Moreover, as recently pointed out [2,12], Px hemichannels are unaffected by La^{3+} and heptanol, which block CxHcs and impair injury-induced Ca^{2+} entry in the intact endothelium of rat aorta [26,27]. Accordingly, our preliminary data indicate that probenecid, a widely employed Px blocker, does not significantly affect the Ca^{2+} response to mechanical injury in rat aortic endothelium. It is worth of noting that Cx-mimetic peptides, either separately or in combination, caused an increase in the $InsP_3$-dependent initial Ca^{2+} peak. A recent study reported that CxHcs may mediate $InsP_3$ efflux into the extracellular space [83]. It is, therefore, conceivable that the prolonged pre-treatment with Cx-mimetic peptides prevented $InsP_3$ produced at the wound edge from moving out of the cytosol, thus increasing the extent of Ca^{2+} release in the first raw of cells.

Conclusion

In conclusion, this study provides the first clear-cut evidence that arterial damage activates surviving ECs to produce NO by inducing Ca^{2+} entry via Cx37Hcs,

Cx40Hcs, and Cx43Hcs. Our data indicate that the membranal compartmentalization of CxHcs and eNOS depends on is enabled by caveolae. Experiments are under way in our laboratory to assess the role played by CxHcs-induced NO synthesis in the regeneration of rat aortic endothelium. These results outline the importance of designing novel prosthetic devices able to release NO after vascular interventions, such as arterial bypass grafting and intravascular stent deployment [84]. Indeed, the currently employed drug-eluting stents may result in late arterial occlusion and, eventually, in patient death due to their reported capability to inhibit endothelial regeneration [11]. Alternatively, the signalling cascade leading to NO production that we have described in the present work might be the alternative target of novel drug-eluting stents. The cardiological practice has unveiled a variety of compounds, such as ZP123 or rotigaptide and (2S,4R)-1-(2-aminoacetyl)-4-benzamidopyrrolidine-2-carboxylic acid hydrochloride (GAP-134), which increase CxHc conductance and, therefore, might be exploited to increase Ca^{2+} influx at the lesion site [2,12]. These substances have successfully been probed as orally-active and anti-arrhythmic drugs in Phase I and II clinical trials conducted on patients suffering either from atrial fibrillation or from unstable angina or myocardial infarction [85,86]. In perspective, these molecules might be locally released by drug-eluting stents to improve CxHc-mediated signalling and boost NO synthesis after surgical interventions on diseased vessels [2,12].

Competing interests
The authors declare that they have no competing interests.

Authors' contributions
RBR: conceived the study, carried out the experiments, analyzed and interpreted the data, drafted the manuscript. JEAC: conceived the study, carried out the experiments, analyzed and interpreted the data. AR: conceived the study, carried out the experiments, analyzed and interpreted the data. ADC: critically revised the manuscript. MPC: critically revised the manuscript. SM: critically revised the manuscript. GG: conceived the study and critically revised the manuscript. FM: conceived the study, analyzed and interpreted the data and drafted the manuscript. FT: conceived the study, analyzed and interpreted the data, critically revised the drafted manuscript. All authors read and approved the final manuscript.

Authors' information
RBR: Professor of Physiology at Benemérita Universidad Autónoma de Puebla. JEAC: Researcher at University of Pavia. AR: Postdoctoral Fellow at University of Calgary. ADC: Assistant Professor of Cardiac Surgery at Second University of Naples. MPC: Assistant Professor of Anatomy at University of Naples "Federico II". SM: Full Professor of Anatomy at University of Naples "Federico II". GG: Assistant Professor of Anatomy at University of Molise. FM: Assistant Professor of Physiology at University of Pavia. FT: Associate Professor of Physiology at University of Pavia.

Acknowledgements
The work was supported by FAR (Fondo d'Ateneo per la Ricerca, University of Pavia, Italy) and CONACYT (Consejo Nacional de Ciencia y Tecnología, Mexico). Grant No. 115230 to RBR.

Declarations
Publication charges for this article were covered by research funds of the project Bando Faro 2012 - Finanziamenti per l'Avvio di Ricerche Originali, cofounded by the Compagnia di San Paolo and by the Polo per le Scienze e le Tecnologie per la Vita of the University Federico II in Naples.
This article has been published as part of *BMC Surgery* Volume 13 Supplement 2, 2013: Proceedings from the 26th National Congress of the Italian Society of Geriatric Surgery. The full contents of the supplement are available online at http://www.biomedcentral.com/bmcsurg/supplements/13/S2

Authors' details
[1]School of Medicine, Department of Biomedicine, Benemérita Universidad Autónoma de Puebla, 13 Sur 2702, Colonia Volcanes, 72000 Puebla, Mexico. [2]Department of Biology and Biotechnology "Lazzaro Spallanzani", Laboratory of Physiology, University of Pavia, via Forlanini 6, 27100 Pavia, Italy. [3]Department of Pharmacology and Therapeutics, Faculty of Medicine, University of Calgary, Calgary, Alberta, Canada. [4]Department of Cardiothoracic Sciences, Second University of Naples, Naples, Italy. [5]Department of Public Health, University of Naples "Federico II", via Pansini 5, 80131, Naples, Italy. [6]Department of Medicine and Health Sciences, University of Molise, via F. De Sanctis, 86100, Campobasso, Italy.

References
1. Tesfamariam B, DeFelice AF: Endothelial injury in the initiation and progression of vascular disorders. *Vascular Pharmacology* 2007, 46(4):229-237.
2. Moccia F, Billington RA, Santella L: Pharmacological characterization of NAADP-induced Ca2+ signals in starfish oocytes. *Biochemical and Biophysical Research Communications* 2006, 348:329-336.
3. Vanhoutte PM: Endothelial Dysfunction - The First Step Toward Coronary Arteriosclerosis. *Circulation Journal* 2009, 73(4).
4. Yoder M, Rounds S: Bad blood, bad endothelium: ill fate? *Blood* 2011, 117(13):3479-3480.
5. Dragoni S, Laforenza U, Bonetti E, Lodola F, Bottino C, Berra-Romani R, Bongio GC, Cinelli MP, Guerra G, Pedrazzoli P, et al: Vascular Endothelial Growth Factor Stimulates Endothelial Colony Forming Cells Proliferation and Tubulogenesis by Inducing Oscillations in Intracellular Ca2+ Concentration. *Stem Cells* 2011, 29(11):1898-1907.
6. Sanchez-Hernandez Y, Laforenza U, Bonetti E, Fontana J, Dragoni S, Russo M, Avelino-Cruz JE, Schinelli S, Testa D, Guerra G, et al: Store-Operated Ca2+ Entry Is Expressed in Human Endothelial Progenitor Cells. *Stem Cells and Development* 2010, 19(12):1967-1981.
7. Lodola F, Laforenza U, Bonetti E, Lim D, Dragoni S, Bottino C, Ong HL, Guerra G, Ganini C, Massa M, et al: Store-operated ca(2+) entry is remodelled and controls in vitro angiogenesis in endothelial progenitor cells isolated from tumoral patients. *PloS one* 2012, 7(9):e4254.1.
8. Moccia F, Dragoni S, Lodola F, Bonetti E, Bottino C, Guerra G, Laforenza U, Rosti V, Tanzi F: Store-Dependent Ca2+ Entry in Endothelial Progenitor Cells As a Perspective Tool to Enhance Cell-Based Therapy and Adverse Tumour Vascularization. *Current Medicinal Chemistry* 2012, 19(34):2561-2580.
9. Piscopo S, Moccia F, Di Cristo C, Caputi L, Di Cosmo A, Brown ER: Pre- and postsynaptic excitation and inhibition at octopus optic lobe photoreceptor terminals; implications for the function of the 'presynaptic bags'. *European Journal of Neuroscience* 2007, 26:2196-2203.
10. Moccia F, Bonetti E, Dragoni S, Fontana J, Lodola F, Berra Romani R, Laforenza U, Rosti V, Tanzi F: Hematopoietic Progenitor and Stem Cells Circulate by Surfing on Intracellular Ca2+ Waves: A Novel Target for Cell-based Therapy and Anti-cancer Treatment? *Current Signal Transduction Therapy* 2012, 7(2).
11. Zargham R: Preventing restenosis after angioplasty: a multistage approach. *Clinical Science* 2008, 114(3-4):257-264.
12. Moccia F, Di Cristo C, Winlow W, Di Cosmo A: GABA(A)- and AMPA-like receptors modulate the activity of an identified neuron within the central pattern generator of the pond snail Lymnaea stagnalis. *Invertebrate Neuroscience* 2009, 9(1):29-41.
13. Siddique A, Shantsila E, Lip GYH, Varma C: Endothelial progenitor cells: what use for the cardiologist? *Journal of angiogenesis research* 2010, 2:6-6.
14. Finn AV, Nakazawa G, Joner M, Kolodgie FD, Mont EK, Gold HK, Virmani R: Vascular responses to drug eluting stents - Importance of delayed healing. *Arteriosclerosis Thrombosis and Vascular Biology* 2007, 27(7).
15. Otsuka F, Finn AV, Yazdani SK, Nakano M, Kolodgie FD, Virmani R: The importance of the endothelium in atherothrombosis and coronary stenting. *Nature Reviews Cardiology* 2012, 9(8).
16. Testa D, Guerra G, Marcuccio G, Landolfo PG, Motta G: Oxidative stress in chronic otitis media with effusion. *Acta oto-laryngologica* 2012, 132(8):834-837.
17. Cattaneo F, Iaccio A, Guerra G, Montagnani S, Ammendola R: NADPH-oxidase-dependent reactive oxygen species mediate EGFR transactivation by FPRL1 in WKYMVm-stimulated human lung cancer cells. *Free radical biology and medicine* 2011, 51(6):1126-1136.
18. Conti V, Russomanno G, Corbi G, Guerra G, Grasso C, Filippelli W, Paribello V, Ferrara N, Filippelli A: Aerobic training workload affects human endothelial cells redox homeostasis. *Medicine and science in sports and exercise* 2013, 45(4):644-653.
19. Mancardi D, Pla AF, Moccia F, Tanzi F, Munaron L: Old and New Gasotransmitters in the Cardiovascular System: Focus on the Role of Nitric Oxide and Hydrogen Sulfide in Endothelial Cells and Cardiomyocytes. *Current Pharmaceutical Biotechnology* 2011, 12(9):1406-1415.
20. Al-Sa'doni HH, Ferro A: S-nitrosothiols as nitric oxide-donors: Chemistry, biology and possible future therapeutic applications. *Current Medicinal Chemistry* 2004, 11(20):2679-2690.
21. Yao XQ, Huang Y: From nitric oxide to endothelial cytosolic Ca2+: a negative feedback control. *Trends in Pharmacological Sciences* 2003, 24(6):263-266.
22. Moccia F, Berra-Romani R, Tanzi F: Update on vascular endothelial Ca(2+) signalling: A tale of ion channels, pumps and transporters. *World journal of biological chemistry* 2012, 3(7).
23. Sbaa E, Frerart F, Feron O: The double regulation of endothelial nitric oxide synthase by caveolae and caveolin: A paradox solved through the study of angiogenesis. *Trends in Cardiovascular Medicine* 2005, 15(5):157-162.
24. Xu Y, Bulikema H, van Gilst WH, Henning RH: Caveolae and endothelial dysfunction: Filling the caves in cardiovascular disease. *European Journal of Pharmacology* 2008, 585(2-3):256-260.
25. Poppa V, Miyashiro JK, Corson MA, Berk BC: Endothelial NO synthase is increased in regenerating endothelium after denuding injury of the rat aorta. *Arteriosclerosis Thrombosis and Vascular Biology* 1998, 18(8):1312-1321.
26. Berra-Romani R, Raqeeb A, Torres-Jacome J, Guzman-Silva A, Guerra G, Tanzi F, Moccia F: The Mechanism of Injury-Induced Intracellular Calcium Concentration Oscillations in the Endothelium of Excised Rat Aorta. *Journal of Vascular Research* 2012, 49(1):65-76.
27. Berra-Romani R, Raqeeb A, Avelino-Cruz JE, Moccia F, Oldani A, Speroni F, Taglietti V, Tanzi F: Ca2+ signaling in injured in situ endothelium of rat aorta. *Cell Calcium* 2008, 44(3):298-309.
28. Verma V, Hallett MB, Leybaert L, Martin PE, Evans WH: Perturbing plasma membrane hemichannels attenuates calcium signalling in cardiac cells and HeLa cells expressing connexins. *European Journal of Cell Biology* 2009, 88(2).
29. De Bock M, Culot M, Wang N, Bol M, Decrock E, De Vuyst E, da Costa A, Dauwe I, Vinken M, Simon AM, et al: Connexin channels provide a target to manipulate brain endothelial calcium dynamics and blood-brain barrier permeability. *Journal of Cerebral Blood Flow and Metabolism* 2011, 31(9).
30. De Bock M, Wang N, Bol M, Decrock E, Ponsaerts R, Bultynck G, Dupont G, Leybaert L: Connexin 43 Hemichannels Contribute to Cytoplasmic Ca2+ Oscillations by Providing a Bimodal Ca2+-dependent Ca2+ Entry Pathway. *Journal of Biological Chemistry* 2012, 287(15).
31. Park JH, Lee MY, Heo JS, Han HJ: A potential role of connexin 43 in epidermal growth factor-induced proliferation of mouse embryonic stem cells: Involvement of Ca2+/PKC, p44/42 and p38 MAPKs pathways. *Cell Proliferation* 2008, 41(5):786-802.
32. Gabriels JE, Paul DL: Connexin43 is highly localized to sites of disturbed flow in rat aortic endothelium but connexin37 and connexin40 are more uniformly distributed. *Circulation Research* 1998, 83(6):636-643.
33. Griffith TM: Endothelium-dependent smooth muscle hyperpolarization: do gap junctions provide a unifying hypothesis? *British Journal of Pharmacology* 2004, 141(6):881-903.

34. Berra-Romani R, Rinaldi C, Raqeeb A, Castelli L, Magistretti J, Taglietti V, Tanzi F: The duration and amplitude of the plateau phase of ATP- and ADP-evoked Ca2+ signals are modulated by ectonucleotidases in in situ endothelial cells of rat aorta. *Journal of Vascular Research* 2004, 41(2):166-173.

35. Berra-Romani R, Raqeeb A, Guzman-Silva A, Torres-Jacome J, Tanzi F, Moccia F: Na+-Ca2+ exchanger contributes to Ca2+ extrusion in ATP-stimulated endothelium of intact rat aorta. *Biochemical and Biophysical Research Communications* 2010, 395(1):126-130.

36. Moccia F, Bertoni G, Pla AF, Dragoni S, Pupo E, Merlino A, Mancardi D, Munaron L, Tanzi F: Hydrogen Sulfide Regulates Intracellular Ca(2+) Concentration in Endothelial Cells From Excised Rat Aorta. *Current Pharmaceutical Biotechnology* 2011, 12(9):1416-1426.

37. Pupo E, Pla AF, Avanzato D, Moccia F, Cruz J-EA, Tanzi F, Merlino A, Mancardi D, Munaron L: Hydrogen sulfide promotes calcium signals and migration in tumor-derived endothelial cells. *Free Radical Biology and Medicine* 2011, 51(9):1765-1773.

38. Koyama T, Kimura C, Park SJ, Oike M, Ito Y: Functional implications of Ca2+ mobilizing properties for nitric oxide production in aortic endothelium. *Life Sciences* 2002, 72(4-5):511-520.

39. Hartell NA, Archer HE, Bailey CJ: Insulin-stimulated endothelial nitric oxide release is calcium independent and mediated via protein kinase B. *Biochemical Pharmacology* 2005, 69(5):781-790.

40. Dedkova EN, Blatter LA: Nitric oxide inhibits capacitative Ca2+ entry and enhances endoplasmic reticulum Ca2+ uptake in bovine vascular endothelial cells. *Journal of Physiology-London* 2002, 539(1):77-91.

41. Rogers C, Parikh S, Seifert P, Edelman ER: Endogenous cell seeding - Remnant endothelium after stenting enhances vascular repair. *Circulation* 1996, 94(11):2909-2914.

42. Orford JL, Selwyn AP, Ganz P, Popma JJ, Rogers C: The comparative pathobiology of atherosclerosis and restenosis. *American Journal of Cardiology* 2000, 86(4B).

43. Rogers C, Tseng DY, Squire JC, Edelman ER: Balloon-artery interactions during stent placement - A finite element analysis approach to pressure, compliance, and stent design as contributors to vascular injury. *Circulation Research* 1999, 84(4):378-383.

44. Schalper KA, Palacios-Prado N, Orellana JA, Saez JC: Currently used methods for identification and characterization of hemichannels. *Cell Communication and Adhesion* 2008, 15(1-2):207-218.

45. Evans WH, De Vuyst E, Leybaert L: The gap junction cellular internet: connexin hemichannels enter the signalling limelight. *Biochemical Journal* 2006, 397:1-14.

46. Moccia F, Berra-Romani R, Baruffi S, Spaggiari S, Signorelli S, Castelli L, Magistretti J, Taglietti V, Tanzi F: Ca2+ uptake by the endoplasmic reticulum Ca2+-ATPase in rat microvascular endothelial cells. *Biochemical Journal* 2002, 364:235-244.

47. Christ GJ, Spektor M, Brink PR, Barr L: Further evidence for the selective disruption of intercellular communication by heptanol. *American Journal of Physiology-Heart and Circulatory Physiology* 1999, 276(6):H1911-H1917.

48. Moses S, Dreja K, Lindqvist A, Lovdahl C, Hellstrand P, Hultgardh-Nilsson A: Smooth muscle cell response to mechanical injury involves intracellular calcium release and ERK1/ERK2 phosphorylation. *Experimental Cell Research* 2001, 269(1):88-96.

49. Martin PEM, Wall C, Griffith TM: Effects of connexin-mimetic peptides on gap junction functionality and connexin expression in cultured vascular cells. *British Journal of Pharmacology* 2005, 144(5):617-627.

50. Okamoto T, Akiyama M, Takeda M, Gabazza EC, Hayashi T, Suzuki K: Connexin32 is expressed in vascular endothelial cells and participates in gap-junction intercellular communication. *Biochemical and Biophysical Research Communications* 2009, 382(2):264-268.

51. Evans WH, Boitano S: Connexin mimetic peptides: specific inhibitors of gap-junctional intercellular communication. *Biochemical Society Transactions* 2001, 29.

52. Tang EHC, Vanhoutte PM: Gap junction inhibitors reduce endothelium-dependent contractions in the aorta of spontaneously hypertensive rats. *Journal of Pharmacology and Experimental Therapeutics* 2008, 327(1):148-153.

53. Brisset AC, Isakson BE, Kwak BR: Connexins in Vascular Physiology and Pathology. *Antioxidants & Redox Signaling* 2009, 11(2):267-282.

54. Kruger O, Beny JL, Chabaud F, Traub O, Theis M, Brix K, Kirchhoff S, Willecke K: Altered dye diffusion and upregulation of connexin37 in mouse aortic endothelium deficient in connexin40. *Journal of Vascular Research* 2002, 39(2):160-172.

55. Simon AM, McWhorter AR: Decreased intercellular dye-transfer and downregulation of non-ablated connexins in aortic endothelium deficient in connexin37 or connexin40. *Journal of Cell Science* 2003, 116(11):2223-2236.

56. Isakson BE, Damon DN, Day KH, Liao YB, Duling BR: Connexin40 and connexin43 in mouse aortic endothelium: evidence for coordinated regulation. *American Journal of Physiology-Heart and Circulatory Physiology* 2006, 290(3):H1199-H1205.

57. Isshiki M, Anderson RGW: Function of caveolae in Ca2+ entry and Ca2+-dependent signal transduction. *Traffic* 2003, 4(11):717-723.

58. Isshiki M, Ying YS, Fujita T, Anderson RGW: A molecular sensor detects signal transduction from caveolae in living cells. *Journal of Biological Chemistry* 2002, 277(45):43389-43398.

59. Munaron L: Intracellular calcium, endothelial cells and angiogenesis. *Recent Patents on Anti-Cancer Drug Discovery* 2006, 1(1):105-119.

60. Fischell TA, Derby G, Tse TM, Stadius ML: Coronary-artery vasoconstriction routinely occurs after percutaneous trans-luminal coronary angioplasty - a quantitative arteriographic analysis. *Circulation* 1988, 78(6):1323-1334.

61. Yoder MC: Human endothelial progenitor cells. *Cold Spring Harbor perspectives in medicine* 2012, 2(7).

62. Schwartz SM, Benditt EP: Clustering of replicating cells in aortic endothelium. *Proceedings of the National Academy of Sciences of the United States of America* 1976, 73(2):651-653.

63. Parthasarathi K, Ichimura H, Monma E, Lindert J, Quadri S, Issekutz A, Bhattacharya J: Connexin 43 mediates spread of Ca2+-dependent proinflammatory responses in lung capillaries. *Journal of Clinical Investigation* 2006, 116(8):2193-2200.

64. Schalper KA, Sanchez HA, Lee SC, Altenberg GA, Nathanson MH, Saez JC: Connexin 43 hemichannels mediate the Ca(2+) influx induced by extracellular alkalinization. *American Journal of Physiology-Cell Physiology* 2010, 299(6):C1504-C1515.

65. Alonso F, Boittin F-X, Beny J-L, Haefliger J-A: Loss of connexin40 is associated with decreased endothelium-dependent relaxations and eNOS levels in the mouse aorta. *American Journal of Physiology-Heart and Circulatory Physiology* 2010, 299(5):H1365-H1373.

66. Straub AC, Billaud M, Johnstone SR, Best AK, Yemen S, Dwyer ST, Looft-Wilson R, Lysiak JJ, Gaston B, Palmer L, et al: Compartmentalized Connexin 43 S-Nitrosylation/Denitrosylation Regulates Heterocellular Communication in the Vessel Wall. *Arteriosclerosis Thrombosis and Vascular Biology* 2011, 31(2):399-U353.

67. Pfenniger A, Derouette J-P, Verma V, Lin X, Foglia B, Coombs W, Roth I, Satta N, Dunoyer-Geindre S, Sorgen P, et al: Gap Junction Protein Cx37 Interacts With Endothelial Nitric Oxide Synthase in Endothelial Cells. *Arteriosclerosis Thrombosis and Vascular Biology* 2010, 30(4):827-U445.

68. Rath G, Dessy C, Feron O: Caveolae, caveolin and control of vascular tone: nitric oxide (no) and endothelium derived hyperpolarizing factor (edhf) regulation. *Journal of Physiology and Pharmacology* 2009, 60:105-109.

69. Schubert AL, Schubert W, Spray DC, Lisanti MP: Connexin family members target to lipid raft domains and interact with caveolin-1. *Biochemistry* 2002, 41(18):5754-5764.

70. Saliez J, Bouzin C, Rath G, Ghisdal P, Desjardins F, Rezzani R, Rodella LF, Vriens J, Nilius B, Feron O, et al: Role of caveolar compartmentation in endothelium-derived hyperpolarizing factor-mediated relaxation - Ca2+ signals and gap junction function are regulated by caveolin in endothelial cells. *Circulation* 2008, 117(8):1065-1074.

71. Weber C: Platelets and chemokines in atherosclerosis - Partners in crime. *Circulation Research* 2005, 96(6):612-616.

72. Lee PC, Salyapongse AN, Bragdon GA, Shears LL, Watkins SC, Edington HDJ, Billiar TR: Impaired wound healing and angiogenesis in eNOS-deficient mice. *American Journal of Physiology-Heart and Circulatory Physiology* 1999, 277(4):H1600-H1608.

73. Guo JP, Panday MM, Consigny PC, Lefer AM: Mechanisms of vascular preservation by a novel no donor following rat carotid-artery intimal injury. *American Journal of Physiology-Heart and Circulatory Physiology* 1995, 269(3):H1122-H1131.

74. Murohara T, Asahara T, Silver M, Bauters C, Masuda H, Kalka C, Kearney M, Chen DH, Chen DF, Symes JF, et al: Nitric oxide synthase modulates angiogenesis in response to tissue ischemia. *Journal of Clinical Investigation* 1998, 101(11):2567-2578.

75. Amano K, Matsubara H, Iba O, Okigaki M, Fujiyama S, Imada T, Kojima H, Nozawa Y, Kawashima S, Yokoyama M, *et al*: **Enhancement of ischemia-induced angiogenesis by eNOS overexpression.** *Hypertension* 2003, **41**(1):156-162.

76. Dimmeler S: **Regulation of Bone Marrow-Derived Vascular Progenitor Cell Mobilization and Maintenance.** *Arteriosclerosis Thrombosis and Vascular Biology* 2010, **30**(6).

77. Isakson BE, Ramos SI, Duling BR: **Ca2+ and inositol 1,4,5-trisphosphate-mediated signaling across the myoendothelial junction.** *Circulation Research* 2007, **100**(2):246-254.

78. Sanchez HA, Orellana JA, Verselis VK, Saez JC: **Metabolic inhibition increases activity of connexin-32 hemichannels permeable to Ca2+ in transfected HeLa cells.** *American Journal of Physiology-Cell Physiology* 2009, **297**(3):C665-C678.

79. Sanchez HA, Mese G, Srinivas M, White TW, Verselis VK: **Differentially altered Ca(2+) regulation and Ca(2+) permeability in Cx26 hemichannels formed by the A40V and G45E mutations that cause keratitis ichthyosis deafness syndrome.** *Journal of General Physiology* 2010, **136**(1):47-62.

80. Schalper KA, Palacios-Prado N, Retamal MA, Shoji KF, Martinez AD, Saez JC: **Connexin hemichannel composition determines the FGF-1-induced membrane permeability and free Ca2+ (i) responses.** *Molecular Biology of the Cell* 2008, **19**(8):3501-3513.

81. Sorensen CM, Salomonsson M, Braunstein TH, Nielsen MS, Holstein-Rathlou N-H: **Connexin mimetic peptides fail to inhibit vascular conducted calcium responses in renal arterioles.** *American Journal of Physiology-Regulatory Integrative and Comparative Physiology* 2008, **295**(3): R840-R847.

82. Shestopalov VI, Panchin Y: **Pannexins and gap junction protein diversity.** *Cellular and Molecular Life Sciences* 2008, **65**(3):376-394.

83. Gossman DG, Zhao H-B: **Hemichannel-Mediated Inositol 1,4,5-Trisphosphate (IP3) Release in the Cochlea: A Novel Mechanism of IP3 Intercellular Signaling.** *Cell Communication and Adhesion* 2008, **15**(4):305-315.

84. Varu VN, Tsihlis ND, Kibbe MR: **Nitric Oxide-Releasing Prosthetic Materials.** *Vascular and Endovascular Surgery* 2009, **43**(2):121-131.

85. De Vuyst E, Boengler K, Antoons G, Sipido KR, Schulz R, Leybaert L: **Pharmacological modulation of connexin-formed channels in cardiac pathophysiology.** *British Journal of Pharmacology* 2011, **163**(3).

86. Salameh A, Dhein S: **Pharmacology of Gap junctions. New pharmacological targets for treatment of arrhythmia, seizure and cancer?** *Biochimica Et Biophysica Acta-Biomembranes* 2005, **1719**(1-2).

24

Lumbar herniation following extended autologous latissimus dorsi breast reconstruction

Sheila Margaret Fraser[*], Hiba Fatayer and Rajgopal Achuthan

Abstract

Background: Reconstructive breast surgery is now recognized to be an important part of the treatment for breast cancer. Surgical reconstruction options consist of implants, autologous tissue transfer or a combination of the two. The latissimus dorsi flap is a pedicled musculocutaneous flap and is an established method of autologous breast reconstruction.
Lumbar hernias are an unusual type of hernia, the majority occurring after surgery or trauma in this area. The reported incidence of a lumbar hernia subsequent to a latissimus dorsi reconstruction is very low.

Case presentation: We present the unusual case of lumbar herniation after an extended autologous latissimus dorsi flap for breast reconstruction following a mastectomy. The lumbar hernia was confirmed on CT scanning and the patient underwent an open mesh repair of the hernia through the previous latissimus dorsi scar.

Conclusion: Lumbar hernias are a rare complication that can occur following latissimus dorsi breast reconstruction. It should be considered in all patients presenting with persistent pain or swelling in the lumbar region.

Background

Breast reconstruction is an important part of the surgical treatment of breast cancer, and is usually performed following a mastectomy. Surgical options for reconstruction include implants, autologous tissue transfer or a combination of both. Autologous tissue transfer is often the preferred option as it can give a more natural appearance to the breast compared to implants alone [1,2]. The latissimus dorsi (LD) flap is an established method of autologous breast reconstruction with relatively few contraindications and complications [3-5].

Lumbar hernias are an unusual type of herniation of the postero-lateral abdominal wall. The majority of this hernia type is acquired, rather than congenital and occurs after surgery or trauma. The diagnosis is usually suspected on clinical grounds and confirmed by CT scanning [6,7].

Lumbar herniation after an LD flap is an uncommon complication that patients are not routinely warned about during the counseling and consent for the procedure. There have been very few published reports over the past 20 years regarding the incidence, detection and management of this complication [8,9].

We present the rare case of lumbar herniation following a latissismus dorsi reconstruction for breast cancer and the consequent diagnosis and treatment.

Case presentation

A 63-year old female with a past medical history of bronchiectasis was diagnosed with a grade 3 ductal breast cancer. She initially underwent breast conservation surgery in the form of a right wide local excision and sentinel lymph node biopsy. Due to the proximity of the carcinoma to the surgical resection margins she subsequently had a skin sparing mastectomy and extended autologous latissimus dorsi flap reconstruction.

On her first post-operative outpatient visit she had a large seroma in relation to the tumour site, which was drained in clinic. She was seen two weeks later and was found to have a large seroma over the back wound (LD site); this was aspirated and drained 650 mls serous fluid. On two consecutive outpatient visits at fortnightly intervals she had recurrent large seromas at the LD site. On each occasion these were aspirated and over a litre of serous fluid drained.

On her fourth visit, following aspiration of the seroma there was a residual fullness in the lower region of the LD donor site. On palpation this felt like a separate firm

* Correspondence: sheilafraser@doctors.org.uk
Department of Breast & General Surgery, Leeds General Surgery, Great George Street, Leeds LS1 3EX, UK

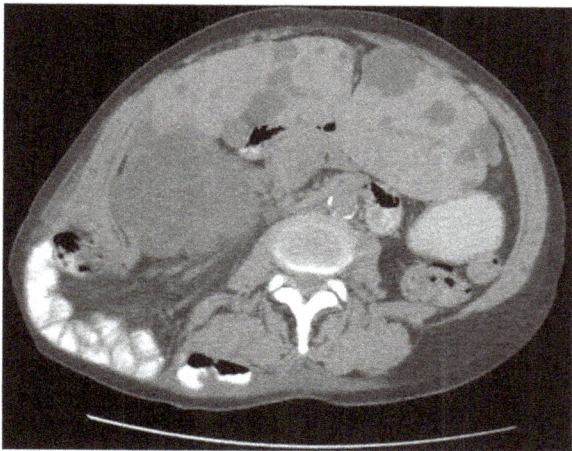

Figure 1 Axial CT scan demonstrating incisional lumbar hernia.

lump, clinically in keeping with a possible lumbar hernia. An urgent CT scan of the abdomen and pelvis confirmed the diagnosis of a lumbar hernia containing the majority of the small bowel and right colon (Figures 1 and 2). The CT scan also demonstrated an incidental finding of an enlarged polycystic liver.

She accordingly underwent an open repair of the lumbar hernia using the previous LD scar for access (Figure 3). Small bowel loops within the hernia sac were freed from

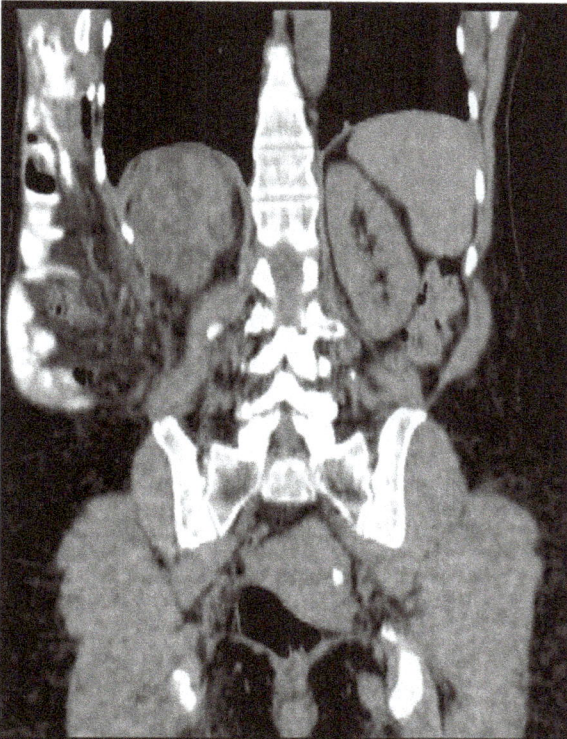

Figure 3 Intra-operative view of lumbar hernia, through previous latissimus dorsi scar.

adhesions and the small bowel and caecum reduced into the intra-abdominal cavity. The edges of the defect were closed with interrupted PDS, and a 30 × 30 cm onlay prolene mesh was used for reinforcement.

Postoperative recovery was uneventful and she was commenced on adjuvant hormonal and herceptin therapy.

Discussion

Breast conservation surgery is an established method of treatment for early breast cancer. In the majority of patients this method of surgery, in combination with radiotherapy, provides effective oncological therapy and long-term survival as compared to mastectomy [10]. However over 30% women in the UK still require a mastectomy for the treatment of breast cancer. Reasons for mastectomy include large cancers, those directly behind the nipple, multi-focal cancers, patient preference and increasingly prophylactic mastectomies due to an improved understanding of the genetics of breast cancer [11,12].

Mastectomy is known to be associated with significant psychological consequences including a distorted body image, loss of self-esteem and sexual dysfunction. Breast reconstruction should be offered to virtually all women undergoing a mastectomy and is an integral part of the surgical treatment of breast cancer. The benefits of an

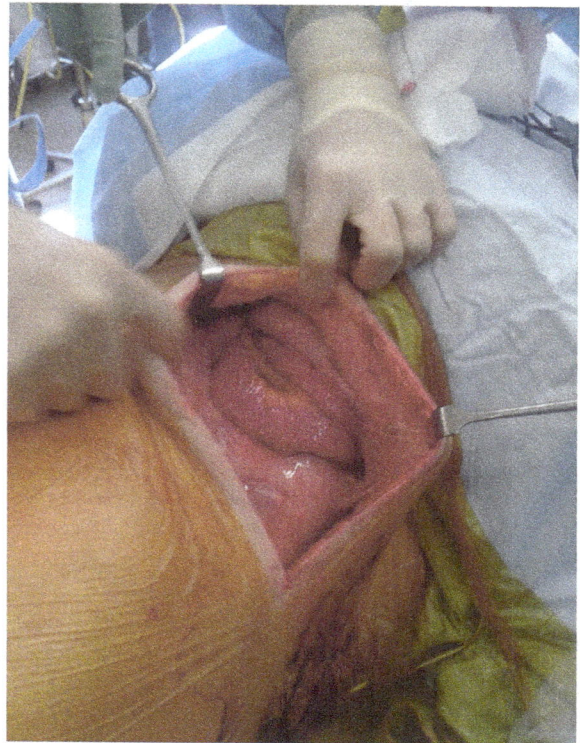

Figure 2 Coronal CT scan demonstrating incisional lumbar hernia.

immediate or delayed breast reconstruction are well recognized, for both emotional and physical well being [4]. Furthermore reconstruction techniques have been shown to be safe with minimal morbidity and no affect on local recurrence rates [5,13].

The aims of reconstructive surgery are to correct the anatomical defect after mastectomy and restore the shape and symmetry of the breasts. Surgical reconstruction options consist of implants, autologous tissue transfer or a combination of the two. In comparison to implants, autologous tissue transfer is considered to give a better aesthetic look [1,2,14].

The latissimus dorsi flap is a pedicled musculocutaneous flap, first used in the late 19th century to cover chest wall deformities following mastectomy complications. The current use of the latissimus dorsi flap was developed in the 1970s for breast reconstruction following mastectomy in patients with radiation damage to the skin and chest wall [15-17]. There are relatively few absolute contraindications to latissimus dorsi breast reconstruction. Complications can be split into flap complications and donor site complications, the most common being mastectomy skin flap necrosis and donor site seroma [18].

Lumbar hernias are an uncommon type of hernia, only 20% present as a congenital condition, the majority are acquired following surgery, trauma or inflammation [7]. Lumbar hernias typically are wide necked and therefore less likely to be prone to strangulation or obstruction. Lumbar hernias usually occur in 2 weak sites in the posterolateral abdominal wall – the superior (Grynfeltt-Lesshalft) and the inferior (Petit) lumbar triangles. However in large incisional defects the hernia can affect the entire lumbar region [6,19].

Due to its rarity there is no standardized surgical technique for lumbar hernia repair. When there is clinical suspicion of a lumbar hernia CT is recommended to get exact information on the size and content of the hernia and to plan for surgical repair [19].

Our patient had pre-disposing factors that in hindsight contributed to the development of a lumbar hernia, despite preservation of the lumbar fascia during the operation. The co-morbidities of bronchiectasis and a polycystic liver both reduced the intra-abdominal compartment size and increased the intra-abdominal pressure. This caused herniation of abdominal contents through a weakened area of the abdominal wall. On further questioning she admitted to a post-operative chest infection with associated coughing and had received oral antibiotics from her GP.

We currently do not routinely image seromas occurring in post-operative breast reconstruction patients. However there was clinical suspicion following recurrent aspiration, due to the residual fullness and the anatomical site of the seroma, that raised the suspicion of a lumbar hernia.

Conclusion

Lumbar herniation is a rare complication that can occur following LD breast reconstruction. It should be clinically suspected in patients with a persistent swelling or pain in the lumbar region and subsequent CT scanning should be performed. Surgical repair is recommended in suitable patients; due to the large size these hernias can reach and related patient discomfort. Pre-existing co-morbidities should be carefully considered in all patients undergoing breast reconstruction.

Abbreviations

CT: Computerized tomography; LD: Latissimus dorsi.

Competing interests

The authors declare that they have no competing interests.

Authors' contributions

SMF wrote the background and discussion and revised the manuscript. HF wrote the case presentation. RA is the Consultant Surgeon who operated on the patient and gave final approval of the version to be published. All authors read and approved the final manuscript.

Acknowledgements

Funding for this manuscript was provided by the Leeds Teaching Hospitals NHS Trust.

References

1. Rawson AE, McClellan WT: **Current concepts in breast reconstruction.** *W V Med J* 2009, **105**(3):16–22.
2. Rozen WM, Ashton MW: **Improving outcomes in autologous breast reconstruction.** *Aesthetic Plast Surg* 2009, **33**(3):327–335.
3. Perdikis G, Koonce S, Collis G, Eck D: **Latissimus dorsi myocutaneous flap for breast reconstruction: bad rap or good flap?** *Eplasty* 2011:11–39.
4. Eric M, Mihic N, Krivokuca D: **Breast reconstruction following mastectomy; patient's satisfaction.** *Acta Chir Belg* 2009, **109**(2):159–166.
5. Reefy S, Patani N, Anderson A, Burgoyne G, Osman H, Mokbel K: **Oncological outcome and patient satisfaction with skin-sparing mastectomy and immediate breast reconstruction: a prospective observational study.** *BMC Cancer* 2010, **10**:171.
6. Cavallaro G, Sadighi A, Paparelli C, Miceli M, D'Ermo G, Polistena A, *et al*: **Anatomical and surgical considerations on lumbar hernias.** *Am Surg* 2009, **75**(12):1238–1241.
7. Salemis NS, Nisotakis K, Gourgiotis S, Tsohataridis E: **Segmental liver incarceration through a recurrent incisional lumbar hernia.** *Hepatobiliary Pancreat Dis Int* 2007, **6**(4):442–444.
8. Evans MD, Thomas C, Williams GL, Stephenson BM: **Latissimus dorsi flap herniation: is it really that rare?** *Surgery* 2011, **150**(1):139.
9. Mickel TJ, Barton FE Jr, Rohrich RJ, Daniel LB, Conner WC: **Management and prevention of lumbar herniation following a latissimus dorsi flap.** *Plast Reconstr Surg* 1999, **103**(5):1473–1475.
10. Fisher B, Anderson S, Bryant J, Margolese RG, Deutsch M, Fisher ER, *et al*: **Twenty-year follow-up of a randomized trial comparing total mastectomy, lumpectomy, and lumpectomy plus irradiation for the treatment of invasive breast cancer.** *N Engl J Med* 2002, **347**(16):1233–1241.

11. Lostumbo L, Carbine N, Wallace J, Ezzo J: **Prophylactic mastectomy for the prevention of breast cancer.** *Cochrane Database Syst Rev* 2004, **4**, CD002748.

12. Tuttle TM, Abbott A, Arrington A, Rueth N: **The increasing use of prophylactic mastectomy in the prevention of breast cancer.** *Curr Oncol Rep* 2010, **12**(1):16–21.

13. Giacalone PL, Rathat G, Daures JP, Benos P, Azria D, Rouleau C: **New concept for immediate breast reconstruction for invasive cancers: feasibility, oncological safety and esthetic outcome of post-neoadjuvant therapy immediate breast reconstruction versus delayed breast reconstruction: a prospective pilot study.** *Breast Cancer Res Treat* 2010, **122**(2):439–451.

14. Reiland-Smith J: **Diagnosis and surgical treatment of breast cancer.** *S D Med Spec* 2010:31–37.

15. Bostwick J 3rd, Vasconez LO, Jurkiewicz MJ: **Breast reconstruction after a radical mastectomy.** *Plast Reconstr Surg* 1978, **61**(5):682–693.

16. Olivari N: **The latissimus flap.** *Br J Plast Surg* 1976, **29**(2):126–128.

17. Schneider WJ, Hill HL Jr, Brown RG: **Latissimus dorsi myocutaneous flap for breast reconstruction.** *Br J Plast Surg* 1977, **30**(4):277–281.

18. Chang DW, Youssef A, Cha S, Reece GP: **Autologous breast reconstruction with the extended latissimus dorsi flap.** *Plast Reconstr Surg* 2002, **110**(3):751–759. discussion 60–1.

19. Tobias-Machado M, Rincon FJ, Lasmar MT, Zambon JP, Juliano RV, Wroclawski ER: **Laparoscopic surgery for treatment of incisional lumbar hernia.** *Int Braz J Urol* 2005, **31**(4):309–314.

25

The PRAISE study: A prospective, multi-center, randomized, double blinded, placebo-controlled study for the evaluation of iloprost in the early postoperative period after liver transplantation (ISRCTN12622749)

Erik Bärthel[1,4*], Falk Rauchfuß[1,4], Heike Hoyer[2], Maria Breternitz[3], Karin Jandt[1] and Utz Settmacher[1,4]

Abstract

Background: Liver graft dysfunction can deteriorate to complete organ failure and increases perioperative morbidity and mortality after liver transplantation. Therapeutic strategies reducing the rate of graft dysfunction are of current clinical relevance. One approach is the systemic application of prostaglandins, which were demonstrated to be beneficial in reducing ischemia-reperfusion injury. Preliminary data indicate a positive effect of prostacyclin analogue iloprost on allograft viability after liver transplantation. The objective of the study is to evaluate the impact of iloprost in a multi-center trial.

Methods/Design: A prospective, double-blinded, randomized, placebo-controlled multicenter study in a total of 365 liver transplant recipients was designed to assess the effect of intravenous iloprost after liver transplantation. Primary endpoint will be the primary graft dysfunction characterized as presentation of one or more of the following criteria: ALAT or ASAT level > 2000 IU/ml within the first 7 postoperative days, bilirubine ≥ 10 mg/dl on postoperative day 7; INR ≥ 1.6 on postoperative day 7 or initial non-function. Secondary endpoints are parameters of post-transplant morbidity, like rates of infections, biliary complications, need of clotting factors or renal replacement therapy and the graft and patient survival.

Discussion: A well-established treatment concept to avoid graft dysfunction after liver transplantation does not exist at the moment. If the data of this research project confirm prior findings, iloprost would improve the general outcome after liver transplantation.

Trial Registration: German Clinical Trials Register: DRKS00003514. Current Controlled Trials Register: ISRCTN12622749.

Keywords: Liver transplantation, Primary graft dysfunction, Initial non-function, Ischemia-reperfusion injury, Prostaglandins

* Correspondence: erik.baerthel@med.uni-jena.de
[1]Department of General, Visceral and Vascular Surgery, Jena University Hospital, Erlanger Allee 101, D-07740 Jena, Germany
[4]Center for Sepsis Control and Care, Jena University Hospital, Friedrich Schiller University, Jena, Germany
Full list of author information is available at the end of the article

Background

The incidence of primary graft dysfunction (PDF) after LT is approximately 25% within a range of 9.3 to 43.7% based on different definitions characterizing PDF [1-5]. Initial non-function (INF) develops in up to 6% of all considered cases and requires urgent retransplantation [6].

Risk factors are prolonged cold ischemia time or higher degree of graft steatosis and subsequent development of severe hepatic ischemia/reperfusion injury (IRI) [5,7]. A cascade of cellular events results in microcirculatory flow disturbance. This may be distinguished as "no-flow" indicating capillary perfusion failure on the one hand, or "reflow-paradox" including activation of the leukocyte-endothelium interaction, release of toxic mediators, and impairment of the endothelial barrier on the other hand [8,9]. There are, obviously, further different factors all contributing to an insufficient function of liver grafts and its detrimental effects on the overall outcome after LT: recipient's condition, the donor data, the organ conservation as well as the immunosuppression and the antibiotic regime in the perioperative period. All of these factors may influence the performance of the graft with possible development of graft dysfunction or non-function as undesired outcomes.

Due to the persisting shortage of donor the transplant centers are forced to accept so called marginal organs. The more criteria of a marginal organ are met, the higher is the risk for development of graft dysfunction [10]. Therapeutic strategies reducing the rate of organ dysfunction are of current clinical relevance. One approach is the systemic application of prostaglandin derivatives. In particular, the prostaglandins E_1 (PGE$_1$) and I_2 (PGI$_2$) showed beneficial protective effects with respect to IRI by improvement of tissue perfusion and by protection of endothelial cells studied *in vitro* and *in vivo*. Both prostaglandins induce vasodilatation, inhibit platelet aggregation and activation of leukocytes and exert a variety of "cytoprotective" effects. PGI$_2$ is believed to play a superior role with respect to inhibition of platelet aggregation via PGE$_1$ and also to inhibit the production of inflammatory cytokines. Therefore PGE$_1$ and PGI$_2$ are supposed to attenuate reperfusion injury.

There is a lack of systematic studies on the effects of synthetic PGI$_2$ analogue iloprost. Many authors have reported the clinical use of the iloprost over the last two decades. Based on its ability to induce vasodilatation, it has traditionally been utilized in the treatment of pulmonary hypertension [11]. Off-label use of iloprost as an adjuvant in elective abdominal aortic aneurysm surgery and after reconstructive surgery for acute lower limb ischemia has been reported [12,13]. In these studies, the PGI$_2$ infusion was associated with a significant reduction of morbidity and mortality suggesting an improved systemic perfusion and reduced secondary end-organ damage.

From 2006 to 2008, we evaluated the impact of the PGI$_2$ analogue iloprost in 80 liver transplanted patients in a prospective, randomized (1:1), open-label, single-center pilot study [14]. Our data indicate that intravenous administered PGI$_2$ analogue iloprost (1 ng/kg BW/min) improves the graft function, particularly in the early postoperative period. We observed ten cases of PDF according to the definition of Haller et al. [15]: eight in the control group (n = 8/40, 20%), and two in the iloprost group (n = 2/40, 5%) (relative risk 0.25, 95% confidence interval (0.05, 1.11). The relative risk did not change after adjustment to three or more extended-donor criteria (EDC). Four out of 40 patients of the control group but none of the iloprost group underwent liver retransplantation due to INF (p = 0.12).

The definition of graft dysfunction after LT varies in the literature. There is currently no standardized terminology [7,10,15-17]. Besides, in the last years, there has been a shift toward abandoning the routine use of T-tubes for reconstruction of the biliary tract [18]. Therefore, in a posthoc analysis we applied a distinct definition of PDF, which was recently validated by Olthoff et al. [19]. This definition utilizes objective post-transplant criteria that were highly associated with graft loss and patient mortality. According to Olthoff et al., we observed 27 cases of PDF (treatment group: n = 11/40 (27.5%); control group: n = 16/40 (40%)) resulting in a relative risk of 0.69 with 95% confidence interval (0.36, 1.30).

The results of our pilot study are encouraging, but due to the number of patients enrolled, the effect of iloprost on early graft function did not reach statistical significance. There is, however, preliminary evidence to suggest beneficial effects in this particular clinical scenario. The clinical outcome after LT is affected by various donor and recipient characteristics such as graft steatosis, long ischemic period or renal insufficiency prior to LT. In order to define the specific impact of PGI$_2$ analogue iloprost on liver graft function, a multicenter, randomized, double-blinded clinical trial including an appropriate number of patients is justified [20]. This is the objective of our PRAISE study.

Methods/Design

The PRAISE study is a prospective, multi-center, randomized, double blinded (patients and investigators), placebo-controlled clinical trial according to the German drug legislation for evaluation of iloprost in the early postoperative period after LT.

The investigational medicinal product is iloprost (Ilomedin®, Bayer Vital GmbH, Leverkusen, Germany). The control group receives placebo. Patients will be assigned to treatment at the ratio of 1:1 according to a computer generated randomization list by means of nQuery Advisor software. Randomization will be restricted by blocking with randomly varying block size and stratified by center. An independent statistician, who is not involved in the analyses, will prepare the randomization list. The university pharmacy of Heidelberg, Germany, will provide the trial medication to the participating centers by sequentially numbered sealed identical boxes according to the allocation sequence.

The end of trial for each patient is reached 180 days after LT. The follow-up period will be 6 months with assessments 9 and 12 months after LT.

Study endpoints

The primary endpoint of this trial is the rate of primary graft dysfunction after liver transplantation. It will be characterized as presentation of one or more of the following criteria in accordance with Olthoff et al [19]: ALAT or ASAT level > 2000 IU/ml within the first 7 postoperative days; bilirubin $\geq$ 10 mg/dl on postoperative day 7; INR $\geq$ 1.6 on postoperative day 7 or as occurrence of initial non-function (INF) defined as graft loss, retransplantation or patient death within 14 days after initial LT not secondary to hepatic artery thrombosis (HAT), biliary complication, recurrent disease or acute rejection. Based on the results of previous investigations a relative reduction of PDF incidence of 50% by iloprost compared to placebo will be expected.

Due to the immunologic capabilities even of the liver, graft dysfunction may lead to an increased incidence of hospital acquired infections and/or sepsis. For this reason, the incidence of infectious complications up to 28 days after LT was defined as an important secondary endpoint. Further secondary endpoints are the rate of INF (described above), the graft and patient survival (28, 180 days after LT), the clotting factor substitution up to day 28 after LT, the rate of biliary complications, the requirement for liver dialysis, the postoperative renal replacement therapy (28, 180 days after LT) and the length of intensive care unit (ICU) stay and hospital stay. The change in SOFA score from day 1 to day 7 after LT is used as a surrogate secondary endpoint predictive for morbidity and mortality after LT. The levels of liver enzymes (ASAT/ALAT) may represent the severity of graft injury due to ischemia/reperfusion and the levels of Quick's value/INR and Factor V and the ICG-PDR are important parameters of the synthetic capacity of the graft. Therefore, the course of these laboratory data until day 7 after LT is also fixed as secondary endpoint. Occurrence of bleeding complications, circulatory instability and pulmonary disturbance during trial intervention as well as incidence of adverse events will be assessed for patient safety. During the post-trial follow-up graft and patient survival and biliary complications will be additionally evaluated 9 and 12 months after LT.

Further objectives will be explored within the scope of a scientific supporting program. Liver biopsies, taken during cold ischemia, after reperfusion and seven days after LT will be performed for histopathological and pangenomic gene expression studies. Furthermore, blood samples will be collected for "multiplex"-analysis of cytokines, chemokines and growth factors in order to investigate a possible modulating effect of iloprost on the inflammatory response after LT.

Infection is one of the leading causes of morbidity and mortality after LT. More than 50% of liver transplant recipients have infections in the first year after transplantation, whereas the majority of bacterial infections occur within 2 months after transplantation [21]. As the differentiation between infectious and non-infectious etiology of the so called SIRS (systemic inflammatory response syndrome) often requires complex and long-lasting tests valuable time is often lost until the definitive diagnosis of sepsis can be made. There is a new approach (SIQnature®, SIRS-Lab GmbH, Jena, Germany) that allows an analysis within one working day and facilitates the clinical interpretation according to a score. The data have not yet been established in patients receiving immunosuppression. Therefore, within the study setting blood samples will be taken for the evaluation of the SIQnature®-test.

Study population and setting

Female and male patients aged 18 years and above who are receiving a full-size liver graft are eligible for the trial. Complete inclusion and exclusion criteria are displayed in Table 1. According to the experience from the pilot study [14] about 83% of primarily enrolled patients reached respiratory and circulatory stable conditions after LT as precondition for trial medication. To randomize 356 patients after LT written informed consent has to be obtained from about 430 patients fulfilling the study criteria observable before LT. In case of patients not able to give informed consent by themselves informed consent has to be given by the legal representative. Patients will be recruited in several German transplant centers. Recruitment was started in April 2012.

Intervention

The investigational medicinal product is iloprost (Ilomedin®, Bayer Vital GmbH, Leverkusen, Germany). The control group receives placebo administered in the same dosage and application form. It is the iloprost 10 µg/ml carrier substance (ethanol, tromethamin, sodium chloride, hydrochloric acid, water for injections). Patients will be allocated to the trial medication immediately after entrance into ICU after LT if respiratory and circulatory stability is reached (noradrenaline < 1 µg/kgBW/min and FiO_2 < 0,6). The application of the trial medication must

Table 1 Criteria for inclusion and exclusion of patients

Inclusion criteria	Exclusion criteria
Full-size liver transplantation	Split liver transplantation or living donor related liver transplantation
Informed consent of the patient or legal representative	Participation on other clinical trials 30 days prior to randomization
Age ≥ 18 years	Retransplantation or multivisceral transplantation
	Respiratory and/or circulatory instability (noradrenaline > 1µg/kgBW/min and $FiO_2 > 0,6$)
	Conditions in which bleeding complications may be expected from the effect of Iloprost on platelets
	Known allergy or intolerance against trial medication, tacrolimus, mycophenolat mofetil, basiliximab or corticosteroids
	Severe coronary artery disease or unstable angina pectoris
	Myocardial infarction within the past 6 months prior to randomization
	Acute or chronic heart failure (NYHA II-IV)
	Cardiac arrhythmias relevant for the prognosis
	Suspected pulmonary artery congestion
	Women of child-bearing potential except women with the following criteria:
	○ post menopausal
	○ sterilization 86 weeks after bilateral ovarectomy
	○ using an effective method of contraception during the trial
	○ sexual abstinence or vasectomised partner
	Pregnancy/lactation

start at the latest within the first three hours after graft reperfusion.

The trial medication will be administered continuously over a period of seven days intravenously with an infusion pump. The dosage will be body weight adapted (1 ng/kgBW/min).

During LT a marked decrease in systemic blood pressure following liver reperfusion is frequently observed [22]. This could be aggravated by iloprost due to its vasodilatatory effect. In our pilot study, clear hemodynamic alterations under iloprost application were not observed. But we recorded a higher number of pulmonary complications i.e. pleural effusion or respiratory impairment. This might be explained by a PGI_2 induced increased intrapulmonary shunt fraction [23]. Therefore, the trial medication should be reduced in patients, who present with bleeding

complications, respiratory disturbances and/or appearance of hypotension episodes.

The immunosuppressive treatment will be standardized for both groups to minimize the effects of different immunosuppressive treatment within this trial. The trial-related immunosuppression is based on retard release Tacrolimus (Advagraf®) in combination with Basiliximab (Simulect®) and Mycophenolate Mofetil. Corticosteroids might be given only as perioperative intravenously bolus.

Study schedule

A schematic view illustrates the Figure 1. All patients or their legal representatives must give written informed consent to participate. The screening visit is defined as assessments made after definition of need for transplantation to confirm eligibility of a particular patient for entry into this trial. During the screening the following assessments will be performed: Patient information, written informed consent, demographic data of the recipient, check for inclusion and exclusion criteria, especially for existing cardiac and pulmonary diseases.

The baseline visit starts after acceptance of the donor organ. During the baseline the following assessments will be made: concomitant medication, non-drug therapies (renal replacement therapy or liver dialysis), the current baseline data of the recipient (height, weight, lab-MELD etc.), donor criteria (age, height, weight, BMI, cause of death, virology data etc. - all data can be obtained from the Eurotransplant donor protocol) and the key laboratory data of the recipient.

During the backtable preparation, a wedge biopsy of the donor liver will be performed. After reperfusion of the graft (after finishing the bile duct anastomosis), a further liver biopsy will be done. After entrance to the ICU, a checking for circulatory and respiratory stability (noradrenaline < 1 µg/kgBW/min and $FiO_2 < 0,6$) with assessment of catecholamines, mean arterial pressure, heart rate, pulmonary disturbances (blood-gas analysis, FiO_2, PEEP, arterial oxygen saturation, pO_2, pCO_2) is necessary before randomization of eligible patients. After that, the trial medication will be started. For patients not fulfilling the post-LT randomization criteria of circulatory and respiratory stability, the trial is terminated.

In the treatment period, the patients receive the trial medication continuously for seven days. During this period, the following procedures should be performed daily: check for circulatory and respiratory stability, clotting factor substitution (FFP, PPSB or other coagulation factor substrates), infections, appearance of adverse events, concomitant medication, non-drug therapies, liver dialysis, renal replacement therapy, number of applicated packed red cells, the blood chemistry and ultrasound of the graft to assess quality of liver parenchyma and perfusion. In cases of an

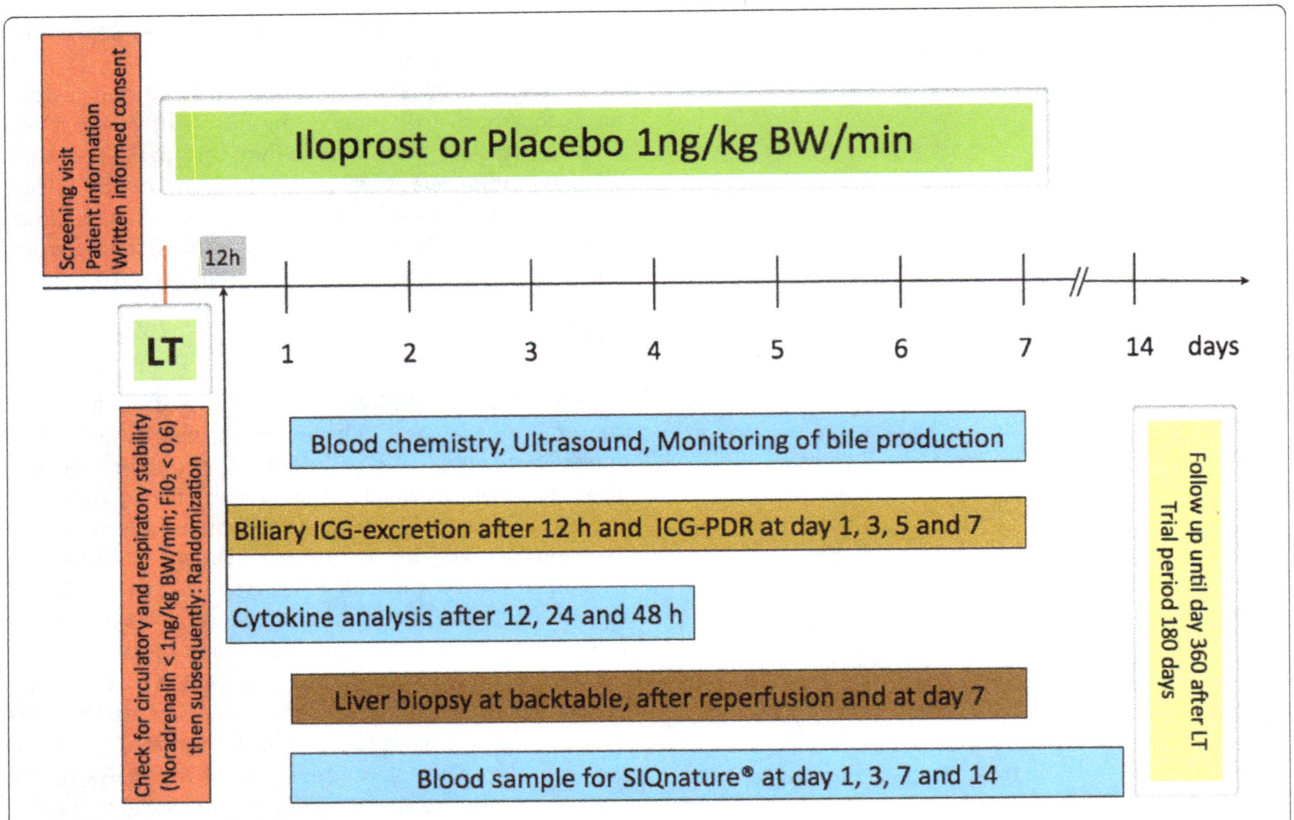

Figure 1 Treatment schedule.

inserted T-tube (or similar) the daily bile production is monitored until the tube is clamped for the first time or at maximum up to day 7 after randomization. An optional measurement of the ICG-PDR with the LiMON-Technology (PULSION Medical Systems AG, Munich, Germany) will be performed.

The blood samples for the cytokine analysis are taken exactly 12 hours after reperfusion, at day 1 and at day 2 after randomization. Further blood samples for the SIQnature® – Test are taken on day 1, 3, 7 and 14 after randomization.

An ultrasound guided percutaneous liver biopsy is performed seven days after LT. In reasonable single cases the percutaneous liver biopsy may be abandoned if the biopsy leads to excessive endangerment of the patient or the graft.

Adverse events (AE) occurring after randomization will be assessed during the trial period up to day 180 after LT. Serious AEs will be managed according to the requirements of the German drug legislation.

Sample size calculation

The hypotheses to be proved for PDF as primary endpoint at a two-sided 0.05 significance level are:

H0: Incidence (PDF) Iloprost = Incidence (PDF) Placebo
HA: Incidence (PDF) Iloprost ≠ Incidence (PDF) Placebo

The PDF definition used for this trial was introduced by Olthoff et al. [19] and validated in a population of 297 liver transplant recipients in the United States who underwent transplantation in 2004-2005 at three centers. PDF incidence was 23.2%. We hypothesize that PDF incidence can be reduced by 50% in patients treated with iloprost compared to placebo (relative risk RR = 0.5). If, according to Olthoff, an incidence of 23% will be used as baseline incidence for the placebo group a two-sided Chi^2-test will have 80% power to detect the clinically relevant relative risk reduction of 50% when the sample size in each group is 169 (nQuery Advisor 6.01). If the baseline incidence of PDF will be 40% as observed in the pilot study on the basis of the Olthoff definition the power will be 98% to detect the postulated effect of RR = 0.5 for the same sample size of 169 in each group. Taking into account a post-randomization dropout rate for primary endpoint data of 5% a total of 356 patients should be randomized.

Statistical analysis

Data will be analyzed for the Clinical Study Report to EC and the regulatory authority when data from the first 180 days post-LT from all patients are declared complete and accurate (end of trial). A follow-up analysis will be performed after all patients complete the follow-up period of 12 months post-LT.

The intention-to-treat (ITT) population as the primary analysis data set includes all randomized patients receiving at least one dose of trial medication. Primary and secondary efficacy data will be analyzed by randomized treatment assignment. The per-protocol (PP) population includes all randomized patients who are most compliant with the protocol. Included patients receive at least 80% of planned trial medication. They complete the study without major protocol deviations. Major protocol deviations will be identified and assignment to PP population will be done at the blind review prior to the 180-day data base lock. The safety analysis population will include all patients who receive at least one dose of trial medication. Safety data will be analyzed by the treatment assignment actually received.

For primary endpoint, the treatment effect will be estimated as relative risk and odds ratio with 95% confidence interval (CI) and will be tested by Chi^2-test. Analysis of PDF will be possibly adjusted for centre by logistic regression with random effects. To evaluate the robustness of results the analysis is repeated for the PP-population. In explorative analyses the treatment effect will be further adjusted to known prognostic donor criteria (donor age and BMI, donor serum peak sodium, cold and warm ischemia time) within a logistic regression model possibly with random center effects.

The secondary endpoint analyses will be performed in the ITT population. Incidence of events by treatment group and relative risks with 95% CI will be estimated for occurrence of any infection, initial non-function, clotting factor-substitution, renal replacement therapy and biliary complications. The Chi^2-test will be used for statistical testing. Length of ICU and hospital stay will be described by quartiles, means and SD. Hodge-Lehmann estimates with 95% CI will be calculated as measure of mean differences, Mann-Whitney U-test is used for significance testing. Rates of graft or patient survival will be estimated by the Kaplan-Meier method at pre-specified time points. Kaplan-Meier curves will be compared by the log-rank test. The hazard ratio with 95% CI is estimated by the Cox regression model assuming proportional hazards. The course of laboratory data over time will be analyzed by linear mixed models using raw or transformed data. Change in SOFA-score will be analyzed by two-sample t-test. Patients with missing secondary endpoint data will be excluded from the respective analysis. There is no interim analysis planned for efficacy. Annual safety reports will be generated for the German Competent Authority and the Data Management and Safety Board.

Ethical and legal aspects

Sponsor of this investigator-initiated trial is the Friedrich Schiller University Jena. The procedures set out in the trial protocol are designed to ensure that all persons involved in the trial abide by ICH-GCP guideline, the ethical principles described in the applicable version of the Declaration of Helsinki and the German drug legislation. The trial was approved by the ethics committee of the Friedrich Schiller University Jena, Faculty of Medicine and the German Competent Authority (BfArM) (EudraCT-Number: 2010-022660-12). The study is registered at the German Clinical Trials Register (DRKS00003514) and in the Current Controlled Trial Register (ISRCTN12622749).

Responsibilities

Coordinating investigator: Prof. Dr. Utz Settmacher, Head of the Department of General, Visceral and Vascular Surgery, Jena University Hospital, Germany.

Trial statistician: Dr. Heike Hoyer, Institute of Medical Statistics, Information Sciences and Documentation, Jena University Hospital, Germany.

Project Management: Department of General, Visceral and Vascular Surgery, Center for Clinical Studies, Jena University Hospital, Germany.

Clinical monitoring, safety and data management: Coordination Centre for Clinical Trials (KKS), University Halle, Germany.

Discussion

Due to the shortage of donor organs, transplant centers are forced to accept so-called marginal organs. Thus, there is a significant interest in the development of new strategies to prevent graft dysfunction and early graft loss. Apart from technical complications (vascular and biliary), acute or chronic rejection, PDF accounts for the majority of indications for re-transplantation [24]. The cause of graft dysfunction is multi-factorial, but IRI plays an important role as being characterized by a severe impairment of organ microcirculation [25]. In several experimental models, prostaglandins (PG) protected the liver from severe damage induced by ischemia and reperfusion [26-29]. Several authors reported a significant decrease of liver enzyme levels after application of PG and a favorable clinical course [30,31]. Nevertheless, its prophylactic administration after LT is still a subject of discussion, because the investigators did not identify a beneficial effect on graft function itself [32,33].

The aim of our study is the investigation of the impact of continuous intravenous administration of PGI_2 analogue iloprost after LT in order to prevent graft dysfunction.

In order to define the specific impact of PGI_2 analogue iloprost on liver graft function, this multi-center study including a larger number of patients and will enable reliable risk stratification according to the MELD score or extended donor criteria. This upcoming trial will be under the patronage of the German Transplantation Society.

Abbreviations
AE: Adverse event; ALAT: Alanin-amino-transferase; ASAT: Aspartat-amino-transferase; BMI: Body mass index; BW: Body weight; EC: Ethics committee; FFP: Fresh frozen plasma; FiO_2: Fraction of inspiratory oxygen; GCP: Good clinical practice; HAT: Hepatic artery thrombosis; ICG: Indocyanine green; ICU: Intensive care unit; INF: Initial non-function; INR: International normalized ratio; IRI: Ischemia/reperfusion injury; ITT: Intention-to-treat; lab-MELD: Laboratory based model for end-stage liver disease; LT: Liver transplantation; pCO_2: Carbon dioxide partial pressure; PDF: Primary graft dysfunction; PDR: Plasma disappearance rate; PEEP: Positive endexpiratory pressure; PG: Prostaglandin/-s; pO_2: Oxygene partial pressure; RR: Relative risk; SIRS: Systemic inflammatory response syndrome; SOFA: Sequential organ failure assessment.

Competing interests
EB received payment for a conference lecture and travel grants from Astellas Pharma GmbH, Munich, Germany. FR received payment for a conference lecture from BAYER Vital GmbH, Leverkusen, Germany. FR and US received travel grants from Astellas Pharma GmbH, Munich, Germany. None of the authors holds any stocks or shares in the funding organizations. There are no patent issues. All authors declare that they have no financial or non-financial competing interests.

Authors' contributions
All authors contributed to the accomplishment of this manuscript. EB wrote the manuscript. EB, FR, MB and HH made substantial contributions to conception and design of the study protocol. EB, FR, MB, KJ and HH wrote the study protocol and revised the manuscript. HH provided the statistical design of the study. US participated in the design and coordination of the trial. All authors read and approved the manuscript.

Funding
Funding for this study is provided by the German Ministry of Education and Research (BMBF, FKZ:01E01002), the Astellas Pharma GmbH, Munich, Germany and the BAYER Vital GmbH, Leverkusen, Germany. They all have no role in the design of the trial and they are not in any way involved in collecting and analyzing data or interpreting of the trial results.

Author details
[1]Department of General, Visceral and Vascular Surgery, Jena University Hospital, Erlanger Allee 101, D-07740 Jena, Germany. [2]Institute of Medical Statistics, Information Sciences and Documentation, Jena, Germany. [3]Center for Clinical Studies, Jena, Germany. [4]Center for Sepsis Control and Care, Jena University Hospital, Friedrich Schiller University, Jena, Germany.

References
1. Schemmer P, et al: Extended donor criteria have no negative impact on early outcome after liver transplantation: a single-center multivariate analysis. Transplant Proc 2007, 39(2):529–534.
2. Pokorny H, et al: Organ survival after primary dysfunction of liver grafts in clinical orthotopic liver transplantation. Transpl Int 2000, 13(Suppl 1):S154–S157.
3. Ploeg RJ, et al: Risk factors for primary dysfunction after liver transplantation–a multivariate analysis. Transplantation 1993, 55(4):807–813.
4. Deschenes M, et al: Early allograft dysfunction after liver transplantation: a definition and predictors of outcome. National Institute of Diabetes and Digestive and Kidney Diseases Liver Transplantation Database. Transplantation 1998, 66(3):302–310.
5. Chen H, et al: Multi-factor analysis of initial poor graft function after orthotopic liver transplantation. Hepatobiliary Pancreat Dis Int 2007, 6(2):141–146.
6. Johnson SR, et al: Primary nonfunction (PNF) in the MELD Era: an SRTR database analysis. Am J Transplant 2007, 7(4):1003–1009.

7. Nanashima A, et al: Analysis of initial poor graft function after orthotopic liver transplantation: experience of an australian single liver transplantation center. Transplant Proc 2002, 34(4):1231–1235.
8. Fondevila C, Busuttil RW, Kupiec-Weglinski JW: Hepatic ischemia/reperfusion injury–a fresh look. Exp Mol Pathol 2003, 74(2):86–93.
9. Tauber S, Menger MD, Lehr H-A: Microvascular in vivo assessment of reperfusion injury: significance of prostaglandin E1 and I2 in postischemic "no-reflow" and "reflow-paradox". J Surg Res 2004, 120(1):1–11.
10. Pokorny H, et al: Influence of cumulative number of marginal donor criteria on primary organ dysfunction in liver recipients. Clin Transplant 2005, 19(4):532–536.
11. Lee SH, Rubin LJ: Current treatment strategies for pulmonary arterial hypertension. J Intern Med 2005, 258(3):199–215.
12. Beirne C, Hynes N, Sultan S: Six years' experience with prostaglandin I2 infusion in elective open repair of abdominal aortic aneurysm: a parallel group observational study in a tertiary referral vascular center. Ann Vasc Surg 2008, 22(6):750–755.
13. de Donato G, et al: The ILAILL study: iloprost as adjuvant to surgery for acute ischemia of lower limbs: a randomized, placebo-controlled, double-blind study by the italian society for vascular and endovascular surgery. Ann Surg 2006, 244(2):185–193.
14. Barthel E, et al: Impact of stable PGI(2) analog iloprost on early graft viability after liver transplantation: a pilot study. Clin Transplant 2012, 26(1):E38–E47.
15. Haller GW, et al: Factors relevant to the development of primary dysfunction in liver allografts. Transplant Proc 1995, 27(1):1192.
16. Heise M, et al: A survival-based scoring-system for initial graft function following orthotopic liver transplantation. Transpl Int 2003, 16(11):794–800.
17. Briceno J, et al: Influence of marginal donors on liver preservation injury. Transplantation 2002, 74(4):522–526.
18. Riediger C, et al: T-Tube or no T-tube in the reconstruction of the biliary tract during orthotopic liver transplantation: systematic review and meta-analysis. Liver Transpl 2010, 16(6):705–717.
19. Olthoff KM, et al: Validation of a current definition of early allograft dysfunction in liver transplant recipients and analysis of risk factors. Liver Transpl 2010, 16(8):943–949.
20. Cavalcanti AB, et al: Prostaglandins for adult liver transplanted patients. Cochrane Database Syst Rev 2011, 11:CD006006.
21. Rubin RH: The direct and indirect effects of infection in liver transplantation: pathogenesis, impact, and clinical management. Curr Clin Top Infect Dis 2002, 22:125–154.
22. Paugam-Burtz C, et al: Postreperfusion syndrome during liver transplantation for cirrhosis: outcome and predictors. Liver Transpl 2009, 15(5):522–529.
23. Honkonen EL, et al: Dopexamine unloads the impaired right ventricle better than iloprost, a prostacyclin analog, after coronary artery surgery. J Cardiothorac Vasc Anesth 1998, 12(6):647–653.
24. Biggins SW, et al: Retransplantation for hepatic allograft failure: prognostic modeling and ethical considerations. Liver Transpl 2002, 8(4):313–322.
25. Kurokawa T, et al: Effects of prostaglandin E1 on the recovery of ischemia-induced liver mitochondrial dysfunction in rats with cirrhosis. Scand J Gastroenterol 1991, 26(3):269–274.
26. Klein M, et al: Preconditioning of donor livers with prostaglandin I2 before retrieval decreases hepatocellular ischemia-reperfusion injury. Transplantation 1999, 67(8):1128–1132.
27. Natori S, et al: Prostaglandin E1 protects against ischemia-reperfusion injury of the liver by inhibition of neutrophil adherence to endothelial cells. Transplantation 1997, 64(11):1514–1520.
28. Totsuka E, et al: Attenuation of ischemic liver injury by prostaglandin E1 analogue, misoprostol, and prostaglandin I2 analogue, OP-41483. J Am Coll Surg 1998, 187(3):276–286.
29. Neumann UP, et al: Reduction of reperfusion injury with prostacyclin I2 after liver transplantation. Transplant Proc 1999, 31(1–2):1029–1030.

30. Kornberg A, *et al*: Impact of selective prostaglandin E1 treatment on graft perfusion and function after liver transplantation. *Hepatogastroenterology* 2004, **51**(56):526–531.
31. Giostra E, *et al*: Prophylactic administration of prostaglandin E1 in liver transplantation: results of a pilot trial. *Transplant Proc* 1997, **29**(5):2381–2384.
32. Henley KS, *et al*: A double-blind, randomized, placebo-controlled trial of prostaglandin E1 in liver transplantation. *Hepatology* 1995, **21**(2):366–372.
33. Klein AS, *et al*: Prostaglandin E1 administration following orthotopic liver transplantation: a randomized prospective multicenter trial. *Gastroenterology* 1996, **111**(3):710–715.

26

Determining the use of prophylactic antibiotics in breast cancer surgeries: a survey of practice

Sergio A Acuna[1,5†], Fernando A Angarita[1,5,6†], Jaime Escallon[2,3], Mauricio Tawil[1,4] and Lilian Torregrosa[1,4*]

Abstract

Background: Prophylactic antibiotics (PAs) are beneficial to breast cancer patients undergoing surgery because they prevent surgical site infection (SSI), but limited information regarding their use has been published. This study aims to determine the use of PAs prior to breast cancer surgery amongst breast surgeons in Colombia.

Methods: An online survey was distributed amongst the breast surgeon members of the Colombian Association of Mastology, the only breast surgery society of Colombia. The scope of the questions included demographics, clinical practice characteristics, PA prescription characteristics, and the use of PAs in common breast surgical procedures.

Results: The survey was distributed amongst eighty-eight breast surgeons of whom forty-seven responded (response rate: 53.4%). Forty surgeons (85.1%) reported using PAs prior to surgery of which >60% used PAs during mastectomy, axillary lymph node dissection, and/or breast reconstruction. Surgeons reported they targeted the use of PAs in cases in which patients had any of the following SSI risk factors: diabetes mellitus, drains *in situ*, obesity, and neoadjuvant therapy. The distribution of the self-reported PA dosing regimens was as follows: single pre-operative fixed-dose (27.7%), single preoperative dose followed by a second dose if the surgery was prolonged (44.7%), single preoperative dose followed by one or more postoperative doses for >24 hours (10.6%), and single preoperative weight-adjusted dose (2.1%).

Conclusion: Although this group of breast surgeons is aware of the importance of PAs in breast cancer surgery there is a discrepancy in how they use it, specifically with regards to prescription and timeliness of drug administration. Our findings call for targeted quality-improvement initiatives, such as standardized national guidelines, which can provide sufficient evidence for all stakeholders and therefore facilitate best practice medicine for breast cancer surgery.

Keywords: Breast surgery, Surgical site infection, Prophylactic antibiotic

Background

Surgical site infection (SSI) of the breast is a source of postoperative complications that are not just limited to prolonged hospital stay and increased hospital costs, but also includes predisposing patients to additional medical interventions (e.g.: surgical debridement or abscess draining), poor aesthetic results, and psychological trauma [1-4]. More importantly SSI can delay adjuvant

* Correspondence: lilian.torregrosa@javeriana.edu.co
†Equal contributors
[1]Department of Surgery, Hospital Universitario San Ignacio, Pontificia Universidad Javeriana, Bogotá, Colombia
[4]Breast and Soft Tissue Clinic, Centro Javeriano de Oncología, Bogotá, Colombia
Full list of author information is available at the end of the article

treatment [2], which can have a detrimental effect on a patient's overall survival [5,6]. Certainly preventing SSIs in breast cancer patients is a necessary step for assuring high-quality surgical treatment.

In order to reduce SSI rates, the general recommendation is to give prophylactic antibiotics (PAs) one hour before starting surgery and to suspend them within the first twenty-four hours post-surgery [7]. Historically, using PAs in breast surgery was thought to be unnecessary [8] given that the breast is a peripheral soft tissue organ with no direct connection to any major body cavity or visceral structure [9] and that breast surgeries are typically classified as clean surgical procedures. Despite this premise, breast cancer surgery has been reported to have higher SSI rates (1.9 - 50%) than other clean surgical procedures [1,5,6,10-23]. Furthermore there are various studies in the indexed literature describing how PAs can decrease SSI rates in this surgical procedure [7]. Even with this evidence there is still no general consensus in the literature [7] therefore, evaluating current practice patterns amongst breast surgeons can be used to build a framework to establish best practice guidelines at a national level. This study aims to determine the use of PAs prior to breast cancer surgery amongst specialists in Colombia.

Methods

Approval from the research ethics board at Hospital Universitario San Ignacio in Bogota, Colombia was obtained prior to starting this study. An online survey was developed in Spanish using a commercial, Internet-based service (Encuesta Fácil, S.L.). The survey consisted of eleven questions (Table 1) that included the following topics: demographics, clinical practice characteristics, and the use of PA in common breast surgical procedures. The questions were developed in Spanish, but for the purpose of this publication they are provided in English.

Before distributing the survey it was validated for internal congruency and user friendliness by conducting

a small pilot study with five breast surgeons, which were not included in the final data analysis of this study. The survey was distributed between November 2009 and March 2010 exclusively amongst breast surgeons in Colombia. A list of names and contact information (electronic mail) was obtained from the national breast surgery society's database [Asociación Colombiana de Mastología (English: Colombian Association of Mastology)].

Respondents were allowed to modify their answers to previous questions, but were unable to edit or resubmit the survey once it was completed. Answers were automatically kept anonymous. A reminder was sent out to those who had not responded two and four months after the survey was originally distributed. No rewards or incentives were given for completion of this survey. Descriptive statistical analysis was carried out using means, medians, standard deviations, and ranges using SPSS 19.0 (IBM, Chicago, IL).

Results

Surveys were distributed amongst all the eighty-eight breast surgeon members of the Colombian Association of Masology of which forty-seven completed the whole survey (response rate: 53.4%). Demographic information

Table 1 Translated survey questions

Number	Question	Possible answer(s)
1	In what city do you practice?	*Open answer.*
2	What is your specialty?	*Choose one of the following:* breast surgery, surgical oncology, general surgery, gynecology/obstetrics, or plastic surgery.
3	How many years of practice do you have in breast surgery?	*Open answer.*
4	What type of practice do you have?	*Choose one of the following:* Private or private/academic
5	What percentage of your cases corresponds to breast surgery?	*Choose one of the following:* <25%, 25 – 49%, 50 – 75%, or >75%.
6	What is your monthly breast surgery case load?	*Choose one of the following:*<5 cases/month, 5 – 15 cases/month, 16 – 25 cases/month, or >25 cases/month.
7	Indicate from the following list of breast surgical procedures in which cases you administer prophylactic antibiotic:	*Select as many as are appropriate:* breast conserving surgery, wire localized excision, mastectomy, axillary lymph node dissection, sentinel lymph node biopsy, reconstruction with flap, reconstruction with implant, terminal conduct excision, and benign lesion excision.
8	Do you use prophylactic antibiotic in all your breast surgeries?	*Choose one of the following:* yes or no.
9	What prophylactic antibiotic do you use?	*Open answer.*
10	If you use prophylactic antibiotic, how do you administer it?	*Choose one of the following:* single pre-operative fixed-dose, single preoperative fixed dose followed by a second fixed dose if the surgery is prolonged, single preoperative fixed dose followed by one or more postoperative fixed doses for >24 hours, or single preoperative weight-adjusted dose.
11	If you do not administer routine prophylactic antibiotic, in what cases do you use it?	*Select as many as are appropriate:* older age, obesity, cancer, smoking, diabetes mellitus, active skin disease, neoadjuvant therapy, use of drains *in situ*, and surgical re-intervention.

is described in Table 2. All of the surgeons reported that they lived in major urban areas in Colombia. Furthermore, 76.6% of the respondents practiced in academic hospital settings. Approximately forty percent of surgeons reported that they performed between 5 and 15 breast surgeries per month.

Only forty surgeons (85.1%) reported that they administered a PA before breast surgeries. The self-reported PA dosing regimens used by this group of surgeons was as follows: single pre-operative fixed-dose (27.7%), single preoperative fixed dose followed by a second fixed dose if the surgery was prolonged (44.7%), single preoperative fixed dose followed by one or more postoperative fixed doses for >24 hours (10.6%), and single preoperative weight-adjusted dose (2.1%). The antibiotic of choice was unanimously cefazolin.

Surgeons who reported using PAs were then asked about the specific breast surgical procedure in which they used them. The distribution of these surgical procedures is shown in Figure 1. The most common procedures in which PAs were administered included breast reconstruction with implant (87.2%) or flap (80.9%), mastectomy (68.1%), and axillary lymph node dissection (61.7%). Nineteen surgeons (40.4%) reported that they used PAs routinely in all their breast surgeries and the remaining twenty-eight surgeons (59.6%) stated that they used targeted prophylaxis while taking into consideration various,

Table 2 Demographic data of survey respondents

Characteristic	
Type of specialty, N (%)	
Breast surgery	23 (48.9)
Surgical oncology	5 (10.6)
General surgery	6 (12.8)
Plastic surgery	13 (27.7)
Years of practice in breast surgery, mean ± SD (range)	13.2 ± 9.9 (1–45)
Type of practice, N (%)	
Private	11 (23.4)
Private/academic	36 (76.6)
Percentage of cases corresponding to breast surgery, N (%)	
<25	9 (19.1)
25 – 49	9 (19.1)
50 – 75	4 (8.5)
>75	25 (53.2)
Volume of breast surgeries per month, N (%)	
<5 cases	2 (4.3)
5 – 15 cases	19 (40.4)
16 – 25 cases	9 (19.1)
>25 cases	17 (36.2)

specific patient characteristics. The distribution of these patient characteristics is outlined in Figure 2.

Discussion

Appropriately selected and timely prophylactic antimicrobial agents are proven to decrease SSI rates in breast cancer patients undergoing surgical treatment [22-24]. Surgeons may hesitate to follow this recommendation because uncontrolled and injudicious use of PAs may lead to antibiotic resistance [25], adverse effects (e.g.: *Clostridium difficile* infection) [26], and increase medical costs [27] because they decrease SSI symptoms until after the patient has been discharged [28]. Nevertheless, the benefits related to this measure outweigh the sporadic number of complications.

Our study shows that the majority of breast surgeons that responded to this survey use some type of PA in breast cancer patients before surgery whether it is administered routinely in all patients or selectively when dealing with specific high-risk variables associated with SSI. Nonetheless, among those surgeons that reported using PAs the practice pattern is heterogeneous. In the literature there is evidence that this disparity is also common amongst surgeons from other countries. For example, a British survey reported that up to 33% of surgeons who performed wide local excisions, mastectomies and sentinel lymph node biopsy used PAs [29]. Another study carried out in Spain reported that 52% of hospitals used PAs in breast surgery [30] although a more recent multi-centric Spanish study revealed that the rate of use of PAs was much higher (97.81%) [31]. These results must be analyzed cautiously because breast cancer surgeries are not always carried out by breast surgeons or other sub-specialized surgeons so there may be a bias in the way the information is gathered.

Studies have evaluated the impact of PAs, but have showed mixed results. Two studies reported a reduction in SSI rates that ranged from 33 to 88% after using cefotaxime and azithromycin [1,22]. Other researchers have not found any significant reduction in SSI rates [23,28,32]. Nonetheless, a Cochrane review concluded that using preoperative antibiotics significantly reduces the risk of SSI (pooled risk ratio 0.71, 95% confidence interval 0.53-0.94) in patients undergoing surgery for breast cancer when compared with placebo or no treatment [7]. This type of prophylactic intervention is reported to potentially benefit high-risk patients especially when they have any of the following risk factors: neoadjuvant chemotherapy, immediate breast reconstruction, blood transfusion, obesity, and smoking [24].

In our study 80% of surgeons reported that they used PAs in patients undergoing breast reconstruction. In a survey of the members of the American Society of Plastic Surgeons the use of PAs was slightly higher (>90%)

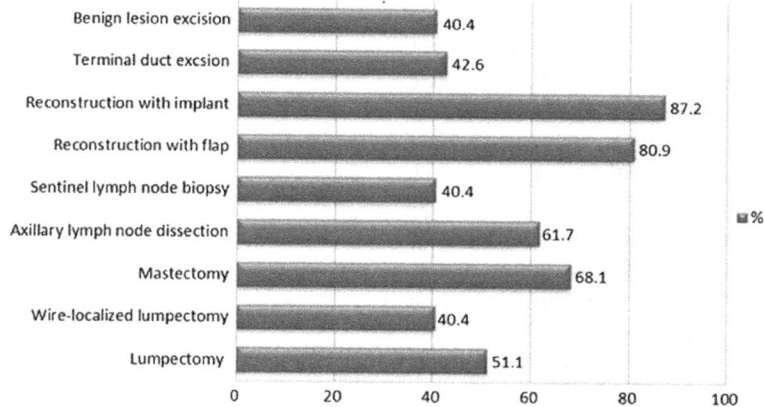

Figure 1 Common breast surgical procedures in which breast surgeons use prophylactic antibiotics. The most common surgical procedures in which surgeons reported they used PAs were breast reconstruction with implant or flap, mastectomy, and axillary lymph node dissection.

[33]. The authors stated that plastic surgeons use PAs in patients undergoing any type of cosmetic or reconstructive breast surgery because a higher rate of SSI would exist if they were not used and also because these types of surgeries *per se* increase the risk of SSI as they have a longer length of duration and use foreign bodies (e.g.: implants). This concept certainly goes along with the recommendation made by the Hospital Infection Control Practices Advisory Committee of the U.S. Centers for Disease Control and Prevention in which clean procedures require antibiotic prophylaxis when implanting foreign material and in any case where an SSI may pose a catastrophic risk [34].

In addition to the standard SSI risk factors inherent to any patient (e.g.: obesity, history of smoking, diabetes, etc.) [34], breast cancer surgery patients have additional, specific risk factors (e.g.: neoadjuvant chemotherapy, re-operations, use of foreign bodies such as implants and drains *in situ*, and post-operative seroma) [14] that increase their susceptibility to post-operative infections.

As a result of this, breast cancer patients exceed the 1.5% SSI rate suggested for elective clean surgery [35,36]. Accordingly, at least 40% of the breast surgeons within our study reported that they administered PAs specifically when their patients had any of these SSI risk factors.

The details of drug choices amongst surveyed surgeons are in line with current recommendations. PAs are typically directed against gram-positive bacteria that comprise normal skin flora (staphylococci and streptococci). Ng *et al.* reported that British surgeons tend to use amoxicillin-clavulonic acid more often than cephalosporins [29]; however at many institutions cefazolin is preferred. For example, Codina *et al.* reported that the majority (36%) of hospitals in Spain prefer cefazolin [30]. Studies evaluating the effectiveness of cephalosporins to reduce breast surgery SSI have had mixed results [20,32,37]. In the past, most breast surgery SSIs were caused by staphylococci and streptococci [5,12,13], but recent data suggests that there are significant rates

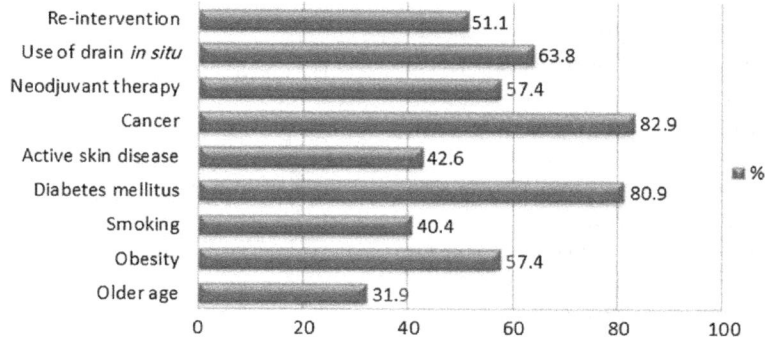

Figure 2 Breast cancer patient characteristics reported to be taken into consideration for targeted prophylactic antibiotic use in breast cancer surgery. Surgeons who reported using targeted prophylaxis considered the following patient characteristics to be the most important ones when considering who should receive PAs: cancer, diabetes mellitus, use of drain *in situ*, neoadjuvant therapy, and surgical re-intervention.

(30–66.2%) of non-staphylococcal infections [35-39]. Additionally, 63% of the staphylococcal isolates have been documented to be resistant to at least one antibiotic [39]. Breast surgeons should be aware of this fact and monitor patients with complicated wounds that do not respond to standardized treatments. In the future there may be a need to change the PAs we are currently using.

Our survey brings to light a couple of issues regarding standardized prescription practices that require improvement in the clinical practice of breast surgeons in Colombia. In this survey only 2.1% of the breast surgeons answered that they actually weight-adjust their preoperative dosing. Although cefazolin is an antibiotic with prolonged half-life, its ability to prevent SSI is significantly affected by sub-optimal dosing therefore in order to assure optimal drug concentrations appropriate weight adjusted dosing and re-dosing is mandatory. On another note, the self-reported timeliness of antibiotic administration is compliant with current recommendations [40] in 89.4% of the breast surgeons we surveyed. Despite the fact that the majority of breast surgeons in this cohort understand the essential role of when and how long PAs should be administered to actually prevent SSIs, there are a significant number of surgeons that reported they extended the use of PAs beyond the first 24 hours post-surgery exclusively with the intention to reduce the risk of SSI. A similar practice pattern has been reported in Spain in which 9% of surveyed hospitals self-reported that their surgeons prolonged the use of PAs for over 24 hours when performing breast surgeries [30]. Randomized studies have shown that administering PAs for only 24 hours is enough to prevent SSIs and that prolonging its use does not provide any additional benefit [41], but instead increases the risk of generating resistant bacterial strains [42], nosocomial infection [42], diarrhea [26], higher health-care costs [27], and increased work load for health-care staff [43].

Conclusion

SSIs, which are commonly associated with breast cancer surgery, require extreme attention amongst breast surgeons because they can take several specific actions to decrease the incidence. One of the preventative measures is appropriately administering PAs. Our study shows that although our cohort of breast surgeons is aware of their importance, variation exists in terms of how PAs are prescribed, specifically with regards to dosing and timeliness. Findings such as the ones described in this study call for the development of targeted quality-improvement initiatives, such as guidelines, that can ensure best practice medicine for breast cancer surgery in Colombia.

Competing interests
The authors declare that they have no competing interests.

Authors' contributions
FAA conceived the study, carried out the survey, participated in the statistical and data analysis and the design of the study, and helped to draft the manuscript. SAA carried out the survey, participated in the data analysis and the design of the study, and helped to draft the manuscript. JE participated in data analysis and helped to draft the manuscript. MT participated in the design of the study and data analysis and helped to draft the manuscript. LT conceived the study, carried out the survey, participated in its design and was the main coordinator. All authors read and approved the final manuscript.

Acknowledgements
The authors would like to thank the Asociación Colombiana de Mastología for providing the contact information of their members as well all of those who responded the questionnaire. The authors would also like to thank Kathryn Ottolino-Perry for editing this manuscript.

Author details
[1]Department of Surgery, Hospital Universitario San Ignacio, Pontificia Universidad Javeriana, Bogotá, Colombia. [2]Department of Surgery, University of Toronto, Toronto, ON, Canada. [3]Department of Surgical Oncology, Princess Margaret Hospital, Toronto, ON, Canada. [4]Breast and Soft Tissue Clinic, Centro Javeriano de Oncología, Bogotá, Colombia. [5]Current address: Division of Experimental Therapeutics, Toronto General Research Institute, University Health Network, Toronto, ON, Canada. [6]Current address: Institute of Medical Science, University of Toronto, Toronto, ON, Canada.

References
1. D'Amico DF, Parimbelli P, Ruffolo C: Antibiotic prophylaxis in clean surgery: breast surgery and hernia repair. J Chemother 2001, 13 Spec No 1:108–111.
2. Coello R, Glenister H, Fereres J, Bartlett C, Leigh D, Sedgwick J, Cooke EM: The cost of infection in surgical patients: a case–control study. J Hosp Infect 1993, 25:239–250.
3. Tejirian T, DiFronzo LA, Haigh PI: Antibiotic prophylaxis for preventing wound infection after breast surgery: a systematic review and metaanalysis. J Am Coll Surg 2006, 203:729–734.
4. Smyth ET, Emmerson AM: Surgical site infection surveillance. J Hosp Infect 2000, 45:173–184.
5. Rotstein C, Ferguson R, Cummings KM, Piedmonte MR, Lucey J, Banish A: Determinants of clean surgical wound infections for breast procedures at an oncology center. Infect Control Hosp Epidemiol 1992, 13:207–214.
6. Recht A, Come SE, Henderson IC, Gelman RS, Silver B, Hayes DF, Shulman LN, Harris JR: The sequencing of chemotherapy and radiation therapy after conservative surgery for early-stage breast cancer. N Engl J Med 1996, 334:1356–1361.
7. Bunn F, Jones DJ, Bell-Syer S: Prophylactic antibiotics to prevent surgical site infection after breast cancer surgery. Cochrane Database Syst Rev 2012, 1:CD005360.
8. Sheridan RL, Tompkins RG, Burke JF: Prophylactic antibiotics and their role in the prevention of surgical wound infection. Adv Surg 1994, 27:43–65.
9. Vitug AF, Newman LA: Complications in breast surgery. Surg Clin North Am 2007, 87:431–451. x.
10. Hall JC, Hall JL: Antibiotic prophylaxis for patients undergoing breast surgery. J Hosp Infect 2000, 46:165–170.
11. Lipshy KA, Neifeld JP, Boyle RM, Frable WJ, Ronan S, Lotfi P, Bear HD, Horsley JS III, Lawrence W Jr: Complications of mastectomy and their relationship to biopsy technique. Ann Surg Oncol 1996, 3:290–294.
12. Beatty JD, Robinson GV, Zaia JA, Benfield JR, Kemeny MM, Meguid MM, Riihimaki DU, Terz JJ, Lemmelin ME: A prospective analysis of nosocomial wound infection after mastectomy. Arch Surg 1983, 118:1421–1424.
13. Chen J, Gutkin Z, Bawnik J: Postoperative infections in breast surgery. J Hosp Infect 1991, 17:61–65.
14. Tran CL, Langer S, Broderick-Villa G, DiFronzo LA: Does reoperation predispose to postoperative wound infection in women undergoing operation for breast cancer? Am Surg 2003, 69:852–856.

15. Witt A, Yavuz D, Walchetseder C, Strohmer H, Kubista E: **Preoperative core needle biopsy as an independent risk factor for wound infection after breast surgery.** *Obstet Gynecol* 2003, **101**:745–750.
16. Wedgwood KR, Benson EA: **Non-tumour morbidity and mortality after modified radical mastectomy.** *Ann R Coll Surg Engl* 1992, **74**:314–317.
17. Barber GR, Miransky J, Brown AE, Coit DG, Lewis FM, Thaler HT, Kiehn TE, Armstrong D: **Direct observations of surgical wound infections at a comprehensive cancer center.** *Arch Surg* 1995, **130**:1042–1047.
18. Danforth DN Jr, Lippman ME, McDonald H, Bader J, Egan E, Lampert M, Steinberg SM, Swain SM: **Effect of preoperative chemotherapy on mastectomy for locally advanced breast cancer.** *Am Surg* 1990, **56**:6–11.
19. Badr el Din A, Coibion M, Guenier C, Nogaret JM, Lorent I, Van Houtte P, Tueni E, Mattheiem W: **Local postoperative morbidity following pre-operative irradiation in locally advanced breast cancer.** *Eur J Surg Oncol* 1989, **15**:486–489.
20. Thomas R, Alvino P, Cortino GR, Accard R, Rinaldo M, Pizzorusso M, Cesareo E, D'Aiuto G: **Long-acting versus short-acting cephalosporins for preoperative prophylaxis in breast surgery: A randomized double-blind trial involving 1,766 patients.** *Chemotherapy* 1999, **45**:217–223.
21. Canavese G, Catturich A, Vecchio C, Gipponi M, Tomei D, Sertoli MR, Repetto L, Badellino F: **Surgical complications related to peri-operative adjuvant chemotherapy in breast cancer. Results of a prospective, controlled, randomized clinical trial.** *Eur J Surg Oncol* 1997, **23**:10–12.
22. Platt R, Zaleznik DF, Hopkins CC, Dellinger EP, Karchmer AW, Bryan CS, Burke JF, Wikler MA, Marino SK, Holbrook KF, Tosteson TD, Segal MR: **Perioperative antibiotic prophylaxis for herniorrhaphy and breast surgery.** *N Engl J Med* 1990, **322**:153–160.
23. Vilar-Compte D, Rosales S, Hernandez-Mello N, Maafs E, Volkow P: **Surveillance, control, and prevention of surgical site infections in breast cancer surgery: a 5-year experience.** *Am J Infect Control* 2009, **37**:674–679.
24. Penel N, Yazdanpanah Y, Chauvet MP, Clisant S, Giard S, Neu JC, Lefebvre D, Fournier C, Bonneterre J: **Prevention of surgical site infection after breast cancer surgery by targeted prophylaxis antibiotic in patients at high risk of surgical site infection.** *J Surg Oncol* 2007, **96**:124–129.
25. Harbarth S, Samore MH, Lichtenberg D, Carmeli Y: **Prolonged antibiotic prophylaxis after cardiovascular surgery and its effect on surgical site infections and antimicrobial resistance.** *Circulation* 2000, **101**:2916–2921.
26. Jobe BA, Grasley A, Deveney KE, Deveney CW, Sheppard BC: **Clostridium difficile colitis: an increasing hospital-acquired illness.** *Am J Surg* 1995, **169**:480–483.
27. Namias N, Harvill S, Ball S, McKenney MG, Salomone JP, Civetta JM: **Cost and morbidity associated with antibiotic prophylaxis in the ICU.** *J Am Coll Surg* 1999, **188**:225–230.
28. Wagman LD, Tegtmeier B, Beatty JD, Kloth DD, Kokal WA, Riihimaki DU, Terz JJ: **A prospective, randomized double-blind study of the use of antibiotics at the time of mastectomy.** *Surg Gynecol Obstet* 1990, **170**:12–16.
29. Ng D, Trivedi PM, Sharma AK, Banerjee D: **Current use of antibiotic prophylaxis in breast surgery: a nationwide survey.** *Breast* 2007, **16**:68–72.
30. Codina C, Trilla A, Riera N, Tuset M, Carne X, Ribas J, Asenjo MA: **Perioperative antibiotic prophylaxis in Spanish hospitals: results of a questionnaire survey. Hospital Pharmacy Antimicrobial Prophylaxis Study Group.** *Infect Control Hosp Epidemiol* 1999, **20**:436–439.
31. Rodríguez-Caravaca G, de Las Casas-Camara G, Pita-Lopez MJ, Robustillo-Rodela A, Díaz-Agero C, Monge-Jodrá, Fereres J, Grupo de Trabajo INCLIMECC de la Comunidad de Madrid: **Preoperative preparation, antibiotic prophylaxis and surgical wound infection in breast surgery.** *Enferm Infecc Microbiol Clin* 2011, **29**:415–420.
32. Penel N, Fournier C, Giard S, Lefebvres D: **A prospective evaluation of antibiotic prophylaxis efficacy for breast cancer surgery following previous chemotherapy.** *Bull Cancer* 2004, **91**:445–448.
33. Hauck RM, Nogan S: **The Use of Prophylactic Antibiotics in Plastic Surgery: Update in 2010.** *Ann Plast Surg* 2011, : [Epub ahead of print].
34. Mangram AJ, Horan TC, Pearson ML, Silver LC, Jarvis WR: **Guideline for prevention of surgical site infection, 1999. Hospital Infection Control Practices Advisory Committee.** *Infect Control Hosp Epidemiol* 1999, **20**:250–278. quiz 279–280.
35. Vilar-Compte D, Jacquemin B, Robles-Vidal C, Volkow P: **Surgical site infections in breast surgery: case–control study.** *World J Surg* 2004, **28**:242–246.
36. Olsen MA, Lefta M, Dietz JR, Brandt KE, Aft R, Matthews R, Mayfield J, Fraser VJ: **Risk factors for surgical site infection after major breast operation.** *J Am Coll Surg* 2008, **207**:326–335.
37. Bertin ML, Crowe J, Gordon SM: **Determinants of surgical site infection after breast surgery.** *Am J Infect Control* 1998, **26**:61–65.
38. Felippe WA, Werneck GL, Santoro-Lopes G: **Surgical site infection among women discharged with a drain in situ after breast cancer surgery.** *World J Surg* 2007, **31**:2293–2299. discussion 2300–2301.
39. Throckmorton AD, Baddour LM, Hoskin TL, Boughey JC, Degnim AC: **Microbiology of surgical site infections complicating breast surgery.** *Surg Infect (Larchmt)* 2010, **11**:355–359.
40. Dellinger EP, Gross PA, Barrett TL, Krause PJ, Martone WJ, McGowan JE Jr, Sweet RL, Wenzel RP: **Quality standard for antimicrobial prophylaxis in surgical procedures. The Infectious Diseases Society of America.** *Infect Control Hosp Epidemiol* 1994, **15**:182–188.
41. McDonald AH, Cleland HJ, Leung M, Slattery PG: **Ring avulsion injuries.** *Aust N Z J Surg* 1999, **69**:514–516.
42. Goldmann DA, Weinstein RA, Wenzel RP, Tablan OC, Duma RJ, Gaynes RP, Schlosser J, Martone WJ: **Strategies to Prevent and Control the Emergence and Spread of Antimicrobial-Resistant Microorganisms in Hospitals. A challenge to hospital leadership.** *JAMA* 1996, **275**:234–240.
43. Wilcox MH, Cunniffe JG, Trundle C, Redpath C: **Financial burden of hospital-acquired Clostridium difficile infection.** *J Hosp Infect* 1996, **34**:23–30.

Permissions

The contributors of this book come from diverse backgrounds, making this book a truly international effort. This book will bring forth new frontiers with its revolutionizing research information and detailed analysis of the nascent developments around the world.

We would like to thank all the contributing authors for lending their expertise to make the book truly unique. They have played a crucial role in the development of this book. Without their invaluable contributions this book wouldn't have been possible. They have made vital efforts to compile up to date information on the varied aspects of this subject to make this book a valuable addition to the collection of many professionals and students.

This book was conceptualized with the vision of imparting up-to-date information and advanced data in this field. To ensure the same, a matchless editorial board was set up. Every individual on the board went through rigorous rounds of assessment to prove their worth. After which they invested a large part of their time researching and compiling the most relevant data for our readers.

The editorial board has been involved in producing this book since its inception. They have spent rigorous hours researching and exploring the diverse topics which have resulted in the successful publishing of this book. They have passed on their knowledge of decades through this book. To expedite this challenging task, the publisher supported the team at every step. A small team of assistant editors was also appointed to further simplify the editing procedure and attain best results for the readers.

Apart from the editorial board, the designing team has also invested a significant amount of their time in understanding the subject and creating the most relevant covers. They scrutinized every image to scout for the most suitable representation of the subject and create an appropriate cover for the book.

The publishing team has been an ardent support to the editorial, designing and production team. Their endless efforts to recruit the best for this project, has resulted in the accomplishment of this book. They are a veteran in the field of academics and their pool of knowledge is as vast as their experience in printing. Their expertise and guidance has proved useful at every step. Their uncompromising quality standards have made this book an exceptional effort. Their encouragement from time to time has been an inspiration for everyone.

The publisher and the editorial board hope that this book will prove to be a valuable piece of knowledge for researchers, students, practitioners and scholars across the globe.

List of Contributors

Robert Kraemer, Mohammad Kabbani, Christian Herold, Marc Busche, Peter M Vogt and Karsten Knobloch
Plastic, Hand and Reconstructive Surgery, Hannover Medical School, Carl- Neuberg-Strasse 1, 30625 Hannover, Germany

Johan Lorenzen
Department of Nephrology, Hannover Medical School, Carl-Neuberg-Strasse 1, 30625 Hannover, Germany

Ziyad Alharbi, Sultan Almakadi, Christian Opländer, Hans-Oliver Rennekampff and Norbert Pallua
Department of Plastic, Reconstructive and Hand Surgery - Burn Center, Medical Faculty, RWTH Aachen University, Pauwelsstr. 30, Aachen D-52074, Germany

Ziyad Alharbi
Division of Plastic Surgery, Specialist Surgery Center, King Abdullah Medical City, Mecca, Kingdom of Saudi Arabia

Michael Vogt
Two-Photon Microscopy Facility, Interdisciplinary Center for Clinical Research (IZKF), Medical Faculty, RWTH Aachen University, Aachen, Germany

Hao Zhang, Fang-da Li, Hua-liang Ren and Yue-hong Zheng
Department of Vascular Surgery, Peking Union Medical College Hospital, Peking Union Medical College and Chinese Academy of Medical Sciences, No, 1 Shuaifuyuan, Dongcheng district, Beijing 100730, P.R China

Claire L Nockolds and Paul S Rooney
Royal Liverpool Hospital, Prescot Street, Liverpool, Merseyside, L7 8XP, UK

Jason P Hodde
Cook Biotech Incorporated, 1425 Innovation Place, West Lafayette, IN 47906, USA

Zhiyong Hou, Yingze Zhang and Wei Chen
Department of Orthopaedic Surgery, Third Hospital of Hebei Medical University, Shijiazhuang, Hebei 050051, China

Jove Graham, Kent Strohecker, Daniel Feldmann and Thomas R Bowen
Department of Orthopaedic Surgery, Geisinger Medical Center, Danville, PA 17822, USA

Wade Smith
Mountain Orthopaedic Trauma Surgeons at Swedish, 701 East Hampden Avenue Suite 515, Englewood, CO 80113, USA

Ulrika Tampe, Rüdiger J Weiss, Zewar Al Dabbagh and Karl-Åke Jansson
Department of Molecular Medicine and Surgery, Section of Orthopaedics and Sports Medicine, Karolinska Institutet at Karolinska University Hospital, SE-17176 Stockholm, Sweden

Birgit Stark and Pehr Sommar
Department of Molecular Medicine and Surgery, Section of Plastic Surgery, Karolinska Institutet, Karolinska University Hospital, Stockholm, Sweden

Jenny Fabiola López, Kristiina Elisa Hietanen, Ilkka Santeri Kaartinen, Minna Tellervo Kääriäinen and Hannu Kuokkanen
Department of Plastic Surgery, Unit of Musculoskeletal Diseases, Tampere University Hospital, Pirkanmaa Hospital District, Teiskontie 35, Tampere 33521, Finland

Toni-Karri Pakarinen and Minna Laitinen
Department of Orthopedics and Trauma, Unit of Musculoskeletal Diseases, Tampere University Hospital, Tampere, Finland

Elroy P Weledji and Pius Fokam
Department of Surgery, Faculty of Health Sciences, University of Buea, Limbe, S W Region, Cameroon

Brian W Wu, Max Berger, George F Hatch III and E Todd Schroeder
Keck School of Medicine, University of Southern California, Los Angeles, CA, USA

Brian W Wu, Jonathan C Sum and E Todd Schroeder
Biokinesiology and Physical Therapy, University of Southern California, Los Angeles, CA, USA

Taro Mikami, Shintaro Kagimoto, Yuichiro Yabuki, Kazunori Yasumura and Jiro Maegawa
Department of Plastic and Reconstructive Surgery, Yokohama City University Hospital, 236-0004 Kanazawa-ku, Yokohama city, Kanagawa prefecture, Japan

Toshinori Iwai
Department of Oral and Maxillofacial Surgery, Yokohama City University Graduate School of Medicine, Yokohama, Japan

Nobuyasu Suganuma, Shohei Hirakawa and Katsuhiko Masudo
Department of General Surgery, Yokohama City University Hospital, Yokohama, Japan

Ming-Kai Hsieh, Lih-Huei Chen, Chi-Chien Niu, Tsai-Sheng Fu, Po-Liang Lai and Wen-Jer Chen
Department of Orthopedic Surgery, Chang Gung Memorial Hospital and Chang Gung University, 5, Fu-Hsin Street, Kweishan Shiang, Taoyuan 333, Taiwan

Chien-Chih Chou, Yi-Yu Tsai, You-Ling Li and Hui-Ju Lin
Department of Ophthalmology, China Medical University Hospital, No. 2 Yuh Der Road, Taichung 404, Taiwan

Hsin-Han Chen
Department of Plastic and Reconstructive Surgery, China Medical University Hospital, Taichung, Taiwan

Hui-Ju Lin
Department of Medical Research, China Medical University Hospital, Taichung, Taiwan
School of Chinese Medicine, College of Chinese Medicine, China Medical University, Taichung, Taiwan

Deo Darius Balumuka
Mbarara University of Science and Technology, Mbarara, Uganda

George William Galiwango
CoRSU hospital, Kisubi, Uganda

Rose Alenyo
College of Health Sciences School of Medicine, Makerere University, Kampala, Uganda

Daniel M Balkin and Mary H McGrath
Department of Surgery, Division of Plastic and Reconstructive Surgery, University of California San Francisco, San Francisco, CA, USA

Quan-Yang Duh
Department of Surgery, Section of Endocrine Surgery, University of California San Francisco, San Francisco, CA, USA

Gabriel M Kind and David S Chang
Department of Plastic Surgery, California-Pacific Medical Center, San Francisco, CA, USA

Yayoi Sakatoku, Masahide Fukaya, Kazushi Miyata, Keita Itatsu and Masato Nagino
Division of Surgical Oncology, Department of Surgery, Nagoya University Graduate School of Medicine, 65 Tsurumai-cho, Showa-ku, Nagoya 466-8550, Japan

Takashi Higuchi, Norio Yamamoto, Katsuhiro Hayashi, Akihiko Takeuchi, Kensaku Abe, Yuta Taniguchi, Yoshihiro Araki, Kaoru Tada and Hiroyuki Tsuchiya
Department of Orthopaedic Surgery, Graduate School of Medical Science, Kanazawa University, 13-1 Takara-machi, Kanazawa 920-8641, Japan

Apostolos Analatos, Mats Lindblad, Ioannis Rouvelas, Peter Elbe, Lars Lundell, Magnus Nilsson, Andrianos Tsekrekos and Jon A. Tsai
Centre for Digestive Diseases, Karolinska University Hospital and Division of Surgery, Department of Clinical Intervention and Technology (CLINTEC), Karolinska Institutet, Stockhom, Sweden

Apostolos Analatos
Department of Surgery, Nyköping Hospital, Nyköping, Sweden

Apostolos Analatos
Centre for Clinical Research Sörmland, Uppsala University, Uppsala, Sweden

Adeodatus Yuda Handaya
Digestive Surgery Division, Department of Surgery, Faculty of Medicine, Universitas Gadjah Mada/Dr. Sardjito Hospital, Jl. Kesehatan No. 1, Yogyakarta 55281, Indonesia

Nova Yuli Prasetyo Budi, Guntur Marganing Adi Nugroho and Aditya Rifqi Fauzi
Faculty of Medicine, Universitas Gadjah Mada/Dr. Sardjito Hospital, Yogyakarta 55281, Indonesia

Jung Woo Chang and M. Seung Suk Choi
Department of Plastic and Reconstructive Surgery, Hanyang University Guri Hospital, Hanyang University College of Medicine, 249-1, Gyomun-dong, Guri-si, Gyeonggi-do 471-701, Korea

Se Won Oh and Jeongseok Oh
Department of Plastic and Reconstructive Surgery, Hanyang University College of Medicine, 17 Haengdang-Dong, 133-792 Seongdong-Gu, Seoul, Korea

Mario Vitacolonna, Florian Herrle, Peter Hohenberger and Eric Dominic Rössner
Division of Surgical Oncology and Thoracic Surgery, Department of Surgery, University Medical Centre Mannheim, Heidelberg University, Theodor Kutzer Ufer 1-3, 68167 Mannheim, Germany

Michael Mularczyk, Hans Haupt and Matthias Oechsner
Center for structural Materials, State Material Testing Institute Darmstadt (MPA), Chair and Institute for Material Science (IfW), Technische Universität Darmstadt, Darmstadt, Germany

Torsten J Schulze
German Red Cross Blood Service, Baden Württemberg-Hessen, Medical Faculty of Mannheim, Institute of Transfusion Medicine and Immunology, Heidelberg University, Mannheim, Germany

Lothar R Pilz
Medical Faculty Mannheim, Heidelberg University, Heidelberg, Germany

Alexander Hallgren, Anders Björkman, Anette Chemnitz and Lars B Dahlin
Department of Clinical Sciences Malmö, Hand Surgery, Lund University, Malmö, Sweden

Francesco Turrà, Simone La Padula, Sergio Razzano, Gisella Nele, Sergio Marlino, Luigi Canta and Fabrizio Schonauer
Unit of Plastic, Reconstructive and Aesthetic Surgery, Federico II University, Via S.Pansini 5, 80131, Naples, Italy

Paola Bonavolontà, Pasquale Graziano and Giovanni Dell'Aversana Orabona
Department of Maxillofacial Surgery, Federico II University, Via S.Pansini 5, 80131, Naples, Italy

Roberto Berra-Romani
School of Medicine, Department of Biomedicine, Benemérita Universidad Autónoma de Puebla, 13 Sur 2702, Colonia Volcanes, 72000 Puebla, Mexico

José Everardo Avelino-Cruz, Francesco Moccia and Franco Tanzi
Department of Biology and Biotechnology "Lazzaro Spallanzani", Laboratory of Physiology, University of Pavia, via Forlanini 6, 27100 Pavia, Italy

Abdul Raqeeb
Department of Pharmacology and Therapeutics, Faculty of Medicine,University of Calgary, Calgary, Alberta, Canada

Alessandro Della Corte
Department of Cardiothoracic Sciences, Second University of Naples, Naples, Italy

Mariapia Cinelli and Stefania Montagnani
Department of Public Health, University of Naples "Federico II", via Pansini 5, 80131, Naples, Italy

Germano Guerra
Department of Medicine and Health Sciences, University of Molise, via F. De Sanctis, 86100, Campobasso, Italy

Sheila Margaret Fraser, Hiba Fatayer and Rajgopal Achuthan
Department of Breast & General Surgery, Leeds General Surgery, Great George Street, Leeds LS1 3EX, UK

Erik Bärthel, Falk Rauchfuß, Karin Jandt and Utz Settmacher
Department of General, Visceral and Vascular Surgery, Jena University Hospital, Erlanger Allee 101, D-07740 Jena, Germany

Heike Hoyer
Institute of Medical Statistics, Information Sciences and Documentation, Jena, Germany

Maria Breternitz
Center for Clinical Studies, Jena, Germany

Erik Bärthel, Falk Rauchfuß and Utz Settmacher
Center for Sepsis Control and Care, Jena University
Hospital, Friedrich Schiller University, Jena,
Germany

**Sergio A Acuna, Fernando A Angarita, Mauricio
Tawil and Lilian Torregrosa**
Department of Surgery, Hospital Universitario San
Ignacio, Pontificia Universidad Javeriana, Bogotá,
Colombia

Jaime Escallon
Department of Surgery, University of Toronto,
Toronto, ON, Canada

Department of Surgical Oncology, Princess Margaret
Hospital, Toronto, ON, Canada

Mauricio Tawil and Lilian Torregrosa
Breast and Soft Tissue Clinic, Centro Javeriano de
Oncología, Bogotá, Colombia

Sergio A Acuna and Fernando A Angarita
Division of Experimental Therapeutics, Toronto
General Research Institute, University Health
Network, Toronto, ON, Canada

Fernando A Angarita
Institute of Medical Science, University of Toronto,
Toronto, ON, Canada

Index

www.ingramcontent.com/pod-product-compliance
Lightning Source LLC
Chambersburg PA
CBHW082011190326
41458CB00010B/3156